The Arc of Conversation

Amy Shaw, PA

The Arc of Conversation

A How-to Guide for Goals
of Care Conversations

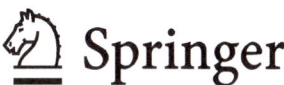 Springer

Amy Shaw, PA
Cheyenne, WY, USA

ISBN 978-3-031-70494-9   ISBN 978-3-031-70495-6   (eBook)
https://doi.org/10.1007/978-3-031-70495-6

This Springer imprint is published by the registered company Springer Nature Switzerland AG
The registered company address is: Gewerbestrasse 11, 6330 Cham, Switzerland

If disposing of this product, please recycle the paper.

To my parents, Cheryle and Joseph Scott, who taught me to read, write, and believe in myself.

Foreword

Most of us will die from progressive chronic diseases. This process will result in major physical, emotional, and spiritual distress for patients and family members. Unfortunately, clinical and academic healthcare institutions do not provide enough education about how to address the suffering of our patients and their loved ones as we approach the end of life. In this context, *The Arc of Conversation* is an invaluable contribution to the education of all healthcare professionals who need to communicate with patients and families at this very critical time of their lives.

Amy Shaw has written a comprehensive but highly enjoyable book covering all major aspects of communication, always from the perspective of the patient and family. All 17 chapters are packed with pearls of wisdom acquired from many years of practice, and they can be applied immediately by clinicians at all levels of practice.

Books written by multiple authors frequently have variable levels of editing and comprehensiveness. This is a single-author book, and the resulting homogenous style makes it very easy to read. The book is written with great empathy for the very difficult experiences of our patients and their loved ones, and it will help countless patients during the most difficult time in their lives.

I was particularly impressed by Amy's description of how her years as a wedding photographer provided her with the experience she later applied to palliative care communication. This made me realize that I had a similar experience. In my case, I had a DJ business that also focused on weddings and other celebrations, and these years greatly influenced the rest of my life as a clinician.

Everyone involved or interested in end-of-life care should read and enjoy this book.

F.T. McGraw Chair in the Treatment of Cancer   Eduardo Bruera, MD
Chair, Department of Palliative, Rehabilitation,
and Integrative Medicine
The University of Texas MD Anderson
Cancer Center,
Houston, TX, USA
April 2024

Acknowledgments

Writing a book is at once an intensely private and public act, both thrilling and terrifying. The notion of *imposter syndrome* cannot be understated. Many times, I pushed through with passion and will, but it was the enthusiasm and support from friends, family, colleagues, and my patients and their caregivers that put the wind in my sails.

Thanks first to Springer-Nature editorial director Richard Lansing and executive editor Gregory Sutorius, whose immediate and welcoming response to my textbook proposal created a foundation of confidence that I deeply valued throughout the process.

Thanks to my parents, Cheryle and Joseph Scott, for instilling in me a fierce sense of self-belief. My father taught me never to take "No" for an answer; my mother, how a truly good and kind person behaves. My sister, Sara Schulz, always has my back; her support over the years has been critical to my survival.

This book would not have reached its present state without a corps of four very passionate and dedicated readers, to whom I am eternally grateful. Their time, attention, dedication, and commitment reminded me that this effort held true purpose.

First, to thank my very astute and diligent copyeditor, Jennifer Moore Ballentine, MA, who read every word, concept, analogy, and turn of phrase with a level of care I cannot begin to capture. When I contacted her to request permission to reprint her Catastrophic Event diagram, I had no idea what a fruitful phone call that would be. When I asked her to serve as a reader for my book, I had no idea the level of effort she would contribute. It was certainly kismet, for before becoming a hospice administrator, she owned a medical publishing company; her editing pen is well-traveled. More like a second writer than a reader, she helped transform a bundle of wheat into a French pastry worthy of the Meilleur Ouvrier de France (MOF) prize, or at least a trip to Paris.

Second, to thank Dr. Jeffrey Chapman, then CMO, who encouraged me to consider my "why" and how I might move from "success to significance" when I shared my desire for a greater role in the healthcare system. That encouragement led me to some bigger thinking: first, to the creation of a strategic initiative for a new role, Director of Compassionate Collaborative Care, to transform the healthcare system with the ideas engendered in this book, and second, to the proposal for this book. His ongoing enthusiasm and a very close reading of my book have been a boon.

Third, to thank neurologist Dr. Mary Kerber, who has sent me many of her patients to care for over the years and who dedicated a close and kind reading of my manuscript—two votes of confidence I keenly acknowledge. A well-loved, well-respected, and well-experienced colleague, her practical, patient-centered, empathetic insights and suggestions were welcomed, embraced, and so very appreciated.

Fourth, to thank David Weiss, who listened to the audiobook version of my manuscript as I read him ten pages a day over several months. His discriminating mind served as the final sieve for my words; his fastidiousness for language and meaning made it impossible for many ill-formed constructs to get through. I especially appreciate his fierce loyalty to my perception of the subject matter; having him in my corner makes me feel as though things are alright in the world.

To those whose expressions of support and belief served as hot air balloons keeping me afloat during the many months of effort; those who remembered to ask how my book was coming along; those who expressed their pride and amazement at my dedication and willingness to the task; those who remained my friends despite my reduced availability; those who helped with the contemplation of an idea here or there; and those who expressed a willingness to purchase a copy of this book when it was finally published: thank you all. Your engaging words reminded me frequently of my ultimate task—to improve the lives of those around us.

There were many who supported me in these ways, including my parents, Cheryle and Joseph Scott, and my sister, Sara Schulz; our beloved Mary Walker, whose sudden death during the writing took us all by surprise; and many others near and dear to my heart, including Dr. Emma Avdic, Madeline Bednar, Stephanie Boster, Lori Brand, Charysse Brown PA-C, Dr. Tracie Caller, Lee Clancy, Riana Davidson, Michal Duller PA-C, Vanda Edington, Grace Ejigiri PA-C, Coleen Haines, Dr. Patricia Judd, Micah Kleit, Jodie Messner, Sarah Perkins, Catherine Reeves, Lisa Spillman, Jackie Van Cleave, Dr. Kristine Van Kirk, Dr. Casey Watkins, Susan Williams, and the University of Wyoming family medicine residents I've precepted and taught over the years.

Finally, I thank my patients, who collectively provided a masterclass in facing ultimate loss with bravery and love. From you, I learned much about how to exit this world gracefully, even if not yet ready, always on one's own terms. Thank you for allowing me to be part of your incredible journeys and enriching my life. The healing was always mutual, and many of you reside yet in my heart, some of you in this book. Because I have loved, I have lived, and I loved every one of you. For that, we shared some space and time, if but briefly, I will remain forever grateful.

About the Book

Intending to fill an important gap in medical training, *The Arc of Conversation* presents an easy-to-learn, standardized approach to having compassionate and collaborative goals of care conversations with patients and families, a skill that can be difficult for clinicians to learn and that is not included as part of standard medical education curricula. Developed by Amy Shaw, PA-C, a palliative care provider, this is the first book to teach everything clinicians need to know to gently guide patients and families through what can often be difficult discussions about illness, disease, end-of-life wishes, and hospice care. The technique taught in *The Arc of Conversation* can be used to discuss any medical diagnosis or treatment, can be employed at any age or stage of an illness, and can be used by healthcare professionals at any level.

Readers will be introduced to the patterns of decline patients follow toward the end of life, criteria for recognizing when a patient's time is limited, ground rules for compassionate communication, and a stepwise method of leading patients and families through difficult goals of care conversations in a collaborative way. The book includes specific questions to ask, and starter language clinicians can use for developing their own patient-friendly talking points about disease progression, the end of life, concerns that a patient's time is limited, advanced directives, code status, and hospice care. An Arc of Conversation Guide, for use when training in this technique, is also included.

The Arc of Conversation makes a compelling case for incorporating the knowledge and techniques taught in this book into medical education to better prepare clinicians to care for patients and their families. Healthcare leaders and systems can incorporate the book's knowledge and techniques by creating programs that embrace a patient- and family-centered approach. Ultimately, *The Arc of Conversation* aims to tackle the challenges faced by the healthcare system in the United States due to a rapidly aging population and increasing financial pressures within the Medicare system.

Guide for Clinicians in Training: Applying *The Arc of Conversation* in Healthcare Settings

The Arc of Conversation serves as a valuable resource for developing course material aimed at educating clinicians across various specialties on effectively engaging with patients and their families. A sample course appropriate for nursing and medical students at all levels of education and training is provided below:

Disease Trajectories (Chap. 4)

Objective: Develop a clinical understanding of the primary disease trajectories patients experience as they approach the end of life.

- Formulate a hypothesis based on a patient's chart review.
- Improve assessment through discussions with the patient and family.

Hospice Criteria (Chap. 5)

Objective: Develop a deep understanding of the hospice criteria for the terminal trajectories patients follow toward the end of life. Specialty providers should focus on learning the criteria relevant to their specialty (e.g., oncology, pulmonology, cardiology, etc.)

- Using a quick reference guide for hospice criteria can be beneficial. Several quick reference guides are accessible online.

Compassionate and Collaborative Conversations (Chaps. 6 and 7)

Objective: Develop the capacity to create a compassionate and collaborative conversational environment for patients and families. Understand the different aspects of a diagnosis, including disease, illness, and sickness. Learn to communicate with patients and their families in a compassionate and empathetic way.

- Learn to recognize the illness and sickness dimensions of a diagnosis. Develop self-awareness of any biases and practice non-judgment.
- Learn to address the disease aspect of a diagnosis in a way that honors patient and family values, priorities, and concerns.
- Develop comfort with patient and family emotions and the ability to recognize and respond to every indication of their emotion.

The Arc of Conversation Technique (Chaps. 8 through 17)

Objective: Learn to guide patients and families through goals-of-care conversations based on the technique taught in *The Arc of Conversation.* Follow the Goals of Care Conversation Guide, included in Chap. 14, while practicing the technique.

- Learn the *investigate-then-educate* technique and the clinician's role as a guide in conversations (Chap. 8).

- The Illness Arc: Learn to investigate the patient and family experience and understanding of illness. Develop an overall assessment of the patient's health status, including identifying the disease driving patient decline and whether the patient meets hospice criteria (Chap. 9).
- The Disease Arc: Learn to investigate the patient and family experience and understanding of the disease driving patient decline. Provide education about the disease to "fill in the gaps of their understanding," and, when appropriate, deliver the news that a patient's time is limited (Chaps. 10 and 15).
- The End-of-Life Wishes Arc: Learn to investigate the patient and family wishes for the end-of-life, including advance directive and code status wishes (Chaps. 11 and 16).
- The Hospice Care Arc: Learn to investigate patient and family experience and understanding of hospice care. Provide education about hospice care, addressing any misconceptions. Ensure a smooth transition to hospice care for those who are ready for hospice care (Chaps. 12 and 17).

Guide for Clinical Staff in Training: Applying *The Arc of Conversation* in Healthcare Settings

The Arc of Conversation serves as a valuable resource for developing training material aimed at educating staff across the healthcare continuum on effectively engaging with patients and their families. A sample course appropriate for clinical and non-clinical staff at all levels of education and training is provided below:

Compassionate and Collaborative Conversations (Chaps. 6 and 7)

Objective: Develop the capacity to create a compassionate and collaborative environment for patients and families.

- Understand the different aspects of a diagnosis, including disease, illness, and sickness. Develop self-awareness of any biases and practice non-judgment.
- Learn to communicate compassionately and empathetically with patients and their families.
- Develop comfort with patient and family emotions and the ability to recognize and respond to every indication of their emotion.

Understanding Patient and Family Experience of Disease (Chaps. 4 and 15)

Objective: Develop an understanding of the primary disease trajectories patients follow as they approach the end of life and how disease can impact patients' and families' lives.

- Understand the most common disease trajectories patients in the United States follow as they approach the end of their lives.
- Understand how illness can impact the lives of patients and their families in ways that may not be apparent in clinical, hospital, or facility settings.

Patient and Family Preferences for End-of-Life Wishes (Chaps. 11 and 16)

Objective: For those responsible for helping patients and families with advance care planning documents, learn to discuss advance directive and code status wishes effectively.

- Learn to discuss the selection of a surrogate medical decision maker.
- Learn to discuss the living will and POLST form.

Hospice Criteria and Hospice Care (Chaps. 5 and 17)

Objective: Understand that there are criteria developed to recognize when a patient's time is limited. Learn the important information about hospice care.

- Learn the important misconceptions about hospice care.
- Learn to represent and discuss hospice care accurately with patients and families.

Guide for Healthcare Leaders: Utilizing *The Arc of Conversation* in Healthcare Institutions

The Arc of Conversation provides a valuable framework for healthcare leaders to promote meaningful conversations, develop expertise, and implement programs within their institutions. By leveraging the content and techniques outlined in the book, healthcare leaders can enhance the quality of care, improve patient outcomes, and foster a culture of compassionate and collaborative communication. Healthcare leadership can also use *The Arc of Conversation* to understand, anticipate, and strategize for the needs of the rapidly aging population.

Promoting Conversations:

- Encourage and Facilitate Training: Healthcare leaders can promote the adoption of *The Arc of Conversation* by encouraging clinicians and healthcare professionals within their institutions to undergo training in the techniques and principles outlined in the book. This can be facilitated through workshops, seminars, and educational sessions led by experts in palliative care and compassionate communication.
- Emphasize the Importance of Compassionate Communication: Leaders should emphasize the significance of compassionate and collaborative communication in patient care. Encouraging open discussions about illness, end-of-life wishes, and hospice care can lead to improved patient satisfaction and better alignment of care with patients' preferences.

Developing Expertise:

- Establish Training Programs: Healthcare leaders can develop structured training programs based on *The Arc of Conversation's* content. These programs can be tailored for clinicians across various specialties to enhance their expertise in engaging with patients and families during difficult conversations.
- Provide Resources and Support: Leaders should ensure that clinicians have access to resources, including *The Arc of Conversation* textbook, and the Arc of Conversation Guide, included in Chap. 14, to help them implement the techniques effectively. Additionally, providing ongoing support and mentorship can help clinicians gain confidence in applying the principles outlined in the book.

Developing Programs:

- Integrate *The Arc of Conversation* into Continuing Education: Healthcare leaders can integrate the concepts from the book into continuing education initiatives within their institutions. This can include incorporating specific modules from the book into existing training programs or developing new courses focused on compassionate communication and end-of-life care. Ensuring that every member of the healthcare community understands hospice care, for example, would better support patient and family needs at the end of life.
- Develop Strategic Patient-Centered Care Initiatives: Healthcare leaders can adopt the patient-centered, compassionate, and collaborative approach outlined in the book by implementing strategic leadership initiatives within their organization. This could include creating a new position within the healthcare system, such as Director of Compassionate Collaborative Care, to integrate the principles from the book across the healthcare system.
- Create Interdisciplinary Initiatives: Leaders can promote interdisciplinary collaboration by bringing together healthcare professionals from diverse backgrounds to learn and apply the principles of *The Arc of Conversation*. This can foster a holistic approach to patient care and improve communication among multidisciplinary teams.
- Create Patient-Centered Care Initiatives: Leaders can promote the development of patient-centered, comprehensive care initiatives to effectively meet the needs of patients and their families navigating challenging disease journeys. These initiatives should prioritize the physical, emotional, and spiritual well-being of patients, ensuring they receive holistic support during their journey. Examples include placing healthcare providers, who have been trained in the techniques taught in this book, in areas of the healthcare system where they are likely to encounter patients with terminal diseases, such as the Emergency Room (ER), Intensive Care Unit (ICU), specialty clinics, primary care clinics, and care facilities. Another example is creating comprehensive disease management programs for the primary terminal trajectories patients in the United States follow at the end of life,

including heart disease, cancer, lung disease, age-related decline, and dementia. Mental health journeys, regardless of terminality, should be prioritized because they often take a significant toll on patients and families.

- Evaluate and Monitor Progress: Healthcare leaders must establish mechanisms for evaluating the impact of integrating *The Arc of Conversation* into their institutions. This may involve monitoring patient satisfaction scores, tracking end-of-life healthcare system utilization (e.g., hospice utilization at the end of life, length of hospice care stay at the end of life, ER visits in the last 6 months of life, and ICU and hospital admissions in the last 6 months of life), and assessing the financial impacts of improving goals of care conversations throughout patient journeys.

Contents

Part II   Ground Rules for Compassionate Conversations

Part III   The Arc of Conversation

About the Author

Amy Shaw is a palliative care physician assistant with 10 years of experience supporting patients with chronic and terminal diseases. In 1999, she graduated from Emory University with a Bachelor of Arts in Psychology. During her time at Emory University, she conducted research on primate behavior and child development in the labs of leading primatologists and completed an honors thesis entitled *One Child's Acquisition of Questions: A Constructivist Account*. Afterward, she established a thriving wedding photography business in San Diego, California. In 2014, she received her Master of Physician Assistant Studies from Chatham University. She currently specializes in providing comprehensive dementia care to patients and their families.

A passionate educator and thought leader in patient-centered care, she is the author of *The Arc of Conversation: A How-to Guide for Goals of Care Conversations*. Learn more at AmyShaw.net.

The techniques taught in this book have helped her improve dementia care in her community. As a result, caregivers have a better understanding of the dementia journey, and patients and their families experience improved quality of life and medical care. This has also led to a reduction in end-of-life healthcare utilization and an increase in the length of hospice care received by patients and families. In 2024, she was featured in a Wyoming PBS documentary titled *A State of Mind: The Caregivers*, focusing on the impact of the dementia journey on caregivers.

In her free time, Amy enjoys visiting art museums, traveling to listen to the world's best symphony orchestras, and hiking with her dog, Juno.

Abbreviations

ABG	Arterial blood gas
ACLF	Acute on chronic liver failure
ACO	Accountable Care Organization
AD	Alzheimer's disease
ADLs	Activities of daily living
AIDS	Acquired immune deficiency syndrome
AKI	Acute kidney injury
ALP	Alkaline phosphatase
ALS	Amyotrophic lateral sclerosis
ALSFRS-R	Revised Amyotrophic Lateral Sclerosis Functional Rating Scale
ALT	Alanine aminotransferase
AMA	American Medical Association
ARDS	Acute respiratory distress syndrome
ART	Antiretroviral therapy
AST	Aspartate aminotransferase
AV	Arteriovenous
BiPAP	Bilevel positive airway pressure
BMI	Body mass index
BUN	Blood urea nitrogen
bvFTD	Behavioral-variant frontotemporal dementia
CABG	Coronary artery bypass graft
CAD	Coronary artery disease
CBD	Corticobasal degeneration
CEA	Carcinoembryonic antigen
CHF	Congestive heart failure
CKD	Chronic kidney disease
CMP	Complete metabolic panel
CMS	Centers for Medicare and Medicaid Services
CMV	Cytomegalovirus
CNA	Certified nursing assistant
CNS	Central nervous system
CO2	Carbon dioxide
COPD	Chronic obstructive pulmonary disease
CPAP	Continuous positive airway pressure

CPR	Cardiopulmonary resuscitation
CrCl	Creatinine clearance
CT	Computed tomography
CTI	Certificate of terminal illness
CVA	Cardiovascular accident
DNR	Do not resuscitate
DPOA	Durable power of attorney
DPOA-HC	Durable power of attorney for health care
ECG	Electrocardiogram
ECMO	Extracorporeal mechanical oxygenation
ECOG	Eastern Cooperative Oncology
EEG	Electroencephalogram
EF	Ejection fraction
eGRF	Estimated glomerular filtration rate
EMT	Emergency medical technician
ER	Emergency room
ESKD	End-stage kidney disease
FAST	Functional Assessment Staging of Dementia
FEV	Forced expiratory volume
FTLD	Frontotemporal lobar degeneration
FVC	Forced vital capacity
GCS	Glasgow Coma Scale
GFR	Glomerular filtration rate
GGT	Gamma-glutamyltransferase
HBsAg	Hepatitis B surface antigen
HCTZ	Hydrochlorothiazide
HD	Hemodialysis
HD	Huntington's disease
HHC	Home health care
HIV	Human immunodeficiency virus
HRS	Hepatorenal syndrome
HTN	Hypertension
IADLs	Instrumental activities of daily living
ICD	Implantable cardioverter-defibrillator
ICD-10	International Statistical Classification of Diseases and Related Health Problems
ICU	Intensive care unit
INR	International normalized ratio
IV	Intravenous
KPS	Karnofsky Performance Scale
LBD	Lewy body disease
LCD	Local coverage determination
MA	Medicare Advantage
MAC	*Mycobacterium avium* complex
MCCM	Medicare Care Choices Model
MDPOA	Medical durable power of attorney

MELD	Model for End-Stage Liver Disease
MI	Myocardial infarction
MMSE	Mini-Mental Status Examination
MoCA	Montreal Cognitive Assessment
MOLST	Medical Orders for Life-Sustaining Treatment
MOST	Medical Orders for Scope of Treatment
NG	Nasogastric
NIPPV	Noninvasive positive pressure ventilation
NP	Nurse practitioner
NYHA	New York Heart Association
OMT	Optimal medical treatment
PA	Physician assistant
PCI	Percutaneous coronary intervention
PD	Parkinson's disease
PE	Pulmonary embolism
PFT	Pulmonary function test
POLST	Physician/Provider Orders for Life-Sustaining Treatment
POST	Physician/Provider Orders for Scope of Treatment
PPS	Palliative Performance Scale
ProQOL	Professional Quality of Life
PSA	Prostate-specific antigen
PSP	Progressive supranuclear palsy
PT	Prothrombin time
PTO	Personal time off
RAAS	Renin-angiotensin-aldosterone system
RBD	REM sleep behavior disorder
RN	Registered nurse
SA-AKI	Sepsis-associated acute kidney injury
SBP	Spontaneous bacterial peritonitis
SEER	Surveillance, Epidemiology, and End Results
SLE	Systemic lupus erythematosus
SLT	Speech and language therapy
SSRI	Selective serotonin reuptake inhibitor
STEMI	ST-elevation myocardial infarction
TB	Tuberculosis
TBI	Traumatic brain injury
TBIL	Total bilirubin
"The Triple C"	Compassionate Collaborative Care Model and Framework
TIA	Transient ischemic attack
TNM	Tumor-node-metastasis
U.S.	United States
UNOS	United Network for Organ Sharing
UTI	Urinary tract infection
VA	Veterans Administration
VP	Ventriculoperitoneal
X-ray	Radiograph

List of Figures

List of Tables

Introduction

1

There is no right answer. Only the answer that is right for you.

I decided to join the Palliative and Hospice Care service after just 2 days of shadowing my predecessor. Something about the way she helped patients and families through discussions of end-of-life care gave me the sense that here was a job that held the promise of meaning. Longing for an area where I could make a contribution, I hoped I'd found my medical calling.

Before joining the Palliative and Hospice Care team in 2019, I couldn't have told you what *palliative* or *hospice care* meant, let alone how they differed. A fairly recent Physician Assistant (PA) program graduate, I hadn't encountered those terms in the classroom or clinic. I was starting from scratch.

With just one month of overlap with the outgoing provider and no training manual to count on, I was left to teach myself this new specialty. Fortunately, my PA school's Problem-Based Learning Paradigm, in which students identify knowledge gaps and work studiously to fill them, prepared me well for this effort. Eager to succeed in my new job, I set out to learn everything I could about the practice of palliative and hospice care.

Although palliative and hospice care are relatively young specialties, the available medical literature on these fields is vast. With many robust resources dedicated to treatment basics, within just a couple of months, I was comfortable with treating constipation, cachexia, cough, and chronic pain, as well as many other symptoms of disease.

But treating symptoms was only one part of my job. An equally, if not more critical, responsibility of palliative care providers is having *goals of care conversations* with patients and families. During these conversations, providers work to discover patient and family values and priorities in order to align patients' wishes with their medical care. Although I searched endlessly for a how-to guide for having these conversations, I repeatedly came up short.

I found articles discussing the disease trajectory patterns patients follow at the end of life, but nothing that taught me how to talk about these trajectories with

A. Shaw, PA, *The Arc of Conversation*,
https://doi.org/10.1007/978-3-031-70495-6_1

patients and families. I had a list of disease-specific hospice criteria, which I used to determine if people were eligible for hospice care, but nothing that taught me how to delicately deliver the concern that the patient's time was limited. Many resources discussed the importance of compassion, empathy, and active listening, and others suggested a few questions or responses to use with patients. Although I could piece together tidbits of advice from one source or another, I needed a comprehensive training manual that taught me everything I needed to know about having difficult conversations with patients and families.

As you can imagine, without this kind of training, talking with patients facing their mortality is a very intimidating task. To the dying individual, the living can represent an element with which they have little left in common. I remember one gentleman asking me how old I was, as though he thought I was too young or couldn't possibly relate to or discuss the concept of dying. Fortunately, when I revealed my age, he visibly relaxed.

Discussions about death and dying can be emotionally fraught for both patients and providers alike. I frequently felt lost in a foreign landscape, without a compass or a map, unable to speak the language. It was difficult to know where to begin and once started, how to progress. Many times, I realized too late that I had pushed patients and families in a way that felt uncomfortable, both for me and for them. When I tried to start again, the magic in the room had disappeared. I also wasn't always confident about what the destination was. Often, I left the conversation without the information I sought, unable to tell the care team what the patient wanted or if the patient and family were genuinely ready for hospice. When I succeeded in eliciting patient wishes, I didn't always understand how I had made it happen. Although I loved my new role, this part of my job felt like a mystery that frequently left me frustrated.

~~~

As I struggled through my first hundred or so goals of care conversations, I began to realize that the best preparation for this work had been the 10 years that I owned a wedding photography studio, working to capture the range of emotions and aspirations of young couples in love, surrounded by their families, not all of whom made for the best table mates or photographic ensembles. Whenever I shared this insight, people would laugh. While amusing, this realization was absolutely true. Without knowing it, owning a business that demanded I know how to usher families through one of the most emotionally charged experiences of a human life, to protect brides from overly enthusiastic bridesmaids, and to successfully capture family portraits full of folks who would rather be sidled up to the bar, taught me a set of lessons I had no idea would come in so handy one day.

Although weddings often share similar elements and traditions, each is a unique reflection of the couple's aspirations, priorities, and preferences. So it is with dying. Whereas patients follow similar disease patterns as they approach the end of life, each patient traverses a unique and profoundly personal terrain that no one else has ever traveled, bringing their private values, beliefs, hopes, and fears.

As a wedding photographer, it was my job to capture the unique richness of each wedding by focusing my camera on the objects and people lovingly selected to represent and bless each couple's new beginning. Afterward, I designed a wedding album to honor the couple's celebration, which they could continue to enjoy in the years ahead.

As a palliative care provider, it is also my job to capture the unique richness of people's lives by compassionately focusing on each patient and family's personal experience and understanding of illness, wishes for the future, and worries and concerns. Acknowledging this inner landscape enables me to honor each stage of a person's journey as I continuously work to align patient and family wishes with their medical care.

To be a good wedding photographer requires patience, compassion, attention to detail, and being fully present and prepared for whatever might happen next. Successful goals of care conversations also depend on these skills, plus the emotional intelligence to read a room and determine when things are going awry.

With weddings, things often go awry. The DJ forgets the playlist, the best man arrives late, and the bride's dress gets torn. Just as wedding hiccups can be stressful, so can the medical detours on a life's journey—an unexpected diagnosis, lengthy hospitalizations, the loss of a spouse or personal independence, even pain and constipation. Photographing weddings for nearly 10 years taught me that people experiencing life's significant milestones deserve compassion, patience, and grace.

Working closely with couples on their wedding day taught me many lessons I use in my current role, which I have come to consider as the "ground rules" for having goals of care conversations. I learned the art of *holding space* for people's suffering, no matter the magnitude, and to refrain from judgment. I learned that sharing my own vulnerability and humanity is a way of building rapport and that respecting everyone's traditions and beliefs is a way of building trust. I learned how to provide a buffer to ease the burden of life's often unfair inclinations with a gentle touch, a tissue, a shared tear, or a well-timed joke.

To ensure my flexibility and emotional solvency, I learned to keep my personal cup full, tending to my inner emotional landscape so that my natural responses would be heartfelt, kind, and centered on the person before me. To be fully present, I learned to leave my personal baggage at the door.

Being a business owner also imparted important lessons about transactions with other people. At its heart, owning a business is about providing a product or service that adds to people's experience and quality of life. This is the underlying truth of the adage, "The customer is always right." With this principle as my guide, I learned the importance of constantly finding ways to say "Yes" to my clients. By remaining flexible and working continuously to accommodate their wishes and priorities, I centered my clients in my service. After all, it was *their* wedding, not mine.

With my patients, I also try to find ways to say "Yes." For example, most people express a strong desire to remain in their homes throughout their lives. Knowing this, I might order home health care to evaluate safety and make recommendations to protect patients from hazards at home, suggest that families privately pay for additional support in the home, or screen patients for Medicaid, which can often send extra help to the home. Guided by the underlying desire always to say "Yes," despite circumstances that might prove challenging, I continually work to improve the quality and experience of a patient's life at every step of their journey.

Owning a business also taught me that providing a service that isn't truly what the client wants is counterproductive. As difficult as it was to be turned down by a couple who had inquired about my work, it was vastly more important that couples loved what I offered so they would end up with photographs they adored. Therefore, it was necessary to ensure that my stylistic and creative vision aligned with the couple's vision for their wedding.

To do this, I developed a conversational approach with potential clients that allowed me to learn their sense of style and vision for their wedding while discussing my service in a manner that would allow clients to arrive at a decision that was right for them without feeling like I was trying to sell them something. Instead, I wanted my clients to know I was offering a service they could choose if they thought it was right for them. Wanting an authentic alignment between my clients' wishes and the photography service they ended up with worked best for everyone.

Early in my work as a palliative care provider, I realized that providers, patients, and their families often assumed it was my job to sell the idea of hospice. Patients unsettled by what felt like a sudden change in course by their physicians, who were hearing about hospice for the first time during my initial visit with them, often expressed their confusion by saying, "So, you're telling me I have to choose hospice?" Providers also often assumed it was my job to sell hospice to patients. Once, a specialist, upset by the news that their patient had chosen hospice care, barked at me, "If you ask people 99 times, on the 100th time, they're going to say 'Yes.'" I have also received more than a few frustrated responses from hospital providers communicating their annoyance when I reported back that a patient or family was not yet ready for hospice care.

Contrary to what is often believed, the role of palliative care is *not* to try to sell hospice care. Rather, our role is to elicit patient and family wishes and then work to align their wishes with their medical care. This pursuit aligns with the medical ethic of respecting *patient autonomy*—the freedom and right for patients to make choices for themselves.

For patients to exercise autonomy, they must be fully informed about the options for care. Patients need information about treatment outcomes (for example, side effects or healing time) and the likelihood of success, which can differ based on factors such as age, recent medical changes, and other diagnoses that might impact outcomes or prognosis. For patients to make choices that are right for them at any point in an illness, they need an appropriate and accurate understanding of their current health status, including how advanced a disease is, how much time they might have left, and what the road ahead will look like.

In its zeal to save lives and treat acute illness, modern medicine often fails to acknowledge the disease trajectory responsible for a patient's decline. Offers for treatment are often made without respect to this critical information.

As one example, most people don't understand that dementia is a progressive disease that follows a predictable and terminal course. Often, patients and families tell me that dementia is *just a little memory loss*, not realizing that dementia eventually robs people of cognitive skills like abstract thinking and logical thought, as well as control of the physical body, including the ability to chew food, swallow safely, and walk. Few understand that the end of dementia is marked by recurrent infections, a sign that the body is no longer able to maintain itself like it once was.

Patients with dementia are often admitted to the hospital with aspiration pneumonia, which occurs when the brain is no longer capable of coordinating the swallow function in a way that protects the lungs from inhaling food or liquid, which can lead to an infection. Failing to appreciate pneumonia as an indication of *end-stage dementia*, families and providers alike often mistakenly believe that antibiotics to treat the pneumonia and a stay in a rehab facility are likely to improve the patient's ability to walk and talk. Patients with limited time at the inevitable end of a dementia journey are often discharged to such facilities, separated from their families and surrounded by strangers, which can be distressing for both the patient and their loved ones.

Even more concerning, loved ones of patients with end-stage dementia who have experienced significant weight loss—a natural part of dementia progression—are sometimes offered feeding tubes to support the patient's nutrition despite the increased risk of aspiration pneumonia that can occur at this stage, not to mention the confusion and anxiety that patients with dementia often experience, which can lead to them pulling on or chewing through their tubes.

In situations like these, patient and family choices are made with incomplete or inaccurate information about the likelihood of treatment success, the advanced nature of the patient's disease, and what is expected ahead. Instead of improving the quality of life and experience of health care for patients and families, treatment decisions made without considering this critical information can lead to increased distress and suffering when patients experience repeated hospital admissions, rehab stays away from their families, and often unsuccessful escalations of care. Importantly, decisions made in the last few months of life are frequently misaligned with what we know patients want at this time of their lives. This is the opposite of respect for autonomy.

In conversations with patients and families about their experiences and understanding of illness, what they expected going forward, and where they thought the patient was in their journey with their health, it became apparent to me early on that our healthcare system was ignoring this vitally important aspect of patient education. Most patients and families had little understanding of disease, why it created the symptoms it did, or how their disease would progress. Without awareness that they were nearing the end of their journey, patients and families were often ill-prepared for this eventuality. Assuming the end was yet far off, many patients and families made decisions that differed wildly from what they told me they would want if they knew their time was limited.

Knowing that patients and families could not make decisions consistent with their values without appropriate education about disease progression, severity, and prognosis, I began to refine my approach to goals of care conversations with the intention of communicating this vital information more effectively so that patient choice could arise from an accurate understanding of health status.

This took a great deal of trial and error and hundreds of conversations. I made many mistakes along the way, which provided valuable input that I used to continually retool my approach. Attending to patient and family feedback (tone of voice, body language, and their willingness to fully participate in the conversation), I learned to detect when I was pushing people too quickly or guiding them into terrain that they weren't prepared to traverse just yet, requiring that I back off, start again, or even stop. By paying close attention to what made patients and families most comfortable, particularly concerning the order of things, I eventually arrived at a stepwise method of having goals of care conversations, which I call *The Arc of Conversation*.

Although *The Arc of Conversation* was developed in the medical setting to discuss patient and family care wishes, the general principles of this methodology can be used to discuss any topic in which there is a need to impart information, from the best way to cook a turkey on Thanksgiving with your teenage son to the likelihood of success of a resuscitation attempt in an 89-year-old. Furthermore, this approach can be learned by medical professionals at any level to be used with patients at any age or stage of an illness to discuss diagnosis, treatment, or wishes. Rooted in compassion, collaboration, and complete information, at its heart, *The Arc of Conversation* is a way of continually centering patients in our care.

<center>~~~</center>

Over the last 50 years, there has been an evolution from a physician-directed approach to medical care to one in which treatment decisions are made in partnership with patients and families, called *patient-centered care*. Involving patients fully in their care requires a shift from simply providing patients with medical options to situating those options within the landscape of a patient's understanding. Too often, I have watched as physicians begin talking about the next steps without first taking the time to understand what patients and families think is going on or what they know about a diagnosis. One only has to notice the glazed look in the eyes of those in the room to understand that nothing the physician says is getting through.

The foundational principle, therefore, of *The Arc of Conversation* is to investigate experience and understanding before providing education. If you take just one thing away from reading this book, make it this:

> *Patients and families will not benefit from education about disease, disease progression, or treatment options if you haven't first taken the time to appreciate what they've been through, how they're making sense of their experiences, what they understand about their diagnosis, and what they believe is going to happen next.*

For this reason, *The Arc of Conversation* begins in the familiar terrain of the patient and family's experience and understanding of *illness*, where they are the experts. I start by asking patients and families to describe how things have been going, which provides a basis for building rapport as I hold space and listen attentively to their stories. As patients recount symptoms and signs of disease, I begin developing an overall assessment of their health status, homing in on the disease trajectory that is driving any decline, and, keeping hospice criteria in mind, I consider whether the patient's time is likely limited. I also ask patients and families how they are making sense of what they have just described to me, allowing them to process what they've been through. I listen for indications of patient and family medical literacy, misperceptions, belief systems, and signs of distress, frustration, and confusion. These insights will inform how I provide education later and serve as opportunities to offer reassurance, compassion, and acceptance, the foundation upon which patients develop trust.

Next, I investigate patient and family experience and understanding of *disease*, focusing on the diagnosis I believe to be responsible for any decline. I ask whether patients and families have seen anyone else go through a similar journey and what they understand about the disease, including why it causes the symptoms it does, what they expect going forward, and what they think the end will look like. I also ask patients and families where they believe the patient is in their overall journey with their health, which tells me how advanced they believe the patient's disease to be and whether they think the patient's time might be limited. This part of the conversation is open-ended, with questions intended to discover the patient and family's medical understanding and beliefs more fully, which serve as a starting point as well as an opportunity to provide value when I fill in the gaps of their medical knowledge with education about the patient's particular disease journey.

Once I have completed my assessment and ascertained what the patient and family understand about the patient's diagnosis, I begin to provide education. I introduce the patterns of decline that people follow toward the end of life and explain the specific disease course the patient is on, including why their symptoms are happening and what they can expect going forward. For patients who meet hospice criteria, I gently deliver this news. This part of the conversation requires the ability to translate complicated medical knowledge into language patients and families can understand and the ability to tactfully and compassionately communicate the concern that the patient's time is limited.

Delivering the news that the patient has reached the end of their journey depends on an accurate assessment of their overall health status, which depends on a working knowledge of the *disease trajectories* patients follow toward the end of life and *hospice criteria*. While many providers base their recommendations for hospice care on a "gut feeling" that the patient is likely to pass within the next 6 months, patients and families deserve more accurate assessments. The hospice criteria used by hospice care teams to determine eligibility for hospice care can be used to more accurately assess when a patient's time is limited.

Like criteria developed to recognize (diagnose) and monitor (stage) disease to direct treatment, hospice criteria were designed to acknowledge the stage of an illness when it is reasonable to believe that the medical community can no longer alter the course of a patient's disease. As such, hospice criteria provide a meaningful and reliable way for physicians to know when to consider and offer the treatment option we call *hospice care*, designed to focus entirely on patient comfort and quality of life.

Delivering timely and accurate information regarding where a patient is in the course of a disease is an essential component of respect for patient autonomy, enabling patients and families to make decisions about medical care that align with their values. Delivering this news too late robs people of precious quality time together and the opportunity to focus on what matters most to them and their families—expressing and experiencing love. Providers intending, albeit nobly, to preserve hope for patients and families, often fail to acknowledge the elephant in the room—disease progression and death—inadvertently providing treatment options that are unlikely to succeed and, in the end, failing patients when they need it the most.

Likewise, providers trained almost exclusively to cure illness and injury may believe that cessation of curative treatment represents personal or medical failure. Not wanting to remove all vestiges of hope, providers preserving their own sense of competence and capacity can inadvertently center themselves in their patient's care instead of centering the patient. Genuine *patient-centered care* requires the shift back to focusing entirely on patient and family values, hopes, and expectations instead of those of the medical community. Respect for patient autonomy demands that patients have the right information at the right time to make decisions that are right for them. So that patients can decide for themselves what is best when they reach the end of their lives, the medical community must develop its working knowledge of disease trajectories, what the end of life looks like, and hospice criteria.

Following education about disease and, when appropriate, delivering the news that the patient meets hospice criteria, the next step in *The Arc of Conversation* is to investigate patient and family *end-of-life wishes*. I ask patients where they want to be at the end of their lives, what they would want their time to look like if they knew their time was limited, and what they are hoping for in whatever time they have left. I also discuss advance directive and code status preferences for patients who either do not meet hospice criteria or who, despite meeting hospice criteria, are not yet ready for hospice care.

Although advance directive and code status preferences should be documented for adults of all ages, I often encounter patients aged 75 and older who have never been asked about their preferences for medical interventions. Instead of waiting until the end of a patient's journey, such documentation should be part of ongoing preventative health maintenance and revisited routinely. I review these topics with my patients annually or whenever their health status changes. Like routine labs or a colonoscopy at age 50, advance directive and code status discussions are important in caring for patients and supporting patient autonomy.

Just as *The Arc of Conversation* begins in the familiar terrain of patient experience of illness, advance directive conversations are best started where patients are comfortable. Regardless of having an advance directive or a living will, most people know what they would want in a situation where interventions are required to keep them alive but without the prospect of improvement. Many people can answer immediately and with certainty that they would not want to be kept alive with such interventions.

Following this usually straightforward consideration, I then move to a discussion of code status. Often, regarding their wishes for resuscitation, patients are asked questions like, "If your heart stops, do you want us to restart it?" or, "If your heart stops beating and you stop breathing, do you want us to do CPR to resuscitate you?" Although well-intentioned to be easy for laypeople to understand, phrasing the question about code status in this way is misleading because it disguises the scant likelihood of a successful outcome by suggesting that restarting someone's heart is as easy as restarting a computer. Furthermore, such language implies that resuscitation attempts are equally successful in all patients when, in reality, the likelihood of success is never great and depends on myriad factors, including who is performing the CPR and where, how advanced a patient's age and disease is, and other health conditions that might impact their prognosis.

Rather, patients need clear language that accurately describes the only circumstance in which cardiopulmonary resuscitation (CPR) is performed—when a person has died. My language is simple, straightforward, and easy for people to process.

If you were to die right now, would you want the medical community to undergo efforts to bring you back to life?

When asked this way, patients are far more likely to make decisions that align with their values. Instead of being misleading, this question asks patients to consider the real possibility of dying, allowing them to think about what they would want for themselves in that situation. This is particularly helpful for patients who have reached the stage of life when they have accepted their mortality and would not want heroic medical interventions of any kind.

For patients and families with questions about the success of a resuscitation attempt, I relate education about likely outcomes to the earlier discussion of their health status, reviewing statistics and specifics of CPR as needed. Doing things in this order, first providing education about where a person is in their health journey and then discussing code status, enables a patient's decision to arise out of an accurate understanding of the options. Having these conversations routinely throughout an illness supports patients and families as their experiences change over the years.

Once discussions of end-of-life wishes are complete, the final step in *The Arc of Conversation* is a discussion of *hospice care*. Although this part of the conversation can be abbreviated for patients who don't meet hospice criteria, I do touch upon this subject with everyone I meet in consultation. Again, I start by asking patients and families about any previous experience with hospice care and their understanding of the word *hospice*. Their answers typically reveal any fears, concerns, or confusion about hospice. When discussing the details that patients need to consider hospice care fully, I will reference their concerns and correct any misconceptions they have.

During this part of the conversation, I carefully monitor patients and families, adjusting and tending to their emotional needs as necessary. Patients and families considering hospice care often need additional time—sometimes days or weeks—to process this new information. During the time that they need to make their decision,

I continue to support them in whatever way I can, addressing their questions and concerns and reassuring them that "There is no right answer, only the answer that is right for them."

The Arc of Conversation

The Arc of Conversation is the textbook I needed when I started in palliative care. It fills an important gap in the medical education curricula by offering a commonsense way of thinking about disease and its progression and a practical strategy (and template language) for goals-of-care conversations with patients and families. It is organized into five sections.

Part I, Acknowledging the Patient's Journey, provides a clinical foundation for understanding terminal disease and its impact on patients and families and for determining when a patient's time is limited. Chapters 2 and 3 follow a single patient case, illustrating the problem inherent to modern medicine, which often misses the forest for the trees and ignores the elephant in the room. Chapter 4 introduces the common terminal disease trajectories patients follow at the end of life, with patient vignettes bringing each trajectory to life. Chapter 5 introduces the hospice criteria used to determine when a patient has reached the end of their journey. The patient vignettes included in this book are faithful representations of actual patient experiences that have been de-identified to protect patient and family privacy.

Part II, Ground Rules for Compassionate Conversation, is a primer on patient-friendly bedside manner. Chapter 6 introduces the three important dimensions of a diagnosis that must be considered and tended to when caring for patients and families. Chapter 7 details the conversational rules of engagement for patient-centered care.

Part III, The Arc of Conversation, teaches a standardized approach to goals-of-care conversations. Chapter 8 introduces the technique and Chapters 9–12 detail the four conversational arcs of The Arc of Conversation.

Part IV, Aligning Patient Wishes With Care: The Goal of Patient-Centered Care, provides a brief conclusion to the book in Chap. 13.

Whereas the first four sections of the book build upon themselves and are recommended to be read in order, Part V can be referenced and read at any point. Chapter 14 is a quick reference guide that can be copied for use as a road map when practicing the technique with patients and families. Chapter 15 provides patient-friendly language for providing education to patients and families about chronic and terminal disease. Chapter 16 provides patient-friendly language for discussing advance directives, including the living will and POLST form. Chapter 17 provides patient-friendly language for discussing hospice care. Those unfamiliar with hospice care may want to start with Chap. 17.

The language of *The Arc of Conversation* is purposefully patient-friendly and intended for use by clinical staff at every level of the healthcare system and of every medical specialty. Patient-centered care that empowers people in their choices requires a clinical team that is knowledgeable and responsive to the needs of patients and families. By codifying the knowledge and conversational technique in *The Arc of Conversation*, I hope to accelerate adoption of compassionate and collaborative care, increase the success of goals-of-care conversations, and improve the experience of medicine for patients, families, and providers alike.

The Arc of Conversation is intended as a starting point for your own evolution as a practitioner. Use it, learn from it, add to its wealth with your own knowledge and experience, and improve upon it continually in your practice.

Part I

Acknowledging the Patient's Journey

The Forest for the Trees: Patient Decline and Acute Illness

2

I remember vividly the first time I told a family member that their loved one was dying of dementia. The patient, who we will call John, was a 93-year-old veteran who lived with his son Greg. When I first met John, he was asleep in his hospital bed. He lay peacefully, connected to the IV line delivering the antibiotics that were fighting the pneumonia that had developed in his lungs.

He was so still and calm that, for a second, when I entered his room, I thought he was dead.

He had the distinct look of the dying—skeletal cheek and eye bones and skin that was waxy and pale. His arms lacked any hint of muscle tone, having long ago lost the muscle mass he'd kept well into old age. It was easy to suspect that this tall, withered man, once strong and capable, had begun the final leg of his journey.

Despite three days of antibiotics, John didn't seem to be improving. A repeat chest X-ray indicated that his pneumonia was clearing up, and daily labs showed that his white blood cell count was almost back to normal. However, the nursing staff was unable to get him to eat, and physical therapy couldn't coax him from bed.

The hospital doctor could not discharge John in his present state. No rehabilitation center in town would accept a patient who wouldn't participate in physical therapy.

I was consulted to speak with Greg about his wishes for his father.

Greg, a retired veteran himself, had dutifully cared for his dad for the last five years. Greg was busy completing a significant bathroom renovation at his home, installing a walk-in bathtub that would make getting his dad in and out of the shower easier. When I met Greg, he was in a hurry to return to his project and was frustrated that his dad didn't seem to be getting better.

Greg was also understandably worried about how he would care for his father at home if his dad could not walk or get himself out of bed. Initially, the hospital doctor assured Greg that John could be discharged to a rehab center, but now Greg was told that might not be possible. He was confused about what would happen next and a bit overwhelmed.

A. Shaw, PA, *The Arc of Conversation*,
https://doi.org/10.1007/978-3-031-70495-6_2

Before my visit, I developed a preliminary assessment of John's overall health status, leading me to believe that John had indeed reached the end of his journey. Concerned that John's time was limited, I imagined he would never use the walk-in tub.

From John's chart, I learned that he had been on memantine and donepezil, medications to treat dementia, for several years. He was also on an antidepressant and something to help him sleep. In the prior 12 months, he had lost 40 pounds, nearly 20% of his total body weight. A recent blood panel mainly showed normal lab values, but his serum albumin was well below normal.

Albumin is a protein made only by the liver that, among other things, attracts and holds onto water molecules in the bloodstream, helping to maintain a person's blood pressure. On a blood panel, albumin provides insight into how well the liver functions and information about a person's nutritional status.

When a person's body can no longer repurpose digestion byproducts into new proteins, their albumin level drops, as does their muscle tone and body mass. John's low albumin explained the significant weight loss he had experienced in the prior year. His body could no longer use his nutrition to maintain itself like it once had.

Unsurprisingly, the bedside nurse informed me that John was bowel and bladder incontinent, that his speech was limited to one- or two-word answers, and that he needed help with eating, toileting, and bathing.

Alongside his pneumonia, these details painted a very clear picture of end-stage dementia.

Although this assessment seemed evident to me (and had required less than 20 minutes of investigation), I could not find *any* mention of dementia in the notes for John's current admission.

Initially, the hospital doctor described John as a "poor historian," documenting the need to speak to his son, Greg, for information about John's condition. The doctor identified three problems in John's assessment: pneumonia, failure to thrive, and dehydration. Treatment plans included IV antibiotics, IV hydration, and a consultation with a dietician to evaluate John's weight loss. Plans for discharging John from the hospital were already being anticipated: "As acute care needs are fulfilled, the patient is expected to be discharged either to home or short/long-term rehab depending on the physical/occupational therapy recommendations."

John's immediate issues were well-documented and being addressed. Although his pneumonia was resolving, John's overall condition wasn't improving.

When I asked Greg to paint a picture of how things had been going for his father over the last few years, he readily described the predictable and gradual decline seen with Alzheimer's disease, the most common type of dementia.

Initially, Greg noticed that John had problems remembering a word or the name of someone he knew and would repeat the same story two or three times during the same phone call or visit. At first, Greg chalked this up to old age, but eventually, he began to worry.

John had always been handy, able to repair anything that needed fixing. But a few years before Greg's mom died, John started doing odd things around the house. Once, when the deadbolt on the garage door became loose, John removed it and refused to put it back on despite always worrying about the possibility of someone breaking in. When Greg's mom couldn't convince John to reinstall the lock, she called Greg for help. Over the years, Greg found himself fixing his dad's "handiwork" more and more often.

After his mom died, Greg noticed a dramatic decline in his father. His mom had been the one to cook, clean, and manage the house, and after her death, John let everything go. He wore the same clothes day after day, rarely took a shower, and forgot to trim his beard. He mainly ate frozen dinners, if he ate at all, and stopped caring for the house and mowing the lawn.

One day, Greg noticed that his dad's car had a couple of new dents. When Greg asked about it, John grew angry, insisting nothing had happened.

It was when John stopped paying his bills and taking his medications that Greg realized that his dad could no longer manage on his own. Despite his father's reluctance to give up his independence, Greg insisted that his dad come to live with him. John put up a big fight but, oddly, forgot about it soon after moving in.

Greg watched as his father continued to decline over the years, needing more help to get dressed in the morning and take a shower. As John's appetite grew smaller and the weight fell from his father's once-robust frame, Greg worried that his dad would fall. He removed the rugs from his home, installed grab bars near doorframes, and began the bathroom renovation. Greg also bought his dad a walker and, chuckling, shared how John, instead of leaning on it for support, just dragged it behind him.

Six months earlier, John began having more frequent accidents, and twice, Greg found him urinating in a closet, confused about how to find the bathroom. Now, John wore adult diapers, and Greg kept a portable commode next to his father's bed.

A few weeks earlier, John began coughing during meals. Worried that his dad would choke, Greg started cutting John's food into small pieces and serving things that were easier for him to chew. When his dad started sleeping most of the day, and Greg couldn't wake him up one morning, Greg decided to call 911.

I am always impressed by the level of loving attention caregivers provide to family members with dementia. I knew that Greg was just one of millions of people patiently attending to a parent's or spouse's needs at home, providing for their physical, spiritual, and social well-being. Like Greg, most caregivers dedicate years to ensuring their loved one is fed, bathed, and clothed. And most, like Greg, do it without the benefit of understanding the changes their loved one is experiencing.

When I asked Greg what diagnosis he thought was responsible for the changes his father had experienced, he couldn't say. When I asked Greg where he thought his father was in his overall journey with his health and what he expected for his father going forward, he had no idea.

Greg is not alone. Most family members of patients with dementia have remarkably little understanding of their loved one's illness, why it causes the symptoms it does, or what they could expect in the future.

Often, I am the first provider to offer an in-depth discussion about a loved one's diagnosis, and very frequently, I am the first to communicate the concern that their loved one's time is limited.

At that point, I had been a palliative care provider for just a few months. Previously, I had worked in the hospital as a member of the cardiology team; thus, I was quite familiar with the hospitalists. I greatly respected their work and went out of my way to be helpful to them without stepping on their toes. At that point, I was not in the habit, particularly as a PA, of telling MDs what was really going on with their patients.

John's situation, however, struck me as an opportunity to provide better patient care and service to the hospital team.

I knew that hospitalists and other specialists were focused on pinpointing with precision the acute ailments that caused patients to feel bad (blood clots, bleeds, infections, tumors, fractures, or fluid overload). With John, I began to realize that the near-exclusive focus on acute ailments, in essence, created blinders, causing the greater picture of the patient's health status to go unseen. John's pneumonia might be resolving, and his blood counts recovering, but he wasn't getting "better," and his end-stage dementia meant that he never would.

Once I recognized this pattern, I began to see it everywhere I looked. Across the disease spectrum, I saw the same thing. Patients like John, admitted with pneumonia who had end-stage dementia. Patients with hip fractures who were dying of old age. Patients intubated in the intensive care unit (ICU) after acute episodes of worsening heart failure or chronic obstructive pulmonary disease (COPD) who had met hospice criteria for several months.

A narrow focus on admission diagnosis and acute stabilization was blinding the healthcare system to the *true cause* for the patient's admission—not aspiration, fall, or exacerbation, but rather, *dementia*, *general decline*, or *organ failure*—terminal trajectories with an expected pattern of decline.

With John, I realized that the healthcare system was missing the forest for the trees.

The Elephant in the Room: Disease Progression and Death

3

Palliative care, sometimes called supportive care, is a medical specialty designed to provide *an extra layer of support* to patients and their families living with chronic or life-threatening disease. Palliative care providers are trained to treat physical, mental, emotional, spiritual, and existential symptoms, and to help families navigate the socio-economic realities that can impact how people experience and survive a diagnosis. Because each patient and family is unique, palliative care providers must continually think outside the box to find ways to improve the lives of those they serve.[1]

In the United States, hospice care is a special type of palliative care created for patients with a terminal diagnosis and short prognosis (typically six months or less) that focuses entirely on patient and family comfort and support. Hospice care seeks to improve *quality of life* when a patient's *quantity of life* is diminished.[2]

For the perspective it has given me, I am grateful that in my role as a palliative care provider, I also serve as a member of our hospice care team. In this capacity, one of my primary tasks is to determine whether patients referred to our hospice center meet eligibility for hospice care, expertise that not all palliative care providers possess. To do this, I review patient charts, identify the diagnosis responsible for the patient's decline, and compare lab values and other evidence of disease progression against *hospice criteria* corresponding to the patient's prevailing diagnosis.

By the time I met John, I had become skilled enough at evaluating patients for hospice eligibility to understand the seemingly disconnected details of John's health—his incontinence, inability to walk, difficulty swallowing, and pneumonia—as a clear picture of end-stage dementia.

---

[1] For a thorough discussion of palliative (supportive) care and template language that can be used to discuss palliative (supportive) care with patients and families, see Chap. 11.

[2] For a thorough discussion of hospice care, see Chap. 5. Template language that can be used to teach patients and families about hospice care can be found in Chap. 17.

© The Author(s), under exclusive license to Springer Nature Switzerland AG 2024
A. Shaw, PA, *The Arc of Conversation*,
https://doi.org/10.1007/978-3-031-70495-6_3

Yet, John's dementia diagnosis had been entirely overlooked. This was concerning because Greg's expectations were set in a landscape that left out this important feature.

The narrative that Greg had received, that his father's pneumonia was expected to clear up and that rehab would help him improve, was inaccurate and incomplete because it failed to acknowledge the terminal nature of John's dementia.

Although IV antibiotics might clear up this current lung infection, John's inability to swallow safely, a byproduct of the degradation of his brain, would not improve. He would almost certainly develop another bout of aspiration pneumonia, the most common cause of death for patients with Alzheimer's disease [1].

The treatment team's plan to discharge John to a short- or long-term rehabilitation facility is a classic example of missing the forest (terminal dementia) for the trees (acute condition such as aspiration pneumonia). Physical and occupational therapists are experts at determining the level of a patient's functional status, but without a greater appreciation of where a patient is in the course of a progressive disease like dementia, recommendations for rehab can be misleading. Moreover, they can lead to a misalignment of patients' wishes with end-of-life care and even a reduction in quality of life when a patient arrives at the end of a journey.

For John, given the advanced nature of his disease, physical therapy was unlikely to be effective and rather more likely to exhaust whatever energy he still had available. Additionally, a stay in a care facility would separate him from his son during the precious time they had left.

It would have been futile for me to talk to Greg about his wishes for his father without guiding him toward the understanding that his father's time was limited. John had reached the point in his journey where, despite medical intervention, his disease had progressed beyond the medical community's ability to alter its course. Moreover, John would continue to experience recurrent infections—*the hallmark of end-stage dementia*—which would require him to continue to return to the hospital.

It was my job to learn what Greg understood his father's wishes would be for his ongoing care, including whether John would want to continue to return to the hospital. If Greg understood that his father would not want to return to the hospital, and particularly if John might prefer to focus on his quality of life and comfort, then it was my job to educate Greg about *hospice care*, a treatment option that enables patients to avoid hospitalizations at a stage in their journey when hospital admissions are expected to recur.

Most people, if given the choice, are eager to avoid hospitalizations. This is particularly true for caregivers of patients with dementia, who understand how distressing hospital stays can be for their loved ones.

As I helped guide Greg further through a conversation about his father's dementia, gently painting a picture of what the end of that journey looks like and where I thought his father was, I could see his shock and dismay.

Not only did Greg not fully understand how seriously ill his father was, but he had no idea that his father's time was limited.

This is not at all uncommon. As happens with many patients, following his diagnosis, John's dementia had mostly gone unmentioned by the medical community over the years. Although Greg ensured that his father never missed an appointment, no one had taken the time to help Greg understand the *why* and *how* of dementia, *where* his father was in his journey, or *what* would happen next.

Without the benefit of this knowledge, Greg had a tough time understanding how a pneumonia diagnosis a few days earlier could so easily signify the end of his father's life.

~~~

Medical doctors hold an honored and revered position in modern society. Surpassing firefighters, nurses, and teachers, doctors routinely top lists of *The Most Respected Profession*, winning people's esteem worldwide.

And for good reason. Doctors save and extend people's lives every day. Whether treating a common cold or ushering the world through the COVID-19 coronavirus pandemic, doctors shepherd people through every stage of life and every manner of medical predicament, helping people get back or stay on track to live the lives they want.

Depending on the specialty, doctors dedicate between seven and 15 years (or more) to pursuing medical knowledge and training. Few other professions demand as much from those who wish to serve the public. The health and well-being of societies worldwide depend, in large part, on the medical acumen of their nation's physicians.

Yet, at least here in the United States, when it comes to caring for patients nearing or at the end of life, the medical community is woefully under-skilled.

I had worked in palliative care for just six months when, in a couple of weeks, I was consulted to see two patients with very different cancer diagnoses. Before my visit, both patients had been seen the same day by their specialists in the hospital and told to follow up with them in the outpatient setting in the next two weeks, with no indication that the providers understood that the patients had reached end-stage.

When I arrived to see these patients, they were *actively transitioning toward death.* Each of them died later on the day of my visit.

It seems particularly unfathomable that physicians specializing in terminal diseases would be unable to recognize death when it was right there in front of them.

Though extreme, these examples are hardly exceptional. For every trajectory leading toward the end of life, I have seen patients at the very end of their journey whose terminal approach had been ignored by the medical team taking care of them. With John's case, I recognized a pattern evident across not just my hospital but the entire healthcare system.

As hospital care has shifted from one in which primary care providers care for their patients both in and out of the hospital to one in which hospitalists specialize in providing care for hospitalized patients, we have lost the forest for the trees. Without the benefit of a long-standing relationship with their patients and with the pressure to discharge patients as quickly as possible, ER providers, hospitalists, and consulting specialists understandably focus nearly exclusively on acute stabilization.

As with John, a narrow focus on acute stabilization leads hospital providers to ignore the elephant in the room—disease progression and death.

The reason for this, though surprising, is quite simple. The medical education system does not train clinicians in end-of-life care, considerations, and conversations. Thus, untrained and unable to recognize when the end is near, providers can easily ignore it.

Can we pause for just a moment to imagine a medical community untrained in criteria to diagnose or treat disease? We can't, because that would be unthinkable.

Yet, in my experience, the medical community is almost entirely ignorant when it comes to utilizing hospice criteria to understand progressive disease course.

As a hospital palliative care provider and geriatrics rotation preceptor for the local family medicine residency program, I regularly interact with new providers fresh from their residencies and medical school. I habitually ask these clinicians whether or not they have heard of or been trained in the use of hospice criteria. I also ask seasoned, experienced physicians this same question. To date, no one has answered in the affirmative.

Even specialists who focus on progressive and terminal illnesses like heart failure, chronic obstructive pulmonary disease (COPD), and neurologic diseases like amyotrophic lateral sclerosis (ALS) and Parkinson's disease (PD) do not have a robust appreciation for or even working knowledge of hospice criteria.

In the three years that I worked in cardiology, I cannot recall having heard of or being taught about hospice criteria for heart disease, even though heart failure is one of the hospital's top reasons for admissions and follows a predictable and eventually terminal course. I can recall just one patient whom our service transitioned to hospice care during my time in cardiology, after a failed at-home trial of an IV pressor—a medication whose job it is to force the heart to pump, without which the patient would be expected to die, and which is a treatment usually reserved for the ICU.

Although clinicians are expertly trained to interpret symptoms and signs on the body as indications of disease, they are not prepared to recognize indications of disease progression and decline, including emergency room (ER) visits, hospital admissions, and care facility stays. Current medical education, with its single-minded focus on acute stabilization, results in a lack of appreciation for the bigger picture, often leading to a failure to appreciate the elephant in the room.

Hospice utilization in the United States bears out these observations. Whereas the Medicare hospice benefit, and its commercial analogs, is designed to give people *at least* six months of quality care at the end of life, the median length of stay on hospice in the United States is just 18 days, a number that has barely budged in the last 15 years [2]. Although the vast majority (70%) of Americans want to focus on quality and comfort at the end of their lives [3], in 2019, just over half of Medicare beneficiaries died with hospice care in place [2].

As we will see in the following chapters, hospital admissions of patients with end-stage disease are not surprising. All terminal disease trajectories follow a pattern where *it is only a matter of time* before a patient is hospitalized. Without an alternative option for care, patients come to the hospital seeking symptom management and stabilization. Once there, the cycle repeats itself—failure to focus on disease progression and recognition of the end leads to failure to align patient wishes with care, and one hospitalization leads to the next.

I believe we can do better.

~~~

Although I didn't recognize it then, my conversation with John's son, Greg, was an early success in applying *The Arc of Conversation* technique taught in this book.

Recognizing John's terminal condition, I took my time with Greg, delving deeply into his experience and understanding of his father's condition, making sure that my assessment was spot on. Only once convinced that my hunch was correct did I risk gently guiding Greg toward the realization that his father's time was limited. I knew that if he didn't believe me, he might share his doubt with the hospitalist, who might agree with him!

Fortunately, Greg responded as most caregivers of loved ones with dementia do. With his new appreciation for the dementia journey, recognizing that the disease had greatly diminished his father's quality of life, he readily accepted what hadn't been named for him before and made the decision to transition his father to hospice care.

In helping Greg understand that his father was likely to remain bed-bound for the rest of his life, I explained that all of John's needs could be met in a hospital bed that Medicare would pay for at his house. Greg no longer needed to worry about his father getting well enough to go to rehab.

The hospitalist, though a bit surprised, was grateful to learn that John met hospice criteria and that Greg wanted to take him home. This nicely resolved the discharge dilemma.

John's case became the catalyst I needed to push our palliative care service in a direction that would provide greater value to patients and providers. Recognizing that no other service had the training or the time to dedicate to the task, I made the assessment of disease progression and evaluation against hospice criteria the foundation of our work.

By performing this simple assessment on every patient we see, our service is better positioned to usher patients and families through *goals of care conversations*, leading to a better alignment of patient and family wishes with their care.

Armed with an accurate understanding of where a patient is in the course of an illness and by following *The Arc of Conversation* technique, any provider can successfully guide patients and families with minimal understanding of a loved one's diagnosis at the start of a conversation to an authentic, self-determined decision about care that aligns with their personal values, hopes, and needs.

When we consider the most critical aspect of patient-centered care—*respect for patient autonomy*—it is easy to appreciate that an accurate assessment is the foundation upon which patients and families make medical decisions that are right for them. True patient-centered care cannot exist without it.

References

1. Todd S, Barr AP, Passmore AP. Cause of death in Alzheimer's disease: a cohort study. QJM. 2013;106(8):747–53. https://doi.org/10.1093/qjmed/hct103.
2. National Hospice and Palliative Care Organization. NHPCO Facts and Figures Report, 2021 Edition. [Internet]. 2021. https://www.nhpco.org/wp-content/uploads/NHPCO-Facts-Figures-2021.pdf. Accessed 9 Jul 2022.
3. Hamel L, Wu B, Brodie M. Views and experiences with end-of-life medical care in the U.S. 2017. https://files.kff.org/attachment/Report-Views-and-Experiences-with-End-of-Life-Medical-Care-in-the-US. Accessed 9 Jul 2022.

Approaches to the End of Life: Disease Trajectories

4

Whenever a patient is before us, we are tasked with answering the question:

What is happening?

As health care providers, we must address this inquiry in a way that provides patients and families with the answers they seek.

Some seek symptom management, such as to be free from pain, swelling, or shortness of breath. Others seek a cure, wanting to rid themselves of an ailment so that they can return to the life they love once again. Still others, if we were to ask, merely seek to understand what they already suspect is unfolding.

How we address each patient's question depends on the depth of our inquiry.

On the surface, we can answer the immediate question:

What is happening right now with this patient?

The answer to this might reveal an acute infection, such as pneumonia, located in the lungs and caused by bacteria. Further investigation might identify the specific antibiotic designed to reduce the offending agent so the patient might recover.

When we think of the trees in the forest of a patient's life and where we, as the medical community, typically exist, we find ourselves mostly at ground level, wandering from tree to tree, addressing specific issues and concerns.

Yet, if we were to expand our perspective and instead fly high overhead, we would peer down and notice that there is a very different question to be asked:

What does what is happening right now with this patient signify?

If we are to help patients and families understand what is happening so that they can make fully informed decisions about what is right for them at a particular juncture in their lives, then this is the question we must continually address.

© The Author(s), under exclusive license to Springer Nature Switzerland AG 2024
A. Shaw, PA, *The Arc of Conversation*,
https://doi.org/10.1007/978-3-031-70495-6_4

To begin to do this requires an understanding of disease as an ever-evolving process, not merely a moment in time. If diagnosis is the snapshot of a patient's medical state, then disease is the motion picture of the patient's life.

The body, as we know, is in constant flux, with systems working continuously to balance each biochemical equation to maintain homeostasis. The bicarbonate buffer system, which balances the pH of the blood and equilibrates the byproducts of respiration (CO_2), is the most well-known and vital example of this process, but there are a plethora of others interlinked.

As organs fail, as metabolism peters out, or as cancer takes over, the harmony of a healthy body is thrown off-kilter. As degraded systems struggle to achieve stasis, the balance becomes upset, and the disease side of the equation predominates, with patients needing care for overwhelming symptoms—the outward manifestation of a system out of whack.

This perpetual shift from stability to instability is the ebb and flow of disease. At times, it is like the tide, and at others, a tsunami, showing up in our diagnosis codes as infections, falls, and respiratory failure and in our utilization reports as emergency room visits and ICU stays.

If stabilization is the immediate task, the next priority is anticipating what comes next. This requires recognizing the specific movie unfolding for the patient before us and learning to interpret the testimony of disease—recurrent infections and admissions, escalations of care, and trips to rehab—as identifiers of a particular trajectory.

Unlike electrons, whose former or future paths cannot be determined by their present state, with large bodies, such determinations are almost always possible. Like the planets, disease follows a fairly predictable course. If we take the time to ask patients and families what they've been experiencing, we can almost always, within the course of a single conversation, accurately determine which trajectory a patient is following and, from there, what is likely to happen next.

As with all things, trends are important to identify because they tend to continue. This is especially true for a patient's functional status—the ability to make it through the day on one's own.

This often-ignored domain, which I believe to be *the most important vital sign*, makes life worth living for many people, particularly older adults. Loss of independence due to functional decline can be so keenly felt as to rob people of their entire *raison d'être*, their purpose for living. Once this is gone, many people willingly give up.

Because patients are far greater than the sum of their lab values and imaging results, the magnification power of our inquiries must be adjusted to take in the whole person sitting before us, rather than to focus solely on the most recent diagnosis. This means prioritizing the human dimension of disease, that is, how the process on the physical body impacts the daily life of the patient and their loved ones.

Ultimately, terminal disease entails a progressive and permanent loss of personal independence. Thus, functional status serves as a primary indicator of disease progression and, as we shall see, a key component of a hospice evaluation. Because it reveals so much, a functional status evaluation should be included as an essential part of ongoing assessment for every patient.

Each of the terminal trajectories follows a unique course, leaving an identifiable signature of symptoms and functional loss in the patient's life. Learning to recognize the shape and duration of each terminal trajectory is the first step in supporting patients and families as they traverse the landscape of disease. Such recognition provides a starting point to help them understand what is happening at the present moment in a deeply meaningful way and, more importantly, to understand what is likely to occur in the subsequent scenes of the movie that is their disease trajectory.

~~~

Most people are somewhat surprised to learn that there are a minimal number of approaches to the end of life. Maybe it's that we want to believe that each of us is unique in the universe, or perhaps it's simply that no one has ever told us otherwise.

If you hold up your right hand and spread your fingers apart, given you've retained all your digits, that's it. There are just five primary patterns of terminal decline [1].

Described in recent decades by various provider-researchers working in palliative and hospice care,[1] the five primary terminal trajectories include Sudden Death, Catastrophic Event, Organ Failure, Cancer, and Frailty/Dementia [1–8]. Two of the trajectories (Sudden Death and Catastrophic Event) are uncommon enough that the vast majority of us (85%) [5] will travel just one of the three remaining paths.

A patient of mine named Tina, who was dying of heart failure, shared an insightful story about her mother, who died of cancer. Early in her mother's illness, Tina asked her mom if she'd ever wondered, "Why me?"

Tina remembered being hurt by her mother's response, "Why not me?"

Believing that her mother should "fight" her disease, the younger Tina heard her mother's words as an effortless capitulation, a giving up. But now, facing her own terminal decline, Tina felt a newfound appreciation for her mother's wisdom.

When I asked her to explain, Tina shared, "None of us is above or below the other guy. God has plans for each of us, and we don't get to decide."

Tina's words were the spiritual equivalent of the statistic I often share with patients and families that nearly all of us will follow just one of three approaches to the end of life. When I shared this information, Tina's eyes widened. When I added that it is primarily the luck of the draw, Tina nodded in agreement.

---

[1] Barney G. Glaser and Anselm L. Strauss first introduced the concept of a *trajectory of dying* in 1965, noting, "the dying trajectory of each patient has at least two outstanding [and variable] properties…duration and shape." [2] Figures describing three disease trajectories (Sudden Death, Steady Death, and Advanced Illness) were introduced by Marilyn J. Field and Christine K. Cassel in 1997 [3]. A 2002 investigation of the patterns of end-of-life decline in 7258 Medicare decedents who died between 1993 and 1998 by June R. Lunney, Ph.D., R.N., Joanne Lynn, MD, MA, MS, and Christopher Hogan, Ph.D. found that the vast majority (92%) of the decedents they studied followed one of four primary trajectories of Sudden Death, Terminal Illness (Cancer), Organ Failure, and Frailty [5]. In 2018, Jennifer Moore Ballentine, MA, described a fifth trajectory, Catastrophic Event, placing events including nonfatal heart attack, stroke, traumatic brain injury, and hip fracture in the elderly within this trajectory framework [1].

Each of us bargains daily with what we believe to be our allotted remaining time, making decisions about seatbelts, vaccinations, exercise, and alcohol according to our perceived ratio of risk and reward. Some of us, hoping to stave off death by one or another cause, take extra vitamins, spend hours at the gym, or play word games or puzzles in our free time.

And yet, barring that daily fifth of vodka, there doesn't seem to be much rhyme or reason for who follows which path toward the end of life. My great-grandmother lived to be 109. Depending on your perspective, she was either fortunate or not. Maybe I'll live that long. But I'm just as likely to die of some form of cancer or organ failure. While most of us *hope* to die painlessly in our sleep after a long life characterized by love and connection, it is simply not up to us. Luck, in many ways, determines much of our lives, and how we die is no exception.

Highlighting the importance of a patient's loss of independence, the five primary disease trajectories can be illustrated with a diagram tracking the decline in functional status over time. When speaking with patients and families, I find that sharing these illustrations allows them to better organize their experiences and understanding of death. Just as I can pull examples of each of these trajectories from my family tree, most people will have seen one or more of these journeys among those they've known.

The patient vignettes that follow are not meant to comprise an exhaustive litany of the presentations of terminal decline. Rather, they are intended to orient the reader to the five primary trajectories and serve as a starting point for developing a greater appreciation and recognition of this critical stage of life.

Sudden Death

Approximately 1 in 10 of us in the United States dies suddenly [1]. We are alive, and then, we simply aren't.

The path described by this trajectory is a sharp, downward plunge, as our life force leaves us in seconds or minutes, with medical intervention unavailable, unsuccessful, or arriving too late to have an impact (Fig. 4.1). In the U.S., common causes of sudden death include sudden cardiac death (most commonly, heart attack), car accidents, gun violence, suicide, homicide, unintentional falls, and poisoning (often due to opioid overdose) [9–11].

In the ninth grade, one of my classmates, thinking that his girlfriend was pregnant, fatally shot himself. Our entire town was stunned. To this day, I can't imagine the trauma his parents experienced as they heard the gunshot shortly after he arrived home, only to find their lives irrevocably altered by such a permanent act.

My great-aunt Margaret accidentally drove her husband's golf cart into a water hazard while on vacation in Florida. Not knowing how to swim, she drowned.

My high school boyfriend, also unable to swim, drowned one summer Sunday afternoon shortly after our graduation. Panicked in the water, he nearly drowned me as well. A very up close and personal experience of his death, this touched me deeply.

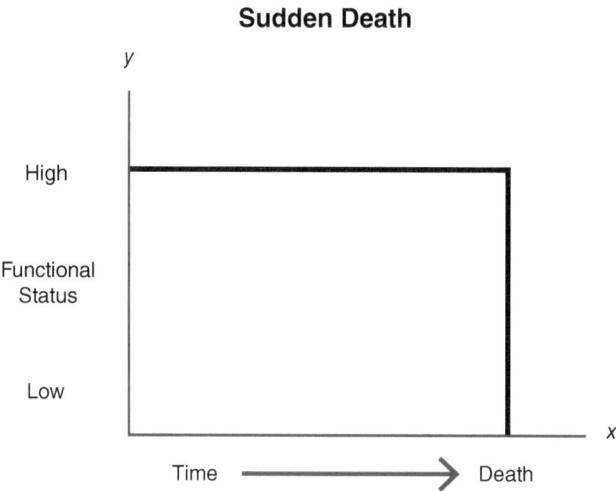

Fig. 4.1 Sudden Death. (Adapted with permission from Lunney et al. (2002). *Profiles of Older Medicare Decedents*. Journal of the American Geriatrics Society [6])

During my emergency medicine rotation in PA school, I encountered a 55-year-old male who had collapsed at home while eating dinner and was rushed into the ER. The first responders had already performed 45 minutes of cardiopulmonary resuscitation (CPR) on the patient by the time he arrived in the ER. A fresh team of medical residents and emergency room staff took over. Still, the patient was pronounced dead after 25 minutes, having succumbed to the most common cause of sudden cardiac death, an acute myocardial infarction (MI, or heart attack).

Sudden death robs victims and loved ones alike of the opportunity to say goodbye. Family is caught unaware, shocked, and left to navigate a world around a sudden and immense void.

Survivor guilt and burdensome existential questions probing, "Why him? Why now?" are common. For victims of violence, additional feelings of anger, blame, helplessness, and rage can impact a loved one's ability to work, sleep, eat, and find peace.

As healthcare providers, our attention and empathy for those left behind—to keep watch for depression, prolonged grief, and even suicide—are important components of our compassionate care. Prescriptions for antidepressants and self-care, as well as referrals to counseling and hospice centers—which provide bereavement support for those left behind—are ways we can help.

Catastrophic Event

On the Catastrophic Event trajectory, the patient experiences a significant traumatic event or medical emergency before their death [1]. Although a person's immediate demise is prevented either by good fortune or by the miracle of modern medicine, the patient is left so functionally and biologically dependent as to have very little remaining quality of life [1] (Fig. 4.2). Families often face the difficult decision to withdraw treatment, allowing the patient to pass in due time.

In 2019, more than 150,000 Americans died following a cerebrovascular accident (CVA or stroke), making it the fifth leading cause of death in the United States [13].

Following the initial trauma, patients and loved ones often experience a cataclysm of emotions, ranging from hope and optimism to hopelessness and despair. Those faced with decisions to withdraw treatment can be plagued by guilt, fear of the unknown, and the heavy weight of "giving up," either on themselves or on a loved one. Depending on the length of time that transpires between the initial event and the patient's death, the shocking emotional impact that accompanies a sudden death may also be experienced. When an extended period follows the catastrophic event, loved ones can suffer the mental, emotional, financial, and physical exhaustion of caregiving. Early and ongoing support by providers trained in the palliative care approach is integral to caring for caregivers.

This trajectory can also take a toll on clinical staff, who can experience the emotional ups and downs of a patient's journey in parallel with the family. The loss of a patient following life-saving heroic medical efforts can be emotionally devastating to care team members, who can feel the emotional weight of what they may believe to be a personal or medical failure. Institutions can mitigate emotional exhaustion and burnout among clinical staff by supporting programs designed to promote compassion, empathy, and collegial support [12].

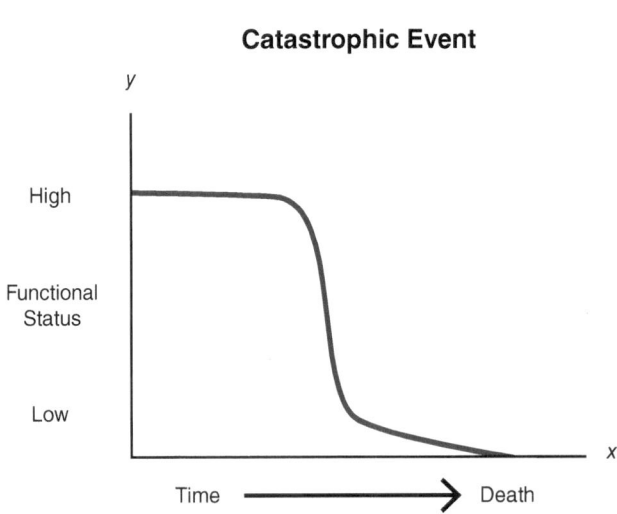

Fig. 4.2 Catastrophic Event. (Adapted with permission from Ballentine, J. M.. (2018). *The Five Trajectories: Supporting Patients During Serious Illness.* CSU Shiley Haynes Institute for Palliative Care [1]. Copyright ©2018, Jennifer Moore Ballentine. All rights reserved)

Although it is impossible to tell exactly what happened, my uncle Craig suffered a terrible bicycle accident one rainy September afternoon. Tourists driving through the State Park where he'd been cycling found him down on the road and called 911 for help. Taken first by ambulance to the local emergency room, he was life-flighted to a trauma hospital in Erie, Pennsylvania, and rushed immediately into the operating room. Exploratory surgery revealed a large hemorrhage. The intracranial bleeding was stopped, and a portion of his skull was removed to alleviate the pressure on his brain.

This intervention saved my uncle's life, but he required subsequent surgeries and escalations of care, including a feeding tube and a breathing machine. Despite the incredible treatment he received, his brain had suffered permanent and devastating damage. He was unable to live on his own without extracorporeal support.

To know my uncle was to know a man who felt most alive outside in the natural world. An avid hunter, fisherman, skier, and cyclist, he would not have wanted to be kept alive by machines if there was no hope that he could once again participate in life in a meaningful way. Nor would he have wanted to burden his family with the task of caring for him in a bed-bound state. Honoring his essence, ten days after his accident, his wife and children made the heartbreaking decision to withdraw treatment and allow him to pass. He died in the ICU with his family at his side.

~~~

During my cardiology days, I cared for a very sweet patient named Walter, who showed up in the clinic for each visit wearing his overalls and accompanied by his engaging, insightful wife, Anita. They eagerly made the 2-hour trek from their tiny Nebraska town twice a year, as they said, to get a visit to the big city of Cheyenne, with a wink and a smile in their eyes.

Walter and Anita were vibrant, warm souls who opened their childless home each year to foreign exchange students and shared the wonders and cultures of the United States with their guests. We swapped stories of travel during Walter's visits, and I always looked forward to seeing his name appear on my schedule.

Thus, it was with a heavy heart, one day, that I saw Anita, more frail and stooped than I could recall, pushing Walter by wheelchair into the clinic waiting room before his appointment.

Back at my desk, I learned from Walter's chart that four months prior, he had suffered a stroke. Despite two months at our hospital's Acute Rehabilitation Unit and six subsequent weeks at a skilled nursing facility, where I knew he had worked upwards of three hours each day with physical, occupational, and speech therapists, he had not regained his ability to walk or swallow. A permanent feeding tube, which had been inserted into his abdomen just two weeks after his stroke, remained.

Although the feeding tube kept Walter's weight in an adequate range, Walter and Anita, too, looked frail, pale, and weak. My heart broke to see the two of them like this, so diminished by what had happened. The strain of caring for Walter was visible on Anita's worn-out face. For Walter's sake, she tried to appear unfazed, but I could tell that his stroke had taken a significant toll on her.

When I asked how they had been since Walter returned home, Anita told me how much Walter missed eating the meals she cooked and how much they both missed their Sunday suppers with their church friends. Anita explained how exhausting it was for Walter to sit upright for so many hours each day while the feeding solution slowly drained from its bag into his stomach. If he slouched or reclined during this procedure, he risked aspirating the liquid nutrition into his lungs.

While Anita spoke, Walter mainly kept quiet. Speaking was a terrible effort for him, his speech a forced whisper, his voice weakened by disuse. I gently touched his knee when he grew frustrated with the effort, reassuring him that it was okay to rest.

Walter had been seen in the ER three times since his stroke, once for aspiration pneumonia and two more times for anxiety. I asked Anita to explain.

She told me that just as Walter couldn't swallow food, he was unable to swallow his own saliva. So much of it collected in his mouth throughout the day that when it pooled toward the back of his throat, he began to feel like he was suffocating. When this happened, and it happened many times each day, he became terribly anxious. Too weak to cough, unable to clear the saliva, he would sometimes begin to panic, and then, as he hyperventilated, the saliva would block his airway. Twice, watching as Walter turned blue during one of these episodes, terrified that he would die in front of her, and not knowing what else to do, Anita called the ambulance.

During the second visit to the ER, the physician gave Walter a prescription for lorazepam, intended to reduce his anxiety. Anita reported that the lorazepam was only mildly helpful, adding that she figured there wasn't a medication on Earth that could calm a person who was convinced he was about to die.

Listening to Walter's lungs, I heard wheezing and congestion. Even without my stethoscope, I could hear the secretions in his throat, which were hampering the airflow to his lungs. His pulse oximeter reading had been 86%, prompting the medical assistant to start supplemental oxygen in the clinic room. All of this pointed to the likelihood that Walter had once again developed pneumonia, and I recommended that he be seen in the ER. Reluctantly, Anita and Walter agreed.

A few days later, I learned from Walter's chart that he and Anita had made what I could only imagine having been a heart-wrenching decision to stop his tube feeding and transition to hospice care. At the time, I wasn't entirely sure what that meant other than knowing that a person without nutrition or fluids would not survive long.

I recall feeling a deep admiration for the bravery and strength of Walter's decision, wondering what I would do in a similar situation. I hoped Walter would have a smooth and peaceful death, free from panic and anxiety, and I wished for Anita the kind of peace she would need to survive the loss of her adoring husband and life partner. Walter passed away two weeks after our visit.

~~~

As a palliative care provider, I met Frank a year and a half before he died. Six months before I was consulted to speak with his wife and daughter about what they thought his medical wishes would be, Frank had suffered a massive stroke while working on the roof of his home. Although he survived falling from his ladder, he had a fitful night, complaining of eye pain, a significant headache, nausea, and weakness. Not understanding that her husband had experienced a medical emergency, it wasn't until morning that Frank's wife, Dottie, brought him to the hospital.

Sadly, the damage to Frank's brain crystallized as the double whammy of the unmitigated, evolving stroke and a fall-induced hemorrhage affected multiple centers of function. In addition to losing his ability to swallow and speak, Frank could not move or control his body in any voluntary way. A feeding tube kept Frank alive, and he spent most of his days immobile in bed. With an indwelling catheter in place, Frank required around-the-clock, personal care for all aspects of living.

Dottie, whose medical literacy was limited by her sixth-grade education, sincerely believed that Frank's brain could recover at any moment. It wasn't so much that she was waiting for a God-given miracle but instead expecting a biological recovery that only she believed possible. At some point along her husband's journey, she had heard a physician mention six months as a timeframe for possible brain healing. She had held that message close to her heart and remained hopeful where no one else felt optimism.

I could sense Dottie's love for her husband as she sat attentively by Frank's side, holding and stroking his hand. When we spoke, I could also see the impact of her limited education, the sometimes frustrating reality of a conceptually immutable belief system that no medical explanation is likely to penetrate.

Although none of the medical providers following Frank believed he had any voluntary capacity remaining, his wife was confident that he moved his eyes meaningfully to her voice and that his occasional grip, believed by the neurologist to be caused by involuntary muscle spasticity, was intentional. Without the benefit of even a rudimentary understanding of cellular biology, Dottie was impervious to the medical team's attempts at explaining the permanence of Frank's brain damage.

Sensitive to her wish for at least six months of potential recovery time, the medical team had waited before involving my team. After a pleasant conversation with Dottie, I reported to the hospitalist caring for Frank that his wife was consistent in her wish to provide his body and brain time to recover. Although six months had come and gone, Dottie sincerely believed that God would intervene on her husband's behalf. Our service would follow him in the outpatient setting and continue to pursue goals of care conversations with Dottie and her family over time.

Over the next 18 months, Frank was hospitalized more than 20 times for aspiration pneumonia, urinary tract infections, and dehydration. Despite receiving an adequate amount of nutrition by the feeding tube, he lost weight, slowly but surely, until his albumin declined precipitously to a number that is consistent with poor wound healing. Pressure points from immobility became ulcers that were unable to heal, leading to cellulitis and sepsis, and additional admissions to the hospital.

Frank's family supported him to the best of their abilities, someone visiting him in the nursing facility where he lived nearly every day. Concerned for his mental and spiritual well-being when the COVID-19 pandemic closed the facility to visitors, his daughter, Anne, took leave from work and moved Frank into her home. Despite making every effort to care for him, Frank's high level of assistance around the clock was too much for Anne to manage. Reluctantly, feeling as though she was letting her father down, she made the difficult decision to move him back to the nursing home.

After one of Frank's hospital admissions, I scheduled a visit with Dottie and Anne to revisit the question of Frank's medical wishes. I was surprised when Anne opened our conversation by letting me know that her mother was ready to change Frank's code status to "Do Not Resuscitate" (DNR) . Recognizing this as a significant development, I asked Anne to explain.

She shared that her mother had accepted that Frank would not recover. Where Dottie had once been hopeful that Frank would return to the active, funny, vibrant man she had married, she now believed that Frank would not want to continue to live like this, dependent on others and separated from his family. Dottie wanted Frank to be comfortable, peaceful, and in a place where the entire family could visit more easily. She did not want Frank to return to the hospital anymore.

Just shy of two years following his incident, Dottie decided to transition Frank to hospice care, remove his feeding tube, and allow him to pass. Frank was transferred to our community's hospice center, where he received continual nursing support during his final weeks of life. Dottie and Anne spent most of their days by his side, and Dottie was there to hold Frank's hand as he took his final breath.

~~~

For Walter, Frank, and my uncle, their fragile physical condition following the initial trauma led to ongoing and intensive medical care, and in my uncle's case, mechanical support for organs no longer able to function on their own.

In contrast, a subset of patients who experience a Catastrophic Event will remain stable at a survivable level of dysfunction for many years and will instead go on to die from a different disease trajectory. This is commonly seen following strokes and other forms of traumatic brain injury (TBI).

Louis, whose car accident more than a decade prior left him wheelchair-bound, incontinent of bowel and bladder, and nonverbal, is still able to feed himself, swallow without incident, and use his arms to power his wheelchair around the nursing facility where he lives. Pleasantly confused, Louis is rarely seen in the ER and hasn't been admitted to the hospital in more than four years, a testament to the excellent care he receives.

Because Louis is at increased risk of developing dementia following his TBI, I carefully watch him for changes in weight and his ability to feed himself, get around on his own, and swallow. Should I notice anything concerning for a transition onto a different trajectory, I will revisit the question of his medical wishes with Louis's family.

Organ Failure

In 2019, approximately 1 in 3 Americans followed the Organ Failure trajectory at the end of their lives [13], with heart and lung disease accounting for the vast majority of organ failure deaths.

This trajectory follows a path of steady loss of function and personal independence punctuated by periods of dramatic disequilibrium, called *exacerbations*, in which patients are frequently hospitalized for stabilization and resolution of symptoms. Functional status tends to decline following each exacerbation, and a return to the former baseline becomes unlikely (Fig. 4.3).

Eventually, patients on this trajectory will reach a point where medical interventions can no longer alter the course of their disease. Without an alternative form of support to aggressively manage and control symptoms (hospice care), it is typically only a matter of time until patients return to the hospital.

At this late stage of disease, escalations of care, including cardiopulmonary resuscitation, intubation, mechanical ventilation, and the use of pressors (drugs that force the heart to pump), become increasingly likely. When disease progresses naturally to requiring such interventions, patients struggle to survive without them. Once these interventions are initiated, patients often find themselves dependent on them, and their quality of life severely diminished. Faced with the decision to withdraw treatment, patients in this circumstance often die in the ICU or on the medical floor.

Because we know that almost everyone wants to spend the end of their lives in comfort and surrounded by loved ones, discussions about end-of-life wishes and education about hospice care must occur long before patients with organ failure get to the point of meeting hospice criteria.

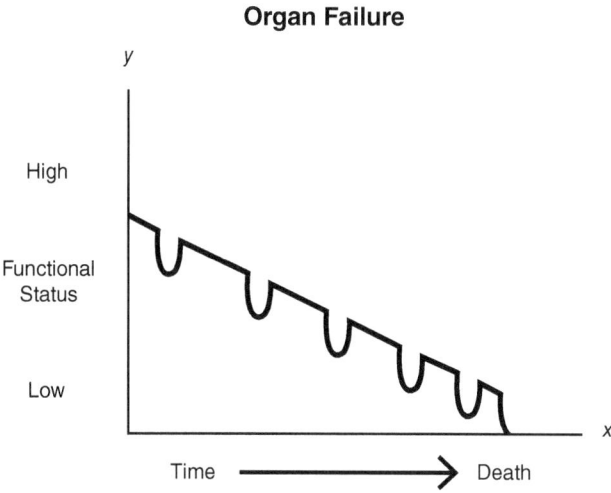

Fig. 4.3 Organ Failure. (Adapted with permission from Lunney et al. (2002). *Profiles of Older Medicare Decedents.* Journal of the American Geriatrics Society [6])

Heart Failure

Heart failure is a progressive and terminal disease that often leads to recurrent hospitalizations. In my hospital, heart and lung failure continually compete for the top reason for admission. In 2018, following septicemia (an infection of the bloodstream), heart failure was the second leading cause of hospital admission in the United States [14]. In 2020, more than 690,000 Americans died of heart disease [15], making it the leading cause of death in the United States [15, 16].

Heart disease comprises various diagnoses involving any of the heart's structural components. Like a house, the heart has rooms (upper chambers called *atria* and lower chambers called *ventricles*), doors (the atrioventricular and semilunar valves), and both an electrical (heartbeat) and plumbing (blood supply) system. Dysfunction in any of these areas can cause heart failure—a decline in the heart's ability to pump.

Derrick's heart had problems with each of its components. Shortly after turning 60, Derrick suffered a major heart attack, requiring open heart surgery to reconstruct his heart's plumbing system. During the heart attack, his heart muscle experienced *ischemia*—poor blood flow due to plaque blocking its arteries—which led to heart failure. Measured as a percentage of the blood pumped forward with each heartbeat is the *ejection fraction (EF)*. Healthy hearts pump 55% or more of the blood that fills the left ventricle forward with each squeeze. Derrick's EF had dropped to just 15% following his heart attack.

After his open-heart surgery, which reconstituted his heart muscle's blood supply using veins harvested from his legs, and with the additional support of medications working to reduce the effort of his heart, his ejection fraction recovered to a normal level within a few months.

When Derrick was 77, one of the vein grafts supplying the left side of his heart muscle failed, clogging with plaque and leading to another heart attack. Derrick received a stent to maintain the patency of the failed graft during a procedure called a *heart catheterization*. His EF had declined again, but despite the stent and optimization of his medications, this time, it did not recover.

When a pump fails, fluid collects upstream. The heart, which has two pumps (the right and left ventricles), pumps blood continuously from its right side to the lungs, on to its left side, then out to the brain and limbs, and back again to the right side. When the left side of the heart fails, blood builds up in the lungs, the right side of the heart, and in the limbs. When the right side of the heart fails, blood builds up primarily in the limbs. Excess blood in the vessels increases hydrostatic pressure, causing water molecules to leak from the vessels into the surrounding tissue. This accumulation of fluid, called *edema* when it occurs in the limbs or the lungs, can lead to uncomfortable swelling, weight gain, or shortness of breath.

Derrick was treated with a diuretic, furosemide, to reduce the extra fluid in his body. Because blood pressure is created in part by the strength of a heartbeat, Derrick's weakened heart, along with the diuretic, caused excessively low blood pressure, making it extra challenging to keep his volume status in check.

When a heart remains constantly in volume overload, the extra fluid stretches the thin-walled upper chambers, and this stretching, called *remodeling*, can become permanent. Remodeled atrial tissue is prone to *ectopy*—spontaneous, inappropriate electrical impulses. When these impulses get transmitted down the electrical wiring system in the heart, they can frequently, erratically, trigger the ventricles to squeeze. As one squeeze interrupts the prior squeeze, forward blood flow is diminished. This arrhythmia, called *atrial fibrillation*, can lead to symptoms of heart failure as well as chest pain and light-headedness as the heart and brain suffer from insufficient blood flow.

It was after Derrick's second heart attack that I met him in the cardiology clinic. He arrived for follow-up, complaining of palpitations. An electrocardiogram (ECG) documenting the electrical activity of his heart showed that he had developed atrial fibrillation.

Despite medications to control the rate and rhythm of his heartbeat and a blood thinner to combat his risk of stroke, Derrick's atrial fibrillation would occasionally become so persistent and rapid that he required hospitalization. During these episodes, his heart failure symptoms worsened, too.

Derrick's near-constant state of volume overload led to damage to the blood vessels in his lungs, leading to *pulmonary hypertension*—elevated blood pressure in the lungs—for which he required supplemental oxygen by nasal cannula. Forced to pump against much higher pressure than it was designed for, the thin-walled muscle of the right side of his heart also began to fail.

Over the two years that I followed Derrick in cardiology, he required various anti-arrhythmic medications, electrical cardioversion, and an ablation procedure to try to control his atrial fibrillation. Eventually, he underwent the insertion of a pacemaker following the destruction of his atrioventricular node, the bundle of tissue that transmits the electrical impulse from the upper to lower chambers. From then on, Derrick's implanted pacemaker device controlled his heart rhythm.

For many patients, this ablation-pacemaker procedure allows a patient's heart function to recover to normal. In Derrick's case, however, his long-standing structural problems had caused permanent remodeling of his heart, and a recovery of its function was no longer possible. Moreover, the permanent stretching of his upper chambers led to stretching, and then failure, of his mitral and tricuspid valves. Imagine a room in your house being expanded so the doors no longer close.

A year into working in palliative care, I started caring for Derrick as one of my patients again. By then, in his early 80s, he lived in an independent living facility, dependent on oxygen and his electric scooter. His near-constant edema, made more difficult to control due to varicose veins and venous insufficiency, led to weeping, wet skin that was prone to infection. I ordered home health care for nursing support to help his leg wounds heal and occasionally treated him with antibiotics for cellulitis.

By this stage in Derrick's journey, he had developed a strong aversion to being hospitalized and had a high threshold for symptom tolerance. Knowing that his heart disease, his constant companion, was incurable and would only get worse and valuing his independence above all other things, he requested palliative care support as a means of avoiding the hospital. I worked closely with Derrick's cardiologist to control his symptoms, and in the last two years of his life, he was admitted just twice for heart failure exacerbations.

A fiercely independent and capable man until his final admission, Derrick was still driving himself to appointments, visiting his men's coffee group on Friday mornings at the mall, putting together 4000+ piece Lego® sets, and reading books about politics and history. He remained as sharp-witted and proactive as ever and, while admitted the final time, requested a hospice consult for himself.

We met to discuss his wishes. Feeling a pang, knowing that Derrick was not long for this world, I asked him to share his wisdom, specifically about how he had arrived at his decision for hospice.

He explained that he never wanted to live dependent on anyone. His dramatic recent decline in energy, inability to move around on his own, and worsening short-ness of breath were the writing on the wall. He knew the end was near. He asked his son to move him to the assisted living floor of the facility where he lived. He was ready for the next step.

I asked Derrick if he was afraid of dying or of being dead. He told me that he was not afraid of either. He had lived a long and fulfilling life.

"It's ages and stages," he explained. "For each age, a different type of living is tolerable to me. After my wife died, with my health declining, I decided to move to the independent living apartment because I knew I couldn't manage on my own, and I didn't want to burden my son. Now, it's time for me to let go, to let happen what will happen."

Derrick's son added that his father only did things on his own terms. The end of his life would be no different from the rest.

Derrick went home the following day with the support of our hospice team. He lived for two more weeks, passing away one Sunday morning, very peacefully in his apartment, just as he wanted.

~~~

In contrast to the steep decline Derrick experienced in his functional and physi-cal status in the last month of his life, Raymond lived a bed-to-chair existence for much of his last two years on account of difficult-to-control heart failure resulting from long-standing cardiovascular disease for which he was no longer a candidate for intervention. During the final two years of his life, Raymond was admitted eight different times for heart failure exacerbations and discharged on five separate occa-sions to a rehabilitation center.

When we met two months before his death, Raymond was short of breath at rest and experiencing intermittent chest pain that was challenging to control despite multiple medications. He wore supplemental oxygen 24 hours a day and, due to his limited mobility, required a hydraulic lift at home to transfer from his living room couch to his bed or bedside commode. He had likely met hospice criteria for many months.

Raymond and his wife spent nearly all of their time within the confines of their ranch-style home, into which they had moved when Raymond's heart problems began impacting his mobility. Very depressed, Raymond was resistant to discussing his diagnosis and wishes with me, seeming to lack any insight into his ongoing decline and the exhaustion that his wife was experiencing.

Despite the apparent toll that caring for Raymond was taking on her, Cheryle remained steadfast in her promise to keep her husband at home until the end of his life. Recognizing that she was experiencing caregiver strain, I prescribed self-care, encouraging her to hire a home health agency for additional support in the home so that she could leave to visit with her friends, run errands without worry, and shift much of her to-do list onto someone else's shoulders. She took my advice, hiring someone six hours daily and eight hours each night, which granted her significant relief and the ability to get a good night's sleep. I was happy she looked more refreshed and relaxed during our next visit.

When Raymond's chest pain became too much for his medications at home to control, Cheryle called 911. At the hospital, an ECG revealed yet another heart attack and further worsening of his heart function from an EF of 25% to just 5%. His kidneys were also failing. Overnight, his severe heart failure led to respiratory failure, which led to intubation and, ultimately, to his wife's difficult decision to withdraw treatment and allow him to pass in the ICU.

Lung Failure

Most commonly caused by chronic obstructive pulmonary disease (COPD)—the sixth leading cause of death in the United States [17]. and the third leading cause of death worldwide [18]—lung failure can develop following any pulmonary insult, including a pulmonary embolism (PE), acute respiratory distress syndrome (ARDS), a stroke or spinal cord injury, pneumonia, or COVID-19. More than 150,000 Americans died of COPD in 2020 [17]. Other causes of lung failure include cystic fibrosis, primary pulmonary hypertension, heart failure, and amyotrophic lateral sclerosis (ALS).

I met Evelyn two years before she passed, one windy day in late October. Sitting in her dining nook, next to French doors overlooking her patio, the blue Wyoming sky provided a magnificent backdrop to our visit.

Evelyn had developed COPD following more than 50 years of smoking. Unable to extract enough oxygen from the atmosphere with each breath, Evelyn depended on supplemental oxygen delivered to her lungs through a nasal cannula, its tubing held in place by her ears and attached at a distance down the hallway to her concentrator.

A tiny, cachectic woman, Evelyn tightened her lips with each exhale, forcing out the air that was trapped in her lungs. Getting up to open the door when I arrived had been quite an effort, and it took nearly 15 minutes for her to breathe comfortably again.

If you inhale a deep breath and then hold that expanded lung position as your new baseline, never allowing your lungs to recoil to a smaller diameter after an exhale, you can experience the exhaustion that accompanies the work of breathing by patients with advanced COPD and other forms of lung failure. Much of their daily energy allowance and caloric intake is dedicated to a biological task most of us take for granted. This can contribute to significant weight loss, called *pulmonary cachexia.*

Evelyn had lost more than 10 pounds in the prior year, and she showed signs of shortness of breath by the need to purse her lips and use her chest muscles to exhale forcibly, even when she was resting comfortably. If she removed her supplemental oxygen, her saturation level would drop as low as 68% after a few minutes, a level that is incompatible with life. Walking even a short distance exhausted her and required her to rest. Evelyn met hospice criteria when I met her.

Over the next two years, I worked hard to keep Evelyn out of the hospital. I reinforced COPD education at every visit, encouraging her to evaluate her physical status every day so that she would recognize when a COPD exacerbation was starting.

Because each patient's exacerbation can present differently, we worked together to recognize her unique hallmark of symptoms. Rather than initially developing a cough, wheezing, or notable shortness of breath, the classic signs of a COPD exacerbation, Evelyn noticed leg weakness and generalized fatigue. I wrote a standing prescription for antibiotics and steroids, which she could request from the pharmacy whenever she felt these symptoms.

During the COVID-19 pandemic, Evelyn's family kept her safe by wearing masks and maintaining a physical distance from her at home. Her son delivered groceries and medications to her house so she wouldn't have to leave for errands, and when Meals on Wheels resumed their operations a few months into the pandemic, she signed up for their daily deliveries. Cooking had become a difficult task.

While I followed Evelyn, I treated her for six COPD exacerbations, for which she did not need hospitalization. Despite my best efforts, however, Evelyn experienced eight admissions for her COPD in the last two years of her life. Over time, the length of her hospital stays increased, as did her need for increasingly invasive respiratory support.

During Evelyn's early admissions, in addition to antibiotics and steroids, her exacerbations required an increase in the amount of oxygen being delivered by nasal cannula. Over the months, her oxygen needs at home increased from three liters per minute to eight, an indication of her worsening pulmonary baseline. Eventually, the nasal cannula was insufficient to support her lungs during an admission. During her last three hospital stays, Evelyn required some form of ventilation support.

At first, a BiPAP machine, which forces air into the lungs through a mask that is strapped in place around the top of the patient's head, was adequate. After a few days of IV antibiotics, with the support of the BiPAP machine, Evelyn's lungs recovered enough for a comfortable return to her nasal cannula.

During her last hospitalization, however, the BiPAP was not enough to support Evelyn's breathing. Despite the BiPAP machine, Evelyn experienced severe respiratory distress and needed to be intubated. Fortunately, she was able to come off the ventilator after just two days. We met in her hospital room a few days later.

This was July of 2020, while the COVID-19 pandemic was raging, and no vaccination was yet available. Evelyn was considering discharging to one of our local nursing facilities for rehabilitation. For the first two weeks, she would be isolated in her room as a precaution against inadvertently bringing the virus with her to the facility. At no point would she be allowed any visitors.

We talked about her wishes going forward. Until then, Evelyn had remained open to any treatment that could help her survive. But this admission had turned a once-theoretical possibility into her new reality. Evelyn understood that if she returned to the hospital again, she might not come off the ventilator the next time. While she was grateful to be alive, she knew she had reached the end of her journey and didn't want any more "heroics."

I asked her to think about going to rehab, where she would not be allowed visitors and would spend the next two weeks mostly alone in her room. We discussed how much energy she had available for participating in physical and occupational therapy and what she felt she might gain at this point in her journey from those interventions. I asked her to think about what she wanted for herself in whatever time she had left; after giving it some thought, she told me that she just wanted to go home.

Evelyn was discharged to her house the following day with hospice support. She survived another month and passed away peacefully in her sleep with her son by her side.

~~~

Unlike Evelyn, Terrence was unable to leave the hospital to pass away at home. Following a fifth admission for exacerbation of his pulmonary hypertension in recent months, Terrence's lungs had declined to the point where he required continuous BiPAP support. Being strapped to the claustrophobia-inducing mask 24 hours each day made talking, eating, and moving around very difficult. Left with little to no remaining quality of life and without the hope of returning home, Terrence and his wife decided to withdraw treatment. After their tearful goodbye, Terrence was given lorazepam and morphine to relax his effort at breathing. Comfortably sedated by these medications, Terrence's body did not struggle as the hospital team transitioned him first from BiPAP to nasal cannula and then to room air. Terrence passed peacefully, less than two hours later, with his wife at his side.

Kidney Failure

Most commonly caused by poorly controlled diabetes mellitus and hypertension, chronic kidney disease (CKD) is the progressive loss of kidney function that ultimately leads to the failure of the kidneys to excrete toxins, electrolytes, and fluid. The final stage of CKD, stage 5, also called *end-stage kidney disease (ESKD)* , results in a wide range of abnormalities and symptoms called *uremic syndrome* [19]. Without hemodialysis (HD), patients at this stage of kidney failure will typically pass within one to three weeks [19].

Despite affecting more than 6 million Americans in 2020, CKD remained the tenth leading cause of death in the United States, accounting for just over 52,000 deaths [20]. While CKD contributes to overall patient decline, ESRD is rarely the primary driver of terminal decline or the primary reason patients with kidney failure elect hospice care. This is because the vast majority (80–90%) of patients with CKD will die of some form of cardiovascular disease—heart failure, stroke, heart attack, or peripheral vascular disease—long before arriving at the point of needing dialysis [19].

Of those who survive long enough to require dialysis, approximately half will also die from cardiovascular disease [19]. Others will die from infection or following the voluntary cessation of dialysis [19].

~~~

Once offered primarily as a bridge to kidney transplant, hemodialysis has become a way of life for many millions of people around the world. Isaac, whose CKD developed because of his diabetes, lived for nearly two decades with the support of dialysis. Until his final year, Isaac enjoyed a deeply satisfying quality of life in the nursing home where he lived. Well-supported by a friendly and engaging staff, for many years, Isaac was well enough to leave the facility on weekends to spend time at home with his wife and children.

A year before he passed, Isaac developed signs of peripheral vascular disease, including painful ischemia in his fingertips. Skin breakdown led to multiple infections that his body was unable to clear, requiring repeated debridement surgeries and, eventually, the amputation of three of his digits. Suffering from incredible pain and unable to heal, Isaac and his family decided it was time to stop dialysis. He passed away at home just two days after his final treatment.

~~~

At age 75, Hank developed CKD in the context of rheumatoid arthritis. A year before we met, Hank was admitted to the hospital for a bladder obstruction caused by a kidney stone blocking one of his ureters. This insult led to an acute and severe worsening of his kidney function, pushing his CKD from a baseline of stage 3 to stage 5.

Hank had always been very clear in his desire never to become dependent on dialysis. He didn't want to be tethered to a schedule requiring so much time and energy to stay alive. He had lived a good life, had raised three successful sons, and held the earnest belief that when it was his time to go, he would try to do so gracefully, without putting up too much of a fight. He was neither afraid of dying nor of being dead, and his deep faith in God assured him that the afterlife would be, in some ways, almost preferable. Given the alternative, he couldn't envision spending three days a week in the dialysis clinic.

Hank's nephrologist was concerned that his kidneys might not recover from the bladder obstruction. Suddenly finding himself in a situation that he had assumed was yet years down the road, Hank agreed to the creation of an arteriovenous (AV) fistula in his left arm to prepare for the possibility of dialysis. Because the fistula would take a few months to mature before it was ready for use, Hank had plenty of time to consider his options. Fortunately, over the next several months, Hank's kidney function returned to its former baseline, and he could continue living dialysis-free.

A year later, however, Hank's health took a significant turn for the worse. Admitted with confusion and fatigue, Hank was once again found to have severe kidney failure, this time in the setting of a urinary tract infection (UTI). Understanding that his confusion was most likely coming from the build up of toxins not being excreted by his kidneys, Hank's family agreed to a trial of dialysis in the hospital. This led to a significant improvement in Hank's mental status, and Hank, himself, not yet ready to let go, agreed to start scheduled dialysis on Tuesdays, Thursdays, and Saturdays.

Hank underwent six dialysis sessions over the next two weeks before again returning to the hospital, this time with shortness of breath. A chest X-ray revealed a pleural effusion (fluid in the lining of the lung) on the right side, and an echocardiogram revealed a moderate drop in his heart function. Hank's mentation was altered enough to prevent him from being able to participate in conversations about his care.

Hank's new problem, heart failure, was responsible for his pleural effusion. Because his failing kidneys, unable to make urine, would not respond to diuretics, a pleural drain was placed to remove the fluid around his right lung. Although dialysis can often help in these situations, because Hank's blood pressure remained dangerously low, removing extra fluid during dialysis was not an option.

Appreciating the fragile state of Hank's health and his now-limited options, honoring his wish for an unencumbered passing, his family decided to forego further interventions and move him to our hospice center.

Hank's family remained by his side around the clock over the next 12 days. On the tenth day, Hank's kidneys ceased making even scant urine, and he fell into a deep, tranquil sleep from which he did not wake. His passing was peaceful, witnessed by his wife and sons, just as he'd hoped it would be.

Liver Failure

Worldwide, liver failure is most frequently caused by alcohol, chronic viral hepatitis (B and C), and nonalcoholic fatty liver disease [21]. Many other conditions, including hemochromatosis, in which too much iron is stored in the body, and schistosomiasis, caused by parasitic worms, can also lead to liver failure. Just over 51,000 Americans died of liver failure in 2020 [22].

Liver cells chronically damaged by disease or alcohol develop fibrosis and regenerative nodules. Once damage progresses beyond the liver's ability to repair itself, a patient is said to have *cirrhosis.*

Most people think of alcohol when they hear the words *liver failure* or *cirrhosis*, and for good reason. In 2015, about half of all deaths in the United States due to cirrhosis were related to alcohol [23].

Every patient I've encountered with alcoholic liver failure has been, beneath their sometimes-spiny exterior, a wounded, diminished soul. The need to self-medicate regularly with the volume of alcohol required to damage one's liver irrevocably indicates a level of spiritual and physical pain and dysfunction I can hardly begin to imagine.

For this reason, whenever I meet a patient with alcohol-induced liver failure, I always make a point of addressing the elephant in their particular room—their alcoholism—early on to set them at ease. Knowing that society's punishment for alcohol and drug abuse, first and foremost, is guilt and shame, I want my patients to know they needn't worry about that with me. "There is no judgment," I reassure. "I understand life is hard, and I'm just here to help."

Darryl arrived at the hospital looking like an emaciated superhero still wearing his costume. His deflated skin and eyes were the color of spring daffodils, the yellowest I had ever seen. His belly was distended by fluid, called *ascites*, when it occurs in the abdomen, and his arms and legs were covered in bruises.

Darryl had called 911 after noticing an alarming amount of dark blood in his stool. He arrived at the hospital feeling weak, light-headed, and scared. His bloodwork revealed a significant drop in his red blood cell and platelet counts and worsening liver function.

The liver is responsible for creating albumin and bile, filtering toxins from the blood, producing components of the coagulation system, storing vitamins and minerals, and processing glucose. As the liver fails, patients can experience a wide range of symptoms.

Without albumin, water molecules leak out of the vessels, causing edema and ascites, leading to pain and discomfort, skin breakdown, and infections. If fluid collects in the pleural cavity, compressing the lungs, patients can experience shortness of breath.

Without bile, which helps absorb nutrients, process fats, and rid the body of bacteria and other chemicals, including yellow-colored bilirubin, patients can experience nausea, diarrhea, malnutrition, and jaundice (yellowing of the skin). If poorly excreted bile salts deposit in the skin, patients can experience generalized itching, called *pruritus*. This typically worsens at night, interfering with sleep, and unconscious scratching can further contribute to skin issues. As toxins, including ammonia, continue to build up in the body and eventually reach the brain, increased confusion, called *hepatic encephalopathy*, can worsen to the point of *hepatic coma*.

Coagulation, one of the body's ultra-critical homeostatic systems, is regulated by various enzymes and factors, many of which originate in the liver. This system carefully controls the delicate balance between bleeding and thrombosis. As liver failure progresses, patients can experience easy bruising and life-threatening clotting or bleeding events.

Having developed jaundice and ascites and now with a presumed hemorrhage in his gastrointestinal tract, Darryl was admitted for the fifth time in seven weeks. When I asked him how things had been going, he told me he wasn't sure he would make it.

He was correct. He was not going to make it.

Patients who drink enough alcohol to severely damage their livers can go on to live fulfilling lives if they stop drinking early enough in the course of their disease. Unlike other organs in the human body, the liver has an amazing capacity for self-repair. *Liver regeneration*, described by scientists for the first time in 2021 [24], allows specific liver cells to divide to replace damaged neighboring tissue. By this process, a liver that has lost up to 90% of its mass can return to a normal size.

Darryl, who told me he had been drinking since the age of 13, had tried to quit many, many times. The longest he was able to stop was 10 years. During that time, he worked for an IT company making six figures. He owned a nice house, had a girlfriend, and had a good life.

But after he hurt his back at work two years earlier, his old demons resurfaced, and this time, they were too strong for him to quell. He started drinking again, and one domino toppled the next. He lost his job, his home, and his girlfriend.

Darryl's former military service provided him with a pension covering rent on his tiny apartment and the cost of one cheap bottle of whiskey daily. He'd started drinking two years earlier, and by now, his liver was well beyond the brink.

The earliest stage of alcoholic liver disease, *steatosis*, in which an unhealthy build-up of fat occurs in the liver, can develop in men consuming 60–80 grams of alcohol daily for 10 years [25]. That is the equivalent of approximately one six-pack of beer, one bottle of wine, or two to five cocktails, depending on their size and stiffness. For women, the threshold is much lower, at one-third to half that amount. Continued drinking will lead to *steatohepatitis* in 1 in 3 patients [26], and with ongoing use, 10% to 20% will develop *cirrhosis* [27].

The risk of cirrhosis increases 25-fold with 160 grams of alcohol intake daily [25]. With just over 300 grams of alcohol in each 750-mL bottle of whiskey, Darryl had ingested nearly twice that amount every day for the last two years. It was little surprise that his body exhibited hallmarks of end-stage liver disease.

With total cessation of alcohol intake, patients can self-heal steatosis and fibrosis, and some with cirrhosis can survive with a liver transplant if they live long enough to be offered a match. Darryl, beyond the point of self-repair and continuing to drink, was out of both options and time. Becoming more frequent and difficult to control, his worsening liver exacerbations pointed to his imminent demise.

The portal vein delivers deoxygenated blood and the byproducts of digestion to the liver from the digestive tract. Cirrhotic liver tissue increases the resistance of this blood flow, causing *portal hypertension*. As blood congests in the digestive tract, increased hydrostatic pressure causes water to leak into the abdomen, contributing to ascites. Portal hypertension, evident in more than 60% of patients with cirrhosis, occurs late in disease and is not reversible [28].

During each of Darryl's previous admissions, his abdomen had been drained by a needle, a procedure called *paracentesis*, and afterward, he had received an infusion of albumin. With each paracentesis, more than five liters of fluid, weighing just over 11 pounds, had been removed from his midsection. But without a naturally replenishing supply of albumin, and now with portal hypertension, he began to experience recurrent ascites, leading him back to the hospital again and again. Recurrent ascites, labeled *refractory*, is a sign that a patient is nearing the end.

Patients at this stage of their journey are at risk of various life-limiting sequelae. Portal hypertension frequently leads to engorged esophageal veins, called *varices*, which carry a risk of hemorrhage. Because a single bleeding event carries up to a 20% risk of mortality [29], routine screening for varices is now part of standard care for patients with cirrhosis. Bleeding varices are treated during upper endoscopy with band ligation, in which a rubber band is applied to cut off the vein's blood supply.

Patients at this point are also at increased risk of developing *spontaneous bacterial peritonitis* (SBP), a life-threatening infection of the ascitic fluid, as well as hepatic encephalopathy and hepatorenal syndrome, in which their otherwise healthy kidneys begin to fail. Each of these events portends a very poor prognosis.

Darryl's severely deranged PT (prothrombin time) and INR (international normalized ratio), lab markers for the liver's ability to build the coagulation factors involved in clotting, put his providers in a challenging situation.

Given his high risk of bleeding during any invasive procedure, the hospitalist was reluctant to offer either further paracentesis for his ascites or band ligation for his presumed hemorrhaging varices. Aside from starting Darryl on a prophylactic antibiotic to try to prevent SBP, the hospitalist had little else to offer. I was consulted to discuss Darryl's wishes.

As with most liver failure patients, Darryl did not understand how the signs on his body—the fluid in his abdomen, his yellow skin, and the blood in his stool—were related to his liver, nor did he appreciate their collective significance. Describing the liver's job, using some of the language provided here, I was able to connect each of these physical changes to his advancing liver disease and, importantly, to help him understand that they were not going to resolve.

I showed Darryl the picture of the organ failure trajectory, explaining that each of his recent hospital visits represented one of the downward dips, or exacerbations, and that without a different kind of support, he could expect to continue to return to the hospital. Explaining that he had reached the point in his journey where the medical community could no longer alter the course of his disease, I explained that any subsequent admission might be his last. Gently letting him know that he had reached the end of his journey, I shared my worry that his time was limited.

Thanks to his newfound understanding of what was happening with his body, Darryl could accept what I explained. When I asked him if the news that his time was limited was surprising, he shook his head, "No."

I asked Darryl what he wanted in the time he had remaining. He told me he wanted to be at home, to be as comfortable as possible, and to watch a few more sunsets from his deck.

Discussing hospice care, I recommended that we place a drain in his abdomen so that the hospice nurse could remove any more fluid that built up in his abdomen at home. When Darryl brought up the hospital doctor's concern for his risk of bleeding, I gently explained that with hospice, we no longer needed to worry about that. The drain would be an essential part of his comfort, our primary goal with hospice care.

Darryl was understandably sad, and like every alcoholic liver failure patient I've met, he was resigned, feeling that he deserved his fate. This always breaks my heart, knowing how people internalize society's judgments. Giving him the fullness of my presence and compassion, I reassured him that we are all human and none of us are perfect, no matter how we appear to others. He nodded, accepting this gift.

Darryl died at home, with the support of our hospice team and his roommate, after a week of brilliant Wyoming sunsets. He passed calmly in his sleep, free from his old demons at last.

~~~

Rarely do patients die from acute liver failure. When this happens in the United States, acetaminophen overdose is frequently the cause, either intentionally, in an attempted suicide, or unintentionally, typically by over-ingesting narcotics that contain an acetaminophen component [30]. Approximately 500 deaths per year in the United States are attributed to acute liver failure due to acetaminophen poisoning [31]. In these cases, the Catastrophic Event trajectory is followed as the kidneys and heart rapidly fail, and patients are taken emergently to the ICU for support.

Cancer

In 2019, approximately 1 in 5 Americans followed the Cancer trajectory at the end of their lives [13]. Accounting for more than 600,000 deaths, cancer was the second leading cause of mortality in the United States in 2020 [32].

Affecting virtually every organ and system, cancer is far from a single diagnosis. Patients can experience a range of symptoms determined by the cancer's location, extent, and pattern of spread. The end of the cancer journey tends to follow a similar pattern of decline, which can be described as a ball rolling off a very steep cliff (Fig. 4.4).

Following a period of functional and physical stability, patients experience a dramatic loss of personal independence and health, usually in a short amount of time. This occurs either because the cancer outpaces the treatment or the treatment results in life-threatening side effects and patient decline.

Many patients' diagnoses are made when they are already well down the cliff. Some are too sick or too old to pursue treatment. Others, following treatment, will

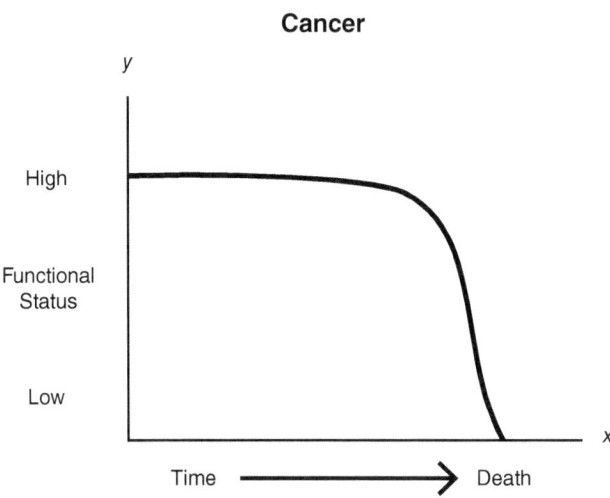

Fig. 4.4 Cancer. (Adapted with permission from Lunney et al. (2002). *Profiles of Older Medicare Decedents.* Journal of the American Geriatrics Society [6])

experience regression or remission of their cancer, remaining on or returning to the plateau of stability, where they may stay for weeks, months, or years. Many fortunate patients will achieve a cure, escaping the Cancer trajectory altogether.

Because the transition from stability to decline can occur abruptly, it is essential that patients with advanced or aggressive cancer receive the extra support of palliative care to help them navigate the emotional, physical, financial, and spiritual upheaval of the cancer journey. Per the 2017 update of the clinical practice guidelines for integrating palliative care into oncology care, released by the American Society of Clinical Oncology, anyone with advanced cancer (defined as distant metastasis at diagnosis, late-stage disease, cancer that is life-limiting, and/or with 6 to 24 months' prognosis) should be referred to palliative care within eight weeks of diagnosis [33].

~~~

Nearly 90 when we met, Richard was a quiet, subdued rancher who didn't mince words or care to belabor a point. He and his wife Arlene had spent their lives raising cattle near the Wyoming-Colorado border. Married for over 65 years, they finished each other's sentences and seemed to exist like two electrons sharing the same orbit, imparting a sense of stability, serenity, and quiet confidence that things were alright with the world.

Five months earlier, Richard had been hospitalized for pancreatitis. Imaging revealed dilated and constricted pancreatic ducts, concerning for cancer. He received a pancreatic stent, which resolved his pain, and the lab reported that the sample collected during the procedure was not malignant.

Two months later, however, again admitted for abdominal pain and pancreatitis, Richard received a second stent, and this time, pathology revealed *adenocarcinoma*, the most common type of pancreatic cancer, which originates in the lining of the pancreatic duct.

When I met Richard, he had not yet seen an oncologist. We discussed his wishes and where he thought he was in his life's journey. He and his wife agreed they had lived a long and happy life, and neither wanted any "heroics" to remain alive. Practical people, they considered cost an important part of their quality-of-life equation. Richard suspected that his time was ending, and he didn't want Medicare paying out substantial amounts trying to keep him around.

Richard reported that most days he was pretty comfortable, other than occasional middle-of-the-night abdominal pain that tended to wake him up, and some nausea now and then. In the prior six months, he had lost 45 pounds, more than 25% of his total body weight, despite Arlene's best effort at keeping him well-fed.

We discussed his weight loss—*cancer cachexia*—as an expected part of the cancer journey [34], which is especially common in patients with pancreatic cancer. Knowing that survival time is indirectly proportional to weight loss [35], I worried that Richard's time was very limited.

Knowing that Richard and Arlene were looking forward to celebrating his birthday later in the summer, I explained that cancer treatment can sometimes improve pain and other symptoms, even if it can't offer the hope of a cure. Wondering aloud if treatment might address his pain, improve his appetite, and prevent further weight loss, I suggested a consultation with an oncologist. Open to learning about his options, particularly if it didn't require a significant investment of either time or money, Richard agreed.

The next time we met, Richard was about to start radiation therapy. Given his age and the risk of side effects, he was not a candidate for a Whipple procedure or chemotherapy. Radiation would be purely *palliative*, with the hope of reducing the size of his tumor and his symptoms, but not expected to stop his cancer's terminal progression.

Richard was skeptical but willing, and Arlene hoped it would help. Not one to take medications, Richard was in the habit of refusing his wife's offer of acetaminophen. He refused anything stronger as well, noting that he didn't want to become addicted. I gently tried to alleviate Richard of that worry on account of his limited life expectancy; still, he wanted nothing to do with narcotics.

After five sessions of radiation therapy, Richard experienced four months with very little pain and, happily, a rebound of his appetite. He gained a bit of weight and felt strong enough to operate his mower, attend church on most Sundays, and celebrate his 90th birthday two days after the Fourth of July with more than 30 friends and family members in attendance.

But just a couple of weeks later, his pain returned with something of a vengeance, unrelieved by acetaminophen or tramadol. Richard gladly accepted my offer of oxycodone and agreed to allow hospice to come in to help. Noting how her husband's symptoms frequently distressed him at night, Arlene was happy to know she would have someone to call anytime she needed support.

Richard passed away in his home just five weeks later, two months after his 90th birthday. Arlene was grateful for the hospice team's support, and although she would miss her dear husband, she was glad that he hadn't suffered very much on his journey.

~~~

Yasmin's pancreatic tumor was large enough at diagnosis to involve her stomach, spleen, liver, and adrenal glands. For two months, she had experienced pain with eating, followed almost always by nausea and vomiting. During that time, she had lost 25 pounds, 18% of her total body weight. Two days before coming to the hospital, her skin had yellowed.

When we met, Yasmin was hopeful for a cure. Just 52 years old, Yasmin spoke confidently, using fighting terms so familiar to our anti-cancer culture, saying assuredly that she was going to "beat this." Her brother, who had recently been diagnosed with brain cancer, had so far survived with chemotherapy and radiation. By her enthusiastic retelling, I knew he represented a beacon in her darkness. She had a deep faith in God and was willing to try any treatment that could be offered.

A PET scan showed involvement of lymph nodes throughout her abdomen, and her thoracic spine showed metastatic lesions. Her liver, affected, was failing, and she had a spot on her left lung. Having spread beyond the organ of origin to involve numerous distant sites, her cancer was advanced, *stage IV*, and incurable.

Although the oncologist explained that treatment would be purely palliative in nature, Yasmin defiantly believed that she would once again return to the activities she loved, including international travel, marathon running, snowshoeing, and hiking. She agreed to platinum-based chemotherapy but required two units of red blood cells on the day she was scheduled for her first treatment, a concerning sign of cancer-related decline [36].

Yasmin received just two chemotherapy treatments. Throughout those weeks, she experienced persistent nausea, vomiting, diarrhea, and weakness. She spent her days in her bed, too weak to walk, and by the last time we spoke, two weeks before she died, she was sleeping almost the entire day.

A week after her final chemotherapy infusion, Yasmin stopped eating. Two days later, unable to rouse her, her family requested hospice care. Yasmin passed away at home the following evening, eight weeks after her diagnosis.

~~~

Rita was diagnosed with stage IV B cell lymphoma after being admitted to the hospital with lower abdominal pain, nausea, and constipation. A CT scan of her abdomen revealed an extensive collection of lymph nodes behind her kidneys abutting her stomach and spleen. A bone marrow biopsy confirmed her cancer diagnosis and a PET scan showed distant involvement of lymph nodes in the chest cavity, as well as in the bones of her sacral, lumbar, and thoracic spine. Her stage IV (metastatic) status carried a poor prognosis.

At 68 years old, Rita had recently moved to town to be closer to her daughters. Like many of my patients, she had spent most of 2020 and 2021 in COVID-19 quarantine, isolated and states away from her family. Eager to reconnect, she looked forward to being a grandmother for the first time.

Rita's cancer diagnosis had come out of left field, and she was in no way willing to capitulate to its ultimate demand. I met Rita three weeks after her diagnosis, just seven months before her death. She reported feeling young at heart, with much life left in her. When we discussed her wishes for care, she was open and willing to try anything.

Rita underwent six cycles of treatment, receiving an infusion of chemotherapy every three weeks. During this period, she was seen in the ER four times and admitted to the hospital once for a fall in which she fractured her left ankle. Fatigued and weakened, initially because of the cancer and, subsequently, the chemotherapy, her functional status declined incrementally over the weeks.

Each cycle of chemo left Rita immunocompromised, preventing her family from visiting, given the risk of COVID-19 or school-year infections. Once again, Rita found herself isolated from her loved ones. With no other support at home following her ankle fracture, Rita was discharged to a rehabilitation facility where she could receive full-time care.

Although Rita's PET scan showed a complete resolution of her cancer following her chemotherapy, her functional capacity did not recover. While in rehab, she was seen in the ER two more times for ongoing back pain. The second visit revealed nodules on her scalp and a newly enlarged lymph node below her left clavicle. A biopsy confirmed a speedy return of her cancer.

A third ER visit resulted in another admission. At this point, Rita could not walk, bathe, or care for herself. A PET scan showed new lymph node involvement in the left axillary (armpit) area. Lab work showed dangerously low levels of red blood cells (anemia) and platelets (thrombocytopenia), for which she received transfusions.

Because Rita's cancer had returned so quickly, she was offered *salvage chemotherapy*, an end-of-the-road option when the standard treatment is unsuccessful.

I have found that most patients have a limited understanding of the comparative likelihood of success of first-, second-, and third-line cancer treatments. Many, like Rita, believe that oncologists reserve their stronger medications for use later, when earlier treatments have failed. Few seem to understand that prognosis declines with second- and third-line options [37].

Despite her incredible weakness and inability to manage herself in any way, Rita agreed to salvage chemotherapy. During the final month of her life, she received two more cycles of treatment, resulting in further *myelosuppression*, reduced bone marrow activity resulting in low blood cell counts, again requiring a transfusion of red blood cells and platelets.

Myelosuppression is the primary reason oncologists stop or limit the dose of chemotherapy [38]. As both standard and salvage chemotherapy were unsuccessful, Rita could be offered nothing further.

Nine days before she died, too frail to come into the clinic, Rita had a phone conversation with her oncologist in which he suggested hospice care. Five days later, she agreed, and four days after that, Rita passed away at the rehabilitation center where she had spent the last two months of her life.

~~~

My uncle Bill's cancer journey began at a checkup for a changing mole on his chest. His melanoma was such a "textbook case" that the physician brought several residents into the clinic room that day to observe its appearance. A PET scan revealed stage IV disease.

This was nearly 25 years ago when few treatments existed for melanoma. The most aggressive form of skin cancer, metastatic melanoma, carried a very poor prognosis at the time, with median survival of less than one year [39].

Bill was offered a promising new treatment called *immunotherapy*, which would trigger the body's immune system to attack the cancer cells. He received routine infusions of *interferon* for nearly a year. The treatment caused incredible fatigue, but on the days that he wasn't sleeping, he was able to work on a limited basis.

To mark the successful completion of his immunotherapy regimen, his extended family gathered for a Celebration of Life. Bill began running again, inspiring his older brother and younger sister to join him for the Los Angeles Marathon in 2001. Bill experienced almost two years of remission, returning to the top of the Cancer trajectory plateau.

His melanoma returned in November of 2002, once again showing up without much fanfare. A low-grade cough that failed to resolve turned out to be a spot on his lung. A few months later, his cancer spread to his bones.

In nearly every memory I have of my uncle, there is a book in his hand. He was an extremely intelligent, avid reader and writer who always kept himself well-informed. A lover of statistics, he did his cancer research, so he was aware of his prognosis. During the last six months of his life, Bill received additional chemotherapy treatments despite knowing that it would not cure his disease. He was hospitalized several times.

The last time I saw him, a month before he passed, he was again admitted to the hospital, very thin and frail. That his time was limited was written in the sadness of his smile and in the tears he shed when my family said our goodbyes. He died a few weeks later, just 46, leaving a wife and teenage son behind.

~~~

Martin's stage III rectal cancer was diagnosed when he was 76 after a bout of rectal bleeding. Following colon resection and placement of a colostomy, Martin began eight cycles of chemotherapy. Affecting his bone marrow's ability to make new blood cells, the first two chemotherapy treatments resulted in anemia and thrombocytopenia, for which Martin required transfusions and a dose reduction for his final six cycles of treatment.

When we met a month after his last infusion, Martin was still very weak. Having lost 70 pounds since his diagnosis, his primary goal was to gain weight and become strong enough to return to the gym. I recommended mealtime support with Meals on Wheels and a medication called mirtazapine, which would improve his appetite, nutritional status, and sleep, essential components of healing. I also provided him with a prescription for physical therapy.

Over the next year, Martin returned to his pre-diagnosis weight. Physical therapy discharged him after a few months, and despite the chemotherapy-induced neuropathy in his hands, he was able to join his friends on the pickleball court again.

Martin follows up with oncology every four months for routine labs, thus far remaining cancer-free. Rarely do I get the opportunity to discharge patients from my care because they have returned to their former baseline. I happily did so with Martin, excited to see him escape the Cancer trajectory. The last time we spoke, he was planning a post-COVID cruise to the Caribbean.

~~~

Denise was not willing to undergo body-altering surgery to ensure her survival. At age 79, Denise was diagnosed with a soft tissue sarcoma of her right leg. Following multiple surgeries to resect the tumor, which returned several years after diagnosis, she was offered definitive treatment with an above-the-knee amputation. Denise categorically refused.

An active outdoorswoman who loved walking her dog, Denise knew that an amputation would not only irrevocably alter her life but also her husband's. She did not want to burden him with the daily demands of caring for her. Weighing her options carefully, Denise decided that life with an amputation was not the right choice for her.

To date, Denise has enjoyed nearly two full, symptom-free years without concerning symptoms or other signs that her cancer is progressing. When this occurs, we will transition her to the higher level of support that hospice provides.

Frailty/Dementia

In the United States, approximately 4 in 10 patients follow the Frailty/Dementia trajectory at the end of their lives [5, 6]; approximately half of these deaths result from frailty, or *age-related* decline [5], and approximately half result from some form of dementia [5].

This trajectory follows a creeping loss of personal independence, so slow and steady as to be nearly imperceptible, with both patients and families incrementally accommodating to their ever-changing reality (Fig. 4.5).

Patients showing age-related decline eventually experience a metabolic shift that impacts their body's ability to maintain itself. A natural transition occurs from a state of maintenance, *anabolism*, in which the body builds more skin, bone, and muscle than it breaks down, to a state of decline, *catabolism*, in which the metabolic scale tips toward tissue breakdown.

As metabolism changes and patients visibly lose weight and muscle mass, internal organ systems are also affected. Organ mass declines in direct proportion to muscle mass, leading to organ dysfunction [40]. The immune system becomes depressed, leaving patients susceptible to infections and poor wound healing [40]. As patients lose muscle tone, muscle mass, and mobility, they are more likely to fall.

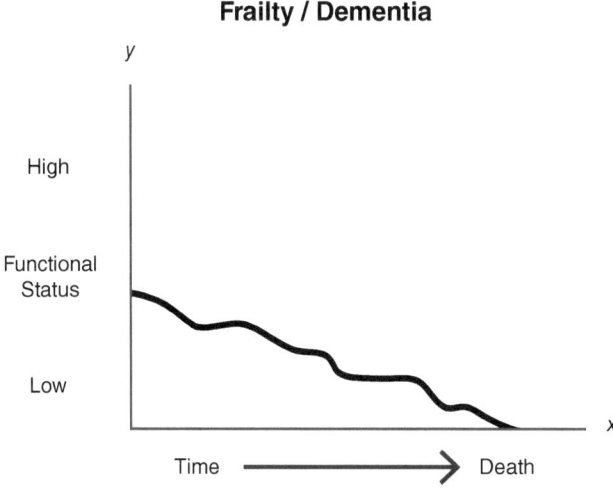

Fig. 4.5 Frailty/Dementia. (Adapted with permission from Lunney et al. (2002). *Profiles of Older Medicare Decedents*. Journal of the American Geriatrics Society [6])

Importantly, this is the context in which many patients fall and break a hip (most commonly a femur). For those with dementia, this metabolic transformation occurs within the context of progressive and eventually terminal brain failure, layering physical decline on top of advanced cognitive and functional deterioration.

A variety of labels are used to refer to this hypercatabolic state, including anorexia-cachexia syndrome, cachexia, protein-calorie malnutrition, marasmus, and protein-energy wasting [34, 40, 41]. While labels differ depending on the presence or type of underlying chronic disease, clinically, it is important to know that cachexia, defined as weight loss of 5% of total body weight in the context of chronic disease or cancer [42], cannot be reversed by nutritional support [43].

A person's metabolic state can be evaluated by monitoring serum albumin level and weight loss. Normal serum album level ranges from 3.5–5.5 g/dL. While albumin level decline is an expected part of aging [44], a level below 3.5 g/dL indicates a metabolic shift toward catabolism [40]. Likewise, involuntary weight loss of more than 10% of total body weight over six months, more than 5% of total body weight over three months, or more than 2% of total body weight over one month is considered clinically significant [45], carrying an increased risk of death [46, 47].

A diagnosis of cachexia can be made with weight loss of 5% or more over 12 months or less or BMI (body mass index) of <20 kg/m², plus three of the following: decreased muscle strength, fatigue, anorexia, low fat-free mass index, and abnormal biochemistry (increased inflammatory markers (CRP, IL-6), anemia (Hg <12 g/dL), low serum albumin (<3.2 g/dL)) [48].

It is important to understand this metabolic shift as both a natural part of disease progression and a harbinger of terminal decline. Occurring in every disease trajectory that patients follow to the end of life, cachexia is particularly common in heart failure (up to 20% of patients), COPD (up to 60% of patients), kidney failure (up to 75% of patients), and cancer (up to 85% of patients) [41]. As we shall see in the following chapter, cachexia, identified by clinically significant weight loss or a declining albumin level, is an element of many of the hospice criteria [49, 50].

~~~

It is caregivers, particularly of those with dementia, who bear the brunt of the Frailty/Dementia trajectory, as loss of independence requires increasing assistance with all aspects of living [1]. As patients lose the ability to make it through their day without help, spouses and other caregivers can experience social isolation, emotional and mental strain, anxiety, depression, physical exhaustion, and new or worsening health concerns of their own [51]. The emotional, physical, and financial burden of caregiving often leads caregivers to neglect their own health maintenance [51], leaving them at increased risk of adverse health outcomes, including death [51–54].

Therefore, for patients on this trajectory, we must widen the scope of our inquiry to include spouses, children, and other caregivers in our concern. Early referral to palliative care or to programs designed to provide comprehensive and ongoing support to patients and families with dementia or other neurodegenerative diseases is a vital aspect of their care.

Frailty

When we say that someone had "died of old age," we are referring to the Frailty trajectory. In this approach, there is no outstanding diagnosis driving patient decline. Rather, patients seem to wither away, losing ground in various domains, including oral intake and body weight, strength and ambulation, energy and wakefulness, and the ability to perform daily tasks.

Because so many patients will follow this trajectory at the end of life [5, 6], we must tune our awareness to the signs of age-related decline. The constellation of changes patients experience can sometimes seem nebulous; thus, routine inquiry into appetite, weight, functional status, falls, and albumin level is vital. As stated previously, trends are important to recognize because they tend to persist.

~~~

Just three months into my job with palliative care, my maternal grandmother died at the age of 94. Six or seven years earlier, she had begun slowly declining. Because I lived out of state and saw her only on holidays, what was nearly invisible to others in my family was much more apparent to me. At the time, I had a meager appreciation for what was happening to her.

Each time I saw her, she seemed to have shrunk a bit more. As her appetite waned, the pounds fell from her sturdy, midwestern frame. I recall naïvely thinking she should eat better, as though her willpower or laziness was the problem.

As my grandmother lost pounds, her skin became thin and easily torn, and she shed muscle mass. Her mobility suffered, and she began falling, breaking her right arm in the same place on two different occasions, years apart.

The second break, two years before she died, refused to heal. Sequential X-rays over six months showed a worsening dislocation, eventually requiring a shoulder replacement. Despite "recovering" from the surgery, she never regained full use of that arm.

Until just one month before she died, my grandmother lived on her own, was able to drive, enjoyed trips to the casino with her closest friend, and handled most of her own affairs.

Around that time, walking began to cause significant pain in her right leg, and the toes on that side darkened, becoming gangrenous and excruciatingly tender. She gave up driving and agreed to let her daughters move her bed into her living room so she wouldn't need to use the stairs.

She was seen in the ER on a couple of occasions for the pain in her foot, and the suggestion was made for her to follow up with vascular surgery for consideration of peripheral angiography, in which a stent could be placed to open the artery supplying blood flow to her right leg.

After reviewing her medical history, the vascular surgeon recommended against any invasive procedure on account of her heart. Ten years earlier, my grandmother had suffered a massive heart attack and had received two stents in her coronary arteries. She remained symptom-free until age 92, when chest pain led to a second heart catheterization, confirming residual atherosclerotic disease that the cardiologist was unable to address due to brittle, tortuous arteries. The vascular surgeon who saw my grandmother in the month before she died worried that her heart would not tolerate another stressful procedure.

A palliative care referral was placed, and a nurse practitioner began to visit my grandmother in her home. Tending to the wounds on her toes, he prescribed morphine to help with the pain. Soon after, he recommended a transition to hospice care. By then, my grandmother barely ate and spent most of her days in bed asleep.

My mother and her two siblings began rotating through eight-hour shifts, caring for their mother around the clock in her living room. My grandmother was not alone when she took her final breath one Friday night in December, peacefully in her sleep.

~~~

When Charles was 92, he suffered a fall while trying to get into his truck, spending five hours on the ground before being found by one of his neighbors. Charles was taken to the hospital, where he was treated for *rhabdomyolysis*, a life-threatening condition resulting from muscle tissue breakdown—in this case, from his hours of immobility—that frequently leads to acute kidney injury. Charles survived and was discharged to a rehabilitation facility, where he spent several weeks recovering his strength before eventually returning home.

Seven months later, Charles was admitted to the hospital with confusion. Found to have a UTI, he was treated with IV antibiotics and expected to be discharged again to the rehabilitation center. When three days of antibiotics didn't clear up his confusion, my team was consulted to discuss his wishes.

In speaking with Charles's son, Howard, I learned that Charles had lost 30 pounds in the previous six months, more than 15% of his total body weight. During that time, Howard had begun helping with meal prep, bathing, and shopping. Charles had stopped driving months earlier and had experienced three falls at home. His albumin on admission was well below normal at 2.4 g/dL.

When I asked Howard where he thought his father was in his overall journey with his health, he told me that he thought his dad had reached the end. I gently shared my agreement, letting him know that his father's weight loss, falls, and functional decline painted a picture of age-related decline, the kind of decline we see when we say that someone is "dying of old age." Given the fact that his father was not responding to the antibiotics, I shared my worry that his time was likely very limited. Howard nodded in agreement.

I asked Howard where he thought his dad would like to be at the end of his life. Howard told me that his mother had passed away at our hospice center, and he was sure that his father would want his final days to be there, too.

That evening, Charles was transferred to the hospice center, where he received close, round-the-clock care for the last nine days of his life. His septic encephalopathy caused restlessness that the nurses treated with lorazepam and morphine. Twice, he received a whirlpool bath, a relaxing experience that soothes skin and relieves pressure points. Like my grandmother in her final days, Charles ate little to nothing and slept nearly the entirety of each day until he, too, passed away peacefully in his sleep.

~~~

Sweet Bernice lived on her own until she was 94 years old. She had no children or other surviving relatives, so a guardianship through a private agency was established to help manage her finances and assist with medical decisions. She qualified for Medicaid assistance, which helped cover the cost of living in a nursing facility.

Bernice had no significant health issues aside from asthma, which would flare up from time to time. Experiencing a high level of care at the facility where she lived, Bernice thrived in the nursing home's social setting, enjoying the beauty salon, bingo, and wheelchair Zumba. She was rarely seen in the ER and experienced no hospitalizations until she turned 100 when she fell and broke her left femur.

Already confined to a wheelchair, Bernice was a frail, tiny woman without the strength at that point to assist in her transfers between her bed, wheelchair, and commode. In the prior year, she had lost 14% of her body weight, dropping from 118 pounds to 102 pounds at the time of her fall. Her albumin at that time was 2.8 g/dL.

The current standard of care for hip fractures involves surgical repair within the first 24 to 48 hours [55]. Although Bernice met hospice criteria at the time of her hip fracture, and although her metabolic state, as indicated by her albumin level, would suggest the risk of poor wound healing, her guardian was offered surgery. Our service was not consulted, and hospice care was not discussed. With no awareness of any alternative, her guardian agreed on Bernice's behalf to proceed with hip replacement surgery.

Surprisingly, Bernice survived the surgery and returned to her nursing home facility, where she lived for another 20 months. She was admitted to the hospital just one additional time for confusion resulting from a UTI that led to sepsis. During that visit, our palliative care service was consulted to discuss wishes with her guardian, who decided to transition Bernice to hospice care at our hospice center, where she remained bed-bound but comfortable until she passed away two months later.

~~~

At age 95, Virginia was living in her own home when she fell and broke her right hip. She arrived at the hospital in a confused state and in pain. In the emergency room, her family was offered surgery as a means of addressing her pain. The following morning, our service was consulted by the hospitalist, who had reservations about the patient's ability to survive surgery.

A chart review revealed that Virginia had lost more than 17% of her body weight in the prior six months. Her albumin was 2.3 g/dL at admission. At under 100 pounds, she was a tiny, frail woman with minimal reserve. She met hospice criteria and likely had for some time.

I met the patient in her room, where she was resting comfortably. Her pain had been significant enough to require frequent doses of IV morphine, which caused sleepiness and increased her confusion. As she dozed, I asked her daughters to paint a picture of Virginia's health in recent months.

Initially, Ellen and Beverly agreed that their mother had been doing well, sharing that she still managed her housework, grocery shopping, driving, and bills.

As I directed my questions toward signs and symptoms of the metabolic shift expected at the end of the Frailty trajectory, asking about Virginia's appetite, weight loss, energy level, and ability to participate in her life, Ellen began to reconsider her answers.

Ellen, who lived down the street from her mother, reported that although she delivered dinner to her mom four or five nights a week, she often found entire portions of the food she had prepared in her mother's refrigerator untouched. The same thing had happened with the Meals on Wheels deliveries Virginia had been receiving, which piled up to the point that Virginia canceled the extra support two months earlier.

Now that she thought about it, Ellen admitted that her mother had recently lost quite a bit of weight, emphasizing how her clothes seemed to hang off her tiny frame. She also noted that her mother spent more time napping throughout the day, something she had never known her mother to do.

Once Ellen shared these observations, Beverly shared her concern that her mother's memory had been slipping. An hour's drive away, Beverly called her mother frequently throughout the day to help keep tabs on her. Recently, Virginia had begun to repeat the same story multiple times each day, often during the same conversation.

Once I felt confident that Ellen and Beverly could see the evidence of Virginia's decline—weight loss, increasing fatigue, and cognitive decline—I asked them how they were making sense of those changes and, importantly, how they were making sense of their mother's hip fracture.

Probably 50% of the family members of patients I encounter on the Frailty trajectory are unable to pin these changes to any particular medical explanation or diagnosis. The other half usually responds by saying, "She doesn't have much time left," or "This is what I would expect as a person gets older."

Virginia's daughters fell into the former group, lacking the insight that their mother had begun a transition toward the end of her life, unable to make sense of the changes she was experiencing. They speculated those changes were happening because Virginia wasn't eating enough or exercising like she once did and, therefore, was becoming deconditioned and weak. Just like I had with my grandmother, Virginia's daughters didn't understand that their mother's weight loss, fatigue, and recent fall reflected a seismic internal metabolic shift that her body was experiencing. Without this realization, Virginia's daughters hoped that after surgery, rehab would help her return to her former level of independence.

Describing their mother as a fiery, feisty, independent woman who called her own shots and was not one to sit down, sit still, or relax, neither Ellen nor Beverly could imagine Virginia enjoying life if she could not walk again. Although I, too, wished that Virginia would be able to walk again and return to living independently, I worried that given her age and the recent decline she had experienced, that might not be possible. I gently shared those exact words, watching Ellen and Beverly for signs of surprise or distress.

After giving them a moment to process what I had just said, I continued, sharing my belief that Virginia had begun to decline in the way that happens when we say that someone is "dying of old age." I paused again, then asked Ellen and Beverly if they had ever seen someone die of old age. To my surprise, despite being in their mid-to-late 60s, neither had.

People who have seen another person die of old age are much more likely to realize by this point in our conversation that their loved one was also following this trajectory. Because Virginia's daughters had not observed this type of decline before, I provided some education. I began by explaining that if we were all fortunate enough to die of old age, each of us would, at some point, make a transition from a state of maintenance, where our body was able to make use of our nutrition to maintain our skin health, bone strength, muscle mass, and immune system, to a state of decline, where despite eating normally, our body was no longer able to make use of our nutrition to maintain itself like it once had. When this happens, a person becomes less interested in eating, loses weight, becomes frail, and can develop mobility issues. This is the context in which many people fall and break a hip. Although many family members think that if only their loved one had not fallen, they would be fine; the reality is that their loved one fell because they had already begun to decline.

I explained that weight loss and a lab value called albumin help assess whether a patient has made this metabolic transition. I explained that Virginia's albumin was well below normal, showing that her body could not make proteins like it once could. Without proteins, the body doesn't function or heal as it should.

I explained that just as the medical community has criteria to diagnose and stage disease, we also have criteria that allow us to recognize when a patient has reached the point where the medical community can no longer alter the course of their disease. The amount of weight that Virginia had lost, along with her declining albumin level, indicated that she had reached the point in her journey where she met what we call *hospice criteria.* I worried that her time was limited.

I paused again, watching Ellen and Beverly's faces for signs of distress or disagreement. Not seeing any, I continued.

Furthermore, when a person gets to this point in their journey, any subsequent insult or injury can be difficult to recover from. I explained that Virginia had experienced a fall and a fracture, which was one insult. Surgery and anesthesia would be two additional major insults. I very much worried that she might not survive surgery.

At that point, I stopped to check in with Ellen and Beverly, asking them if anything I had just said was surprising. Both shook their heads, "No."

Ellen shared that earlier in the day, she and Beverly had asked their mother how she would feel if she didn't survive surgery. Virginia responded, "Well, then it wasn't meant to be."

Ellen told me that she and her sister believed that their mother fully understood and accepted the risk of surgery. They wanted to honor their mother's wishes, even if she might not survive.

Virginia was taken into surgery two hours after our conversation. She survived the operation and was transferred to the ICU, but the strain proved too much for her heart, and she passed away during a cardiac event just five hours later. Although this was not the outcome they hoped for, Virginia's daughters were comforted by the realization that they had supported their mother's final medical wish.

~~~

It is a very delicate matter to lead a family that has already decided to pursue a treatment option like surgery to the realization that their loved one has reached the end of their journey. For the family, a decision to switch directions and choose hospice care can feel antithetical to the idea of seeking medical care in the first place, the equivalent of giving up. This is particularly true in a culture like that of the United States, where we deny and defy death at all costs, indeed often very high costs, and often pursue medical care until our very last breath.

Furthermore, deciding against the medical recommendation of a surgeon can be a tall order for anyone. As we know, patients are in the habit of deferring to physicians on important medical decisions. With their seemingly magical ability to rescue patients from the brink of death, surgeons seem almost God-like at the apex of the medical hierarchy. Understandably, patients put a great deal of faith in their guidance. Going against a surgeon's recommendation can feel like denying a directive from on high.

From my perspective, guiding patients and families toward the knowledge that the end is near in a situation like this can feel like I am casting doubt on the expertise of my surgeon colleagues. This is always an uncomfortable situation, and one that I prefer to avoid, finding that it's typically not a good idea for my team to be consulted after a decision for surgery has already been made.

And yet, I know that many physicians, especially surgeons, are not trained with the knowledge of hospice criteria and, thus, are unprepared to recognize when a patient has reached that point in their journey. Also, busy surgeons do not have the luxury of spending time investigating appetite, weight, and mobility changes as my team does. Surgeons don't mean to harm patients, but they see something broken and know they can fix it. While no surgeon wants a patient to die in their operating room or during the hours after surgery, the larger context is often irrelevant or invisible to them.

Despite wanting to avoid this fraught situation, I experience this predicament regularly with patients on every disease trajectory, not infrequently after they have already been offered treatments that are unlikely to be of benefit or to align with their end-of-life wishes. Often, as happened with both Bernice and Virginia, treatment is offered without respect to the advanced nature of the patient's disease progression.

Thus, I often find myself in the precarious position of needing to provide accurate medical information to enable families to make appropriate decisions comfortably but in a sensitive way that upholds their confidence in the rest of the care team. With Ellen and Beverly, it was my job to ensure that they understood the risk of surgery at that point in Virginia's journey, to elicit from them their understanding of Virginia's wishes for herself, and to do what I could to align her wishes with her care, all while not casting doubt on the competence or wisdom of the surgeon.

By the end of our conversation, I felt satisfied that Ellen and Beverly understood that their mother's time was limited and the reasons why. I was confident that they knew their mother's wishes and were comfortable honoring them and that they accepted the risk to her life that surgery posed. Most importantly, I believed that Virginia's wish for surgery authentically aligned with her essence as a capable, independent person who would not want to live if she was unable to participate in her life fully. Although Virginia died shortly after surgery, I do believe that her wishes were aligned with the medical care she was offered.

~~~

Often, when surrogate decision-makers are helped to understand that a patient's time is limited because of ongoing decline, they will decide to forego surgery and other invasive treatments and choose hospice care. This is especially true for patients who, following surgery, will need to be sent to a rehabilitation center where they will be separated from their spouse or children in whatever precious time they might have left.

While I would not suggest that elderly patients like Bernice and Virginia should not be offered surgery, I feel strongly that medical decision-makers deserve an accurate and complete understanding of a patient's pre-treatment health status. For patients admitted with a hip fracture, the Frailty trajectory must be considered, requiring an investigation of their recent clinical picture and their metabolic state, including weight loss and serum albumin level. Because physicians are not trained to recognize when a patient meets hospice criteria, we can be pretty certain that most elderly patients being offered hip fracture surgery are not benefitting from this type of assessment.

Although it is impossible to know for sure why one patient survives a major intervention like orthopedic surgery, and others do not, it seems reasonable to posit that those who already meet hospice criteria at the time of a hip fracture are likely to have worse outcomes following surgery, for the biological reasons indicated at the beginning of this section.

Surprisingly, little research has been conducted into this question. A 2011 study of patients undergoing surgical procedures showed worse morbidity and mortality in those with a DNR in place before surgery [56]. There are numerous studies looking at 1-year mortality and other outcomes of orthopedic surgery in the frail elderly [57–60]. One study even talks about patients being discharged to hospice settings [61]. But no study I can identify specifically investigates outcomes in the subset of patients who meet hospice criteria at the time of orthopedic surgery.

I suspect this is because physicians are not trained to recognize when patients meet hospice criteria; thus, this information is not routinely documented in patient charts. Moreover, because hospice criteria are not something that providers are taught, researchers are also likely unaware that patients can be defined in this way.

It seems reasonable to suspect that if families were gently guided to the realization that the end was closing in for patients meeting hospice criteria at the time of a fall and hip fracture, and if hospice care was described accurately and offered as a viable option for care, most families would choose hospice care. Further research using hospice criteria for patient classification would be worthwhile.

~~~

Carmen, the wife of a patient of mine, was deeply distressed that she had not been offered hospice care when her husband, Manuel, with advanced dementia, a history of multiple falls, weight loss, and declining albumin, was offered surgery after a fall and hip fracture.

After surgery, Manuel was discharged to a local rehabilitation center. Because of his advanced dementia, he did not understand or remember why he needed to be there, separated from his wife and dogs. Anytime Carmen was not by his side in the facility, he became very tearful and depressed. So weak that he was not able to fully participate in therapy, he developed a worsening UTI that required a catheter, which caused significant pain and additional misery.

Frustrated by Manuel's ongoing challenges, Carmen did some reading online, only to realize that Manuel likely would have been an excellent candidate for hospice care at the time of his fall. She was correct.

I had been following Manuel for several months. In my notes, I documented his near-end-stage dementia, numerous falls, and ongoing weight loss. In the leading portion of my assessment, I had indicated that he was close to meeting hospice criteria. Sadly, this information was not discussed with Carmen when Manuel was seen in the ER. He was not re-evaluated against hospice criteria at the time of his admission, and Carmen was not offered hospice care as a reasonable treatment option.

When I met Carmen at the rehabilitation center to discuss what she thought Manuel's wishes would be, she was distraught to the point of tears at the idea that when it had mattered the most, she had failed to advocate for her husband properly. I did my best to reassure her that she was, in fact, an incredible advocate for him and that he was so fortunate to have her on his side.

When I asked Carmen what she wanted for Manuel in the time that he had left, she told me that she wanted to take him home because that was where he wanted to be. However, she was concerned that in his present weakened state, she would not be able to care for him there. She worried he would need to be stronger so she could help him move around the house. This is a common misconception that many spouses and family members share.

I gently cleared up this confusion by painting a picture for Carmen of what hospice care would look like. I explained that the hospice benefit under Medicare would pay for a hospital bed to be delivered to their home. Given the risk to her health, I would not recommend that Carmen try to help Manuel get in and out of bed anymore, even to use the commode. Instead, she could care for him around the clock in the hospital bed, which could be positioned in their living room so that he could easily visit with family and look out their bay window. I reassured Carmen that most patients at the end of their lives are cared for in this way, sharing the story of my grandmother's final days. With her final concern alleviated, Carmen eagerly agreed to take Manuel home, where he passed peacefully a few weeks later.

Because of Carmen's deep sorrow at the thought of having failed her husband in the moment of his greatest need, I now discuss the possibility of a fall and hip fracture whenever I encounter patients on the Frailty/Dementia trajectory. This provides a stress-free opportunity for loved ones to consider their wishes in advance. Many families have questions about how hospice care could help in that situation, and many have misconceptions or fears about hospice care that I can clear up and address. Providing space for families to consider the option of hospice care outside of acute crisis is a helpful way to prepare family members for difficult decisions ahead.

To further assist my patients and their families, I will document their wishes in the patient's chart. Knowing that busy providers won't always see my notes, I also encourage families to advocate for their loved ones by requesting a consultation with a member of my team in the event of a hospitalization.

For patients hospitalized during my working hours, I will go one step further by contacting the ER, speaking directly with the attending physician, and requesting the consultation myself. In this way, I help ensure that my patients receive ongoing and collaborative support from someone trained in disease progression assessment and hospice criteria and care.

Dementia

Because human intellectual endeavor is only ever, at best, an approximation of describing the truth, it is important to understand that these five disease trajectory diagrams and descriptions are merely a convenient organizational system, a helpful tool for thinking about the end of life.

In truth, the brain is an organ like the heart, lungs, liver, and kidneys. The brain is the most important organ of the human body; without a functioning central nervous system, the other organs cannot function at all.

All of that is to say that dementia, the progressive and eventually terminal failure of the brain, could instead have been assigned to the Organ Failure trajectory. In that way, it would have been neatly arranged with the other trajectories of organs that fail. I debated this decision when writing this book. Should Dementia remain with Frailty, or should it be moved to the Organ Failure trajectory?

I decided to keep it here because the slow and steady decline that patients and families experience with dementia and most of the neurodegenerative diseases is best described by the Frailty/Dementia trajectory diagram (Fig. 4.6). However, conceptualizing dementia as a form of organ failure allows for a better appreciation of its extensive impact.

Many patients and families are confused about the relationship between dementia and Alzheimer's disease (AD), believing that one is worse than the other. I will clear up this confusion, explaining that dementia is the general umbrella term for what we call *brain failure* and that AD is the most common cause or type of dementia.

Frailty / Dementia

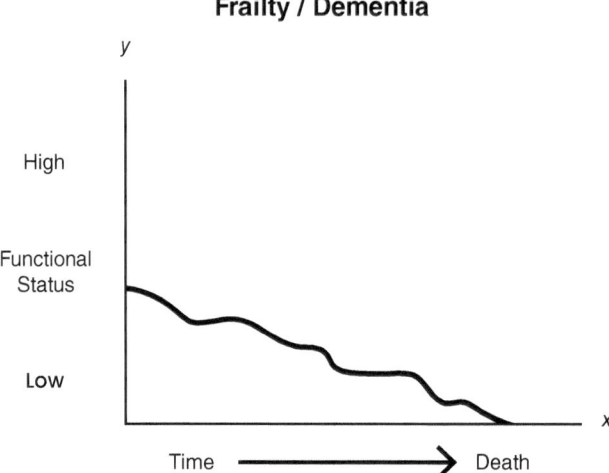

Fig. 4.6 Frailty/Dementia. (Adapted with permission from Lunney et al. (2002). *Profiles of Older Medicare Decedents*. Journal of the American Geriatrics Society [6])

Additionally, many people think of dementia as primarily *memory loss*, when in actuality, dementia is comprehensive brain failure that impacts every domain of a person's life. As a patient goes through a dementia journey, the brain atrophies or shrinks, losing volume and function associated with the affected geographical regions.

I find that it resonates deeply with close caregivers to hear dementia described as "the journey of going from infancy to adulthood, in reverse." When I use this phrase, I can virtually see the light coming on above a caregiver's head. Words have power, and naming a thing validates it, making it real. More times than I can count, I have seen how this particular description of dementia, delivered with compassion and empathy, can lift the burden of guilt and shame from a caregiver's shoulders, helping to make sense of the confusing reality of dementia and at the same time acknowledging and validating the caregiver's lived experience.

If the job of a parent is to raise an independent adult, then dementia's impact is to effectively rob patients of that upbringing. Above all else, dementia is the progressive and total loss of personal independence.

As we grow up, we move through stages of development. One of the first things we learn gives us what I consider to be our *foundational humanity*, our ability to be an emotional being and live in relationship to others.

As infants, we learn to be social and interact with our family members, learning to smile by six to eight weeks, then at two months, learning that essential human connection skill of conversational noisemaking, cooing, and laughing. This is the underpinning of language and emotional relatability, which occurs nearly two years before children learn to comprehend or produce language in any meaningful way. Videos of tiny babies having "conversations" with their parents come to mind.

From birth, infants hone their social awareness and understanding, looking to others for insight into their social and emotional environment, learning to match their parent's facial and vocal expressions by three and one-half months and others by five months [62]. The ability to pick up on cues from facial expression and tone of voice, particularly in the setting of a strong attachment bond with parents, which imparts a sense of safety, allows older infants to work out whether it is okay to go to a stranger's arms or to crawl across a room to play with new toys or a new infant they haven't previously encountered.

As one of the first skills to develop in infancy, our foundational humanity is one of the last skills to leave us on the dementia journey.

As our brains develop, we acquire skills in an upward fashion, moving from the brainstem to the cerebral cortex [63], developing simple motor skills before those that involve higher-level planning and simple concepts before more sophisticated cognitive dexterity. We learn to crawl, then to walk, then to ride a bike. We learn to name the animals before delving into cellular biology and to share toys with other toddlers before learning to cooperate or compete with our mates on the playground.

As we learn to function in the physical and social world, as we build confidence and character, our foundational humanity and sophisticated cerebral cortex enable us to develop intimate relationships—to acquire close friends, get married, or have children or pets—and lead us to meaningful careers, the desire to start a business, to lead a non-profit, or to write a book.

Throughout the complex course of a human lifespan, memory, in its various forms (working, recent, procedural, semantic, etc.), weaves our personal experiences like fibers in fabric into the elegant tapestry of an individual human life.

Dementia is the unraveling of this canvas, one developmental puzzle piece at a time. As the cortex, limbic system, and brainstem atrophy, as cerebral and cerebellar volume is lost, and as areas of function and the different aspects of memory are affected, patients experience an incremental but permanent decline in executive, visuospatial, sensorimotor, and autonomic function, skills that are lost in roughly the reverse order of acquisition, in what leading Alzheimer's researcher, Dr. Barry Reisberg, calls *retrogenesis* [64].

Because these changes are usually subtle, outsiders and onlookers often miss the milestones of the dementia journey. Families, too, are often in the dark about what is happening with a loved one, not understanding the changes they are witnessing and unable to make sense of this complicated, challenging, and often grief-ridden journey.

Stages of Dementia

Generally speaking, dementia progresses through four major stages of loss: Recent Memory, Cognitive Function, Personal Care, and Physical Function.

Recent Memory is diminished first, as the *hippocampus* is impacted by disease. Part of the *limbic system*, the seat of human emotion and memory, the *hippocampus* plays a vital role in our ability to make it through the day, allowing for storage and retrieval of new information about the world around us and our personal experiences. This is a type of long-term memory called *declarative memory*, but what most people refer to as *short-term memory* [65, 66].

As declarative memory degrades, patients experience difficulty with new and recent information of any type, such as recalling where they put their keys (and due to declarative memory loss, they are unable to track back through their day to find them), what was previously said in conversation, who visited the day before, what appointments are ahead, whether they took their morning medications, or what they had for lunch.

As you can imagine, without the ability to encode new bits of information, patients, especially those younger or not yet retired, can experience great difficulty at work, when participating in hobbies, and in social situations. Early on, patients with dementia become poor historians of their own lives because reporting reliably on recent events requires robust recent memory. This stage often goes unnoticed, with many people chalking up short-term memory issues to normal aging or stress.

Cognitive Function declines next, as the cerebral cortex suffers widespread damage and both conceptualization and processing are affected. In addition to sensory and motor regions, much of the cerebral cortex is what is called *association cortex*, vast areas of gray matter dedicated to integrating and manipulating information from neighboring or distant parts of the brain [67].

Most important at this stage is volume loss in the *prefrontal association cortex*, the part of the human brain that makes humans unique in the animal kingdom, giving us the ability to perform complicated cognitive tasks, including logic, reason, abstract thinking, computation, anticipation, planning, and judgment [67]. This part of our brain gives us concentration, motivation and drive, creativity and curiosity, the ability to take another person's perspective, and allows us to delay gratification and control our impulses [67].

The prefrontal cortex is also the hub of *working memory*, the type of short-term memory that allows us to hold information in our minds for brief periods (on the order of seconds) while other cortical regions process it [66].

Intersecting directly with these higher-order tasks is the critical component of *semantic memory* [66, 68], the ability to conceptualize ideas using language, which depends on various cortical regions of the temporal and parietal lobes responsible for word storage, syntax, and semantics, including many regions beyond the well-known Broca's and Wernicke's areas [69].

Loss of volume in these areas can impact language comprehension and conceptualization while reading, writing, or participating in conversation [69]. Finding the right word can be challenging, as patients struggle to express thoughts with a shrinking vocabulary and conceptual inventory [66, 67]. And it goes without saying that conceptualization is necessary for much of our higher-order processing skills, including abstract reasoning, planning and judgment, and the ability to think about the future or the past [66].

Equally crucial to appropriate conceptualization and processing of the world around and within us is reliable sensory input from our auditory and visual cortexes located in the temporal and occipital lobes, respectively [67]. As these and neighboring regions of association cortex become affected, object and face recognition, depth perception, and visuospatial processing (e.g., pattern recognition) can decline [67]. Furthermore, auditory and visual hallucinations can occur [67, 70], profoundly impacting a patient's ability to thrive.

Conceptualization and processing abilities collectively form the basis of human culture—science, religion, art, philosophy, architecture, poetry, and politics [66]. In our day-to-day lives, it is this set of higher-level cognitive skills that enables us to perform *instrumental activities of daily living* (IADLs) [71], those tasks required to live independently in our own homes and engage successfully with society as we cook, clean, drive, shop, and manage our appointments, medications, mealtime, finances, our homes, and pets.

As patients experience a decline in logic and reason, sensory input, and working, recent, and semantic memory, it becomes difficult or even dangerous for them to drive, follow a recipe, manage a house, or respond to telemarketers. Because the stakes can be very high for errors with IADLs, it is at this stage that family members often get involved to help protect loved ones, particularly those who live on their own, by managing their affairs.

Personal Care degrades next, as patients lose the ability to care for their physical bodies, tasks referred to as *basic activities of daily living* (ADLs) [71]. These tasks include getting dressed, bathing, toileting, bladder and bowel incontinence, and feeding oneself. The ADLs are acquired during development between the ages of approximately two and eight years.

Personal care skills rely on *procedural knowledge*, a type of long-term memory that integrates higher-level cognition with motor skills related to a task [66], such as buttering a slice of bread, putting on a button-up shirt, or drying one's hair. Performing procedural skills requires attention, working memory, and higher-order motor planning, all of which rely on a healthy frontal lobe [66]. ADLs also require coordination of sensorimotor abilities, integrating functions of the frontal motor cortex, parietal somatosensory cortex, and cerebellum [67].

At this point in a dementia journey, not only are patients losing procedural skills, but because of deficits in attention, working memory, recent memory, and sensorimotor coordination, patients, for the most part, cannot acquire new skills. Imagine a patient who pulls his walker behind him instead of relying on it for support. Procedural skills that are retained are often learned very early in life and hold deep, personal significance on the order of a personality trait.

Physical Function is impacted last, as voluntary and autonomic control centers decline, ultimately leaving patients unable to walk, sit up on their own, chew food, swallow, verbalize, and smile.

Although bladder and bowel continence are included with the ADLs and indeed rely on procedural knowledge lost during the Personal Care stage, I tend to think of their loss as the leading edge of the final major stage of dementia, when control of the physical body begins to disintegrate. Insofar as appropriate bladder and bowel control requires intact brain function in different regions of the cortex, cerebellum, and brainstem, integrating sensory, motor, and reflex functions; loss in these regions well represents the comprehensive impact of dementia.

Finding one's way to the bathroom requires appropriate visuospatial processing and ambulatory control and coordination. Following the steps of toileting involves procedural memory and motor planning. Voluntary bowel and bladder control requires conscious awareness of the need to evacuate, voluntary sphincter muscle control, and intact brainstem reflexes [72]. And of course, bladder and bowel output are deeply connected to one's awareness of thirst and hunger and one's drive to drink and eat.

Advanced dementia, which impacts diverse regions of the brain, can affect continence in a multitude of ways, resulting in a wide range of disorganized habits, including doing things out of order or in the wrong place, frequency, urgency, or retention, or incontinence of every kind (stress, urge, leak, and overflow) [73, 74]. Loss of voluntary bladder and bowel control (what we tend to think of as frank incontinence) tends to occur after the loss of procedural toileting skills.

During this final, or end-stage, of dementia, the metabolic shift to *hypercatabolism* occurs, with patients becoming less interested in eating and drinking, evidencing weight loss, mobility issues, and frequently, falls. As organs and systems decline further, patients become much more susceptible to recurrent infections—the hallmark of end-stage dementia—including UTIs, sepsis, and aspiration pneumonia, the most common cause of death for patients with Alzheimer's disease [75]. Aspiration results from the loss of brainstem control of the reflex-initiated pharyngeal swallow function and gag response and can be further impacted by declining levels of consciousness [76].

Eventually, patients with dementia will follow a similar transition toward death as patients on the Frailty trajectory, becoming increasingly fatigued, spending more and more time in bed, with dwindling interest in eating or drinking until, at last, if they are fortunate enough to be managed with hospice care at the end of their lives, they pass away in their sleep.

Causes of Dementia

The picture I have just painted describes the journey that most people with a diagnosis of dementia will follow, that of Alzheimer's disease (AD) , which affects 60% to 80% of those with dementia [51]. In 2022, an estimated 6.5 million Americans are living with a diagnosis of AD in the United States [51], meaning 6.5 million families are affected by this devastating disease. This number is expected to nearly double by 2050 as the aging baby boomer generation radically increases the U.S. population of those over 65 over the next 30 years [51]. Incidence of Alzheimer's disease increases with age, affecting approximately 1 in 20 patients by age 65 to 74, 1 in 10 by age 75 to 84, and 1 in 3 over 85 [51]. In 2020, AD was the seventh leading cause of death in the United States [16, 77], accounting for the death of more than 130,000 Americans.

After Alzheimer's disease, vascular dementia, most often caused by strokes, accounts for 5% to 10% of cases, followed by Lewy body disease (LBD) (5% of cases) and frontotemporal lobar degeneration (FTLD) (3% of cases) [51]. Patients who develop neurodegenerative diseases such as Parkinson's disease (PD), amyotrophic lateral sclerosis (ALS), and Huntington's disease (HD) are also at increased risk of developing dementia, as are those with the atypical parkinsonian disorders corticobasal degeneration (CBD) and progressive supranuclear palsy (PSP). All of these etiologies present somewhat differently on account of the regions of the brain impacted by disease.

After a stroke, 1 in 3 patients will develop dementia [78]. This can occur after a single stroke or after multiple strokes over some time. Residual deficits may be apparent and reflect the part of the brain affected by the stroke, often weakness of a limb or one side of the body. As shown in the examples provided earlier in this chapter, many patients will experience devastating functional and physical loss. Those with small vessel disease, which affects the tiny blood vessels deep within the white matter and areas nearer the base of the brain, often initially develop bladder issues, weakness, mobility issues, and falls [79, 80].

Patients with stroke may experience improvement or stabilization in their deficits with rehabilitation, typically within the first six months [79]. After that time, evolving changes may occur, possibly due to the *neighborhood effect* [67]—in which damage to one area of the brain typically leads to damage in neighboring tissue—or to vulnerability caused by the underlying pathologies of AD (plaques and tangles), LBD (Lewy bodies), or FTLD (tau and transactive response DNA-binding proteins) already present.

Lewy body disease is marked by four prominent manifestations occurring across the journey described above, including REM sleep behavior disorder (RBD), fluctuations in cognition, visual hallucinations, and parkinsonism. *REM sleep behavior disorder (RBD)*, in which patients act out their dreams, sometimes violently, often predates the diagnosis of LBD by years or decades. This can be challenging and distressing to patients and spouses, leading to years of interrupted sleep for everyone in the house. *Fluctuations in cognition* can be quite robust, with spouses noting that they never know what type of person they'll be living with from day to day. Of note, I find this to be very common with my Alzheimer's patients as well.

Patients with LBD tend to show two different presentations: those with *visual hallucinations* (usually of people, animals, or insects) followed later by motor deficits characteristic of Parkinson's disease, called *parkinsonism*—tremors, muscle stiffness, and hesitant movement and speech—or those who first show motor deficits and then, later on, visual hallucinations.

I frequently find patients with LBD being separately treated by a sleep specialist, psychiatrist, and neurologist; their families are left confused by the variety of diagnoses unrecognized as the constellation of LBD. Sometimes, I am the first provider to put these puzzle pieces together, helping to make sense of this confusing assortment of symptoms.

Frontotemporal lobar degeneration encompasses three pathologies impacting behavior, conceptualization, language, and speech [81]. Patients with *semantic dementia* and *progressive nonfluent aphasia* will show deficits in conceptual knowledge and language abilities, and speech, respectively, due to damage in the temporal lobes [81].

Patients with *behavioral-variant frontotemporal dementia (bvFTD)* will show wild personality and behavior changes due to loss of frontal lobe mass, which affects impulse control, judgment, foresight, and reason [81]. One of my patients with bvFTD, a 75-year-old family woman previously fond of cooking for her relatives, is now primarily interested in gambling, finding her way to a local casino, and inviting strange men back to her home, much to the distress of her children. Another patient, convinced that her "cheating" husband was trying to kill her, called the police on him several times, causing significant marital distress before her eventual diagnosis and admission to a geriatric-psychiatric facility.

It is relatively easy to differentiate the slow and subtle story of Alzheimer's disease from the more dramatic presentations of Lewy body disease and behavioral-variant frontotemporal dementia. And yet, studies looking at biopsy evidence from deceased patients with dementia show that most people have a mixed picture, with evidence of more than one type of dementia pathology [51]. I find this to be true in practice, with Alzheimer's patients frequently showing hallmarks of Lewy body disease (motor issues or visual hallucinations), semantic dementia (severe language deficits), or small vessel vascular disease (bladder control issues), well before otherwise expected.

Patients also do not always make a linear progression through the major stages I've described. This is particularly true of vascular dementia patients, who tend to show a collection of deficits across the journey or who may show stabilization in one area (procedural memory) while continuing to lose ground in another (sensorimotor control). Furthermore, because of the areas targeted by disease, memory tends to be spared far into the journey for patients with FTLD and further into the journey for LBD patients than for those with AD [51].

Psychiatric Symptoms of Dementia

To complicate things further, patients at any stage of their dementia journey can experience any of the various psychiatric symptoms expected as the brain's biochemical milieu changes. These include *anxiety*, which can be described as an underlying sense of unease; *depression*, affecting 20% of patients with AD and 50% of those with vascular dementia [82]; *agitation*, the physical or verbal expression of anxiety (for instance, picking skin, pacing, pushing, or repeating a question, yelling, or cussing); *apathy*, a near-total loss of motivation, drive and interest in participating in life; *delusions*, beliefs—often paranoid—that other people don't share; *hallucinations*, auditory or visual; *insomnia*, trouble falling or staying asleep; and *sun-downing*, increased confusion as the day progresses.

Additionally, many patients experience *hypnopompic hallucinations*, in which they seem to bring elements from their sleeping reality into their waking state, often believing that a parent or sibling they were dreaming about is still present in their home, similar to a delusion or a visual or auditory hallucination. This likely stems from the confusing residue of a dream maintained in a brain that is losing the sharp boundary between the sleeping and waking states. Patients without the cognitive skills to work out for themselves that they were dreaming often wake up eager to find the person they were "visiting with," and caregivers often report a difficult time in the aftermath.

Psychiatric symptoms can range from mild to moderate to severe or even reach crisis level. Caregivers tend to absorb and experience the brunt of these symptoms, leading to anger, frustration, fatigue, depression, and strain—both physical and emotional. Patients experiencing moderate to severe symptoms need either aggressive outpatient medication management and very close (weekly or more frequent) follow-up to titrate dosing or should be hospitalized for medication management, stabilization, and consideration of placement in a care facility when caregivers are no longer able to manage things at home.

Visual hallucinations and delusions can be quite robust and consistent over time and tend to be the most alarming set of symptoms. Examples from patients I have seen include giant spiders on the wall, dogs running about the house, children playing at the kitchen table, a hooded man breaking into the house each evening to steal the patient's personal effects, a stranger climbing into bed to sleep between the patient and spouse, multiple nefarious strangers standing on the lawn, surveillance chips being inserted into windows, and four different versions of a loved one. Often, the line between hallucination and delusion is blurred.

Surprisingly, patients are not always distressed by these altered realities. The woman whose bed was routinely invaded by a stranger considerately spent the remainder of each night on the floor. Her husband, knowing that she was safe there, regarded this as an acceptable situation, and we did not adjust her medications. In contrast, a bvFTD patient convinced that he had murdered four strangers was so distraught that he needed to be admitted for urgent medication management.

When symptoms cause distress to the point that the patient or family's daily routine is interrupted or when symptoms lead to moderate to severe agitation or aggression, patients can be treated with an antipsychotic. For those with mild to moderate symptoms, an antidepressant is often suitable. For all families, I teach non-pharmacologic strategies for communication. This education is often all that is needed for patients with mild symptoms and helps all caregivers and family members to reduce the frustration and distress that accompanies dementia. Chapter 15 includes language for educating family members about dementia, including non-pharmacologic strategies for communication and management of the patient's environment.

A note on the use of antipsychotics to treat psychiatric symptoms of dementia: While recently discussing my routine use of these medications for patients with moderate to severe psychiatric symptoms of dementia with a physician colleague, they noted the black-box warning and abundant evidence of increased risk of sudden death that accompanies the use of these drugs, adding that these medications are not safe and should not be used. This conversation occurred on a day when a patient shared an observation about the end-of-life care a loved one had received: "Doctors treat quantity, not quality."

I shared with my colleague the incredible distress that severe symptoms can pose to both patients and families and how I frequently witness the significant improvement in both the patient's daily function and caregiver's strain that antipsychotics can provide, but that I had not seen one of my patients taking an antipsychotic die suddenly. When titrating antipsychotics or adding any QT-prolonging medications, we monitor with a follow-up ECG, and when starting patients on an antipsychotic, I review the black-box warning of sudden death with caregivers; rarely does a family member decide against a trial of the medication. Additionally, we "start low, go slow, and stay low," using doses significantly lower than the doses used in the studies that resulted in the black-box warning [83].

Dementia as Criterion for Hospital Admission

For reasons that are unclear to me, dementia tends to be dismissed as a qualifying hospital admission diagnosis. Often, when dementia patients exhibiting a high psychiatric symptom burden who are repeatedly seen in the ER are sent home, their families are told that there is nothing *organically* wrong with them: workups for UTIs and other abnormalities in electrolytes and organ function normal. How striking that psychiatric symptoms of dementia are not considered *organic* and often go unrecognized for what they are—the outward presentation of the underlying organic pathology occurring in the brain.

The fact is that the psychiatric symptoms of dementia are precisely what is expected with brain failure. These symptoms are no less real or distressing to patients and families than the shortness of breath, chest pain, edema, and cough that accompany heart and lung failure.

Furthermore, just as cardiovascular disease treatment relies on optimal medical treatment (OMT) with statins, antiplatelets, beta-blockers, and RAAS (renin-angiotensin-aldosterone system) inhibitors, OMT for dementia includes medications intended to minimize the effects of psychiatric symptoms—antidepressants, antipsychotics, neuroleptics, sleep aids, etc.

The ICD-10 codes for *dementia with behavioral disturbance*[2] are acceptable hospital admission diagnosis codes for which the Centers for Medicare and Medicaid Services (CMS) will reimburse hospitals, and can be used to support a patient's admission for necessary medication management.

The medical community must evolve its understanding and appreciation of the dementia journey, must learn to diagnose more effectively (i.e., earlier, more accurately), and must develop its approach to addressing and treating dementia symptomatology, particularly if we are to prepare for the onslaught of this disease we will experience in the coming decades.

---

[2] There are separate ICD-10 codes for *dementia with behavioral disturbance* specific to Alzheimer's dementia, vascular dementia, frontotemporal dementia, Lewy body dementia, etc.

Why Dementia Often Goes Undiagnosed

Dementia, unlike the other trajectories, intersects with every other disease process, making it difficult for patients to remain compliant, before eventually pulling ahead as the most compelling aspect of a patient's journey, at which point treatments for other conditions may no longer make sense or even be beneficial. It is, therefore, incredibly heartbreaking to know how many patients (and, importantly, their families) go without a diagnosis for so long or without the education needed to make sense of this complicated experience.

Dementia often goes undiagnosed because our *foundational humanity* intersects with another important aspect of our human nature, our *foundational motivation*—the desire to feel *competent, capable*, and *in control*. All of us, whether we have dementia or not, have an innate need to feel successful in social and practical situations [84], and this need, when combined with our ability to read the social cues imparted verbally and nonverbally by people in our social environment, leads us to respond in ways that *convey* our competence, capability, and control.

Suppose you've encountered someone in public whom you are certain you know but cannot recall in which context you met; social norms will probably lead you to engage superficially, if you're brave enough to engage with them at all, in a manner that does not betray your ignorance. You'll say things like, "How's it going? How have you been?" without inquiring about the specific details of their life you cannot recall.

Patients often visit their physicians alone. With a robust ability to read facial expressions and tone of voice, patients, even nearing end-stage dementia, can still work out what words to say in response to a question. We all know how to respond in a way that provides the answer sought and how to engage with minimal verbalization to make it look like we're following along. If you have ever tuned out while on the phone while thinking about 10 other things, you may have noticed that a part of your brain remains engaged enough to enable you to utter the slight indications of surprise, agreement, and concern at just the correct times so that you appear competently engaged.

Patients with dementia retain these skills, too, even when they've lost most of their conceptual and higher-order language capabilities. One of my near-end-stage dementia patients remained socially engaged, meeting and greeting me at the door with her bright smile, taking me by the arm, and leading me back to her kitchen, where she engaged in a babble of sounds expressing clearly her excitement, inquiry, curiosity, and concern but without semantic meaning. I responded in kind, modulating my intonation to provide her with the conversational feedback she sought.

It is by this mechanism of social mimicry that patients go undiagnosed well into the dementia journey, even into the end stage, particularly those with significant *cognitive reserve*—cognitive dexterity to solve problems creatively [85], which enables patients to mask the disease better. Rather than assuming patients intentionally hide their illness, I think it is quite natural for each of us to succeed in our social and physical environment by making use of whatever strategies and capacities we have available to us. If a spouse is not present to confirm whether the patient is providing accurate answers, patients of all levels of cognitive reserve will be motivated to give a history that shows that nothing at all is awry. Patients without issues who seem to follow the conversation raise few red flags.

Because dementia is prevalent in the general population, healthcare professionals should confirm the history gained from an older patient by speaking with individuals who witness the patient's experiences throughout the day—such as spouses, caregivers, others in the home, or staff at the patient's living facility. The increased likelihood that patients of advanced age will have dementia requires an adjustment to our standard history-taking, which often relies solely on communication with the patient.

Four Pillars of Support for Patients with Dementia

Together, our foundational humanity and our foundational motivation elegantly provide the mechanism for honoring and supporting patients with dementia at every stage of their journey, regardless of their level of capacity. Knowing that a patient's dignity derives from the way others navigate the patient's innate need to feel competent, capable, and in control, caregivers should be taught the four pillars of support for patients with dementia: Managing Expectations, Managing Communications, Managing the Patient's Environment, and Self-Care.

Because the dementia journey entails progressive and permanent loss of cognitive and physical capacity, it is caregivers who must adapt to the disease. The four pillars provide a framework for adaptation, ensuring that patients and caregivers alike can share a positive, loving, family-affirming experience across the dementia journey.

Managing Expectations means aligning expectations for the patient's capacity for communicating, thinking, and navigating the physical and social environment with the reality of the disease. Having realistic expectations can prevent frustration. Thus, the first step in helping caregivers is to teach them what cognitive skills are being lost at each stage and how that will show up in the patient's life, allowing caregivers to match their expectations with reality.

As dementia progresses, patients will have a difficult time remembering new information (Recent Memory), managing complicated cognitive tasks (Cognitive Function), navigating procedural tasks (Personal Care), and will eventually require around-the-clock care and support (Physical Function). Caregivers who know what to expect are better prepared to address patient needs in a way that preserves patient dignity.

Managing Communications is easier for caregivers who understand the cognitive skills being affected at each stage of the disease. Communication strategies that account for cognitive losses include the following:

- Asking fewer questions for information finding (Recent Memory),
- Trying not to convince, explain, or change a patient's mind and asking fewer "Why" questions (Cognitive Function), and

- Narrating the present and keeping instructions simple and concrete (Personal Care).

At every stage, it is important that caregivers manage their facial expressions, tone of voice, and body language so as not to communicate negativity, including judgment, condescension, criticism, or frustration.

Keeping a person's innate need for dignity in mind, all communications should attempt to avoid forcing a confrontation with the patient's cognitive deficits, which can cause feelings of shame, embarrassment, or frustration. Questions with the purpose of information finding, comments like "You remember," complicated topics, and complex instructions can make a person with significant cognitive deficits feel incompetent, incapable, and as though things are not in their control. Likewise, practices like reorientation or correction should be discouraged because being told that today is Tuesday is really of no importance to a patient with dementia at any stage, and being corrected again and again will only cause chagrin.

Rather, caregivers can be taught to reassure, step into the patient's reality, change the topic, and try to keep the mood light. It is a rare instance when the very next thing that a person with dementia is about to do will result in bodily harm or injury. Thus, caregivers should prioritize the patient's dignity by being supportive and encouraging rather than restrictive and corrective. While reviewing this manuscript, Jennifer Moore Ballentine, MA, originator of the Catastrophic Event trajectory, shared the following story with me, which perfectly embodies this advice.

> When I was a brand-new hospice volunteer at a small hospice house, I encountered a patient whose dementia led her to believe she was on board a ship, taking a lengthy cruise. Her room was her "berth," the dining room was "the captain's table," the hallway was the "promenade," and the outdoor patio was the "deck." I wasn't sure how to respond to this, so I asked the hospice chaplain what the best approach would be. "Well," he said, "I'll tell you what I do … I just pull up a deck chair and enjoy the salt air!"

Managing the Patient's Environment means that caregivers will need to manage complex tasks, including all of the IADLs (Cognitive Function), simplify the physical and social environment to keep patients safe (Cognitive Function), provide around-the-clock supervision and cueing and management of procedural tasks, including all of the ADLs (Personal Care), and, eventually, provide full care for patients with end-stage disease (Physical Function). Caregivers with varying degrees of physical, emotional, and financial resources will need help in aligning patients' needs with the caregivers' abilities to provide care.

Self-Care, the fourth pillar of support for patients with dementia, encourages caregivers to prioritize their own health and well-being. Self-care is a necessity for all caregivers and should be encouraged by healthcare providers.

To remain loving and patient requires that caregivers work from a full cup. Caregivers should be encouraged to maintain activities and relationships that provide an outlet for creativity, connection, and relaxation. Each caregiver's self-care will look different, and although quantity is less important than quality, routine self-care should be a standard part of caregiver support for loved ones with dementia.

Just like airplane announcements encouraging adult passengers to tend to their own oxygen needs before helping a child, caregivers must first care for themselves to care for others.

The four pillars help caregivers in the challenging but necessary task of reconceptualizing their loved ones with dementia. Although patients with dementia look like the capable people they once were, dementia permanently alters their capacity for thinking, communicating, and navigating their physical and social environments. Caregivers who are successful at adapting to the disease shift their conception of the patient to accommodate this new reality. Just as we would not ask a person with a broken arm to carry in the groceries with that arm, recognizing that certain expectations, communications, and environmental features can unnecessarily tax a patient's cognitive capacities allows caregivers to uphold patient dignity across the dementia journey no matter the patient's capacity. Caregivers who prioritize self-care are better able to remain loving and kind as they do so.

Alzheimer's and Dementia Care Program

Recognizing the sweeping impact of the dementia journey on families, particularly on spouses and caregivers, I was thrilled to be part of a team at my hospital that helped establish a comprehensive dementia support program for our community. Thanks to a grant provided to UCLA by the John A. Hartford Foundation, my hospital became one of the first 15 dissemination sites in the country to implement the Alzheimer's and Dementia Care (ADC) Program designed by Dr. David B. Reuben and Nurse Practitioner (NP), Leslie C. Evertson.

As with most disease trajectories, the dementia journey is often not well understood by patients and families, including why they are experiencing the challenges they face or what they can expect ahead. A significant part of my work is to provide education about dementia, to teach strategies for addressing the day-to-day struggles that accompany a patient's progressive loss of independence, and to help caregivers anticipate and prepare for evolving care needs. Almost all of my work for patients with dementia is in providing support to spouses, children, and other caregivers, normalizing their experience and helping them navigate this challenging journey.

Working closely with families to monitor their loved ones' dementia progression, I continually collaborate with spouses and children to align their wishes with their loved ones' care. Close follow-up allows me to identify when patients transition into meeting hospice criteria. Because I have reinforced dementia education and managed end-of-life expectations continually along the way, spouses and children are typically ready and relieved to transition their loved ones to hospice care when that time arrives. Most patients can be transitioned to hospice care seamlessly in the outpatient setting, avoiding distressing end-of-life hospitalizations and unwanted or non-beneficial escalations of care. Consistent with UCLA's findings [86, 87], this targeted intervention resulted in a significant increase in the average length of hospice stay and a dramatic reduction of hospital utilization in the last six months of life (including hospital admissions, ICU stays, and ER visits), metrics that reflect better alignment of family wishes with patient care and improved quality of life for patients and caregivers.[3]

Patients with dementia will eventually lose their ability to make their own medical decisions, so they must be allowed to specify their end-of-life wishes and identify a surrogate medical decision-maker early in the course of the disease. As is true with the other disease journeys, it becomes much easier for families to decide on hospice care when the patient is provided the opportunity to participate in their advance care planning ahead of time.

~~~

Dale, with no prior hospitalizations, had come to the ER after a fall at home. Too confused to follow his wife's instructions as she tried to help him stand back up, she had called 911 for help. At the hospital, Dale was found to have a UTI that had caused sepsis.

In speaking with the floor nurse, I learned that Dale was presently bowel and bladder incontinent, sleeping most of the day, and reluctant to eat anything he was offered. His chart revealed that he was taking memantine and had a diagnosis of dementia. With an albumin of 2.2 g/dL on admission and little improvement after nearly a week of IV antibiotics, I worried that Dale's time was limited and that he had reached the end of his dementia journey.

The floor nurse shared her insight that Dale's wife, Marian, was very confused about her husband's condition and struggled to make decisions on his behalf. The hospitalist had consulted our service for help.

As I began leading Marian through our conversation, asking her to paint a picture of how things had been at home over the last few years, I could sense her reluctance to divulge the details of her husband's experience, as though she worried she was betraying his trust. When she proudly explained that Dale had been an economist, repeatedly describing him as the "smart one" at home, I understood her hesitation. Having taken an intellectual back seat to her husband for so long, Marian struggled to trust her observations, judgments, and competence.

Dale, once an accomplished university professor, had been forced into early retirement when it became clear that he could no longer keep up with the demands of teaching, writing, and running the research lab that he had helped to found. Devastated, he had fallen into a deep depression, and Marian, unsuccessful at talking him out of his funk, had sought medical advice from multiple specialists over

---

[3] Of the first 200 patients enrolled in the Alzheimer's and Dementia Care (ADC) Program at my institution between March 2021 and October 2023, 47 patients were transitioned to hospice care and five others died during a hospital admission without having been enrolled in hospice care prior to death. The 47 decedents who died with hospice care in place experienced an average of 51 days of hospice care support, an increase of 222% over the average length of hospice stay for patients at my institution (23 days). During the last six months of life, the 52 decedents enrolled in the ADC Program at my institution experienced an average of 0 ICU stays, 0.69 hospital admissions, and 0.54 ER visits, a reduction from 0.51 ICU stays, 1.3 hospital admissions, and 0.86 ER visits during the last six months of life for the average patient at my institution.

the years, seeking a diagnosis that would explain her husband's inability to work. But cognitive assessments repeatedly pointed away from dementia, and Dale, feeling defensive, eventually refused further appointments, leaving Marian to experience his journey without support.

Marian recounted the isolation she felt, with her husband at home for more hours than she had ever seen him, unable to coax him from his study, where he busied himself keeping lists while avoiding conversation, dinner, and outings. Over the years, Marian lost contact with her friends and saw less and less of her own family. In recent years, she reported being entirely on her own.

To set Marian at ease, I gave her my full attention, focusing on her as much patience, kindness, and empathy as I could muster. As she took me through the years of Dale's journey, I frequently responded with sympathy, acknowledging how difficult it must have been for her as I tried to validate and honor her private experience. Marian was the caregiver who taught me, early on in my palliative career, that spouses often suffer in silence, with little insight or understanding of their loved one's illness, going to great lengths of personal sacrifice, often with little acknowledgment or thanks.

To provide Marian with scaffolding for her narrative, I targeted my line of questions to focus on the changes Dale would have experienced as he progressed through the stages of loss—Recent Memory, Cognitive Function, Personal Care, and Physical Function—asking about memory issues for recent activities or conversations; difficulty handling finances, medications, driving, appointments, and housework; difficulty remembering to shower or change clothes, and issues with dressing, bathing, and toileting; and finally, concerns about continence, swallowing, ambulation, appetite, and weight loss.

In the 10 years since Dale retired, he had moved very predictably through the expected stages of decline. Early on, as he began having problems with Recent Memory, Dale relied on list-making, sticky notes, and other reminders to make it through the day.

As Dale began exhibiting issues with Cognitive Function, Marian started managing aspects of their lives that had not formerly fallen under her purview, including their home, automobiles, and finances. She found herself learning new skills in areas where she lacked prior experience, including how to fix a toilet, light the pilot on the furnace, and how frequently to schedule an oil change. I could detect her pride and accomplishment as Marian reported her management successes.

By this point in our conversation, Marian had grown comfortable enough with me to reveal some of her more intimate struggles with Dale. When Dale began exhibiting issues with Personal Care three years earlier, and Marian needed to remind him to take a bath, shave, and change his clothes, Dale's anger surfaced, and he began routinely yelling and swearing at her. Sometimes, their disagreements grew physical, and Dale lashed out on more than one occasion, bruising Marian. As Marian recounted this part of their story, I felt her shame and embarrassment and reached out to offer a tissue as I told her how sorry I was that she had experienced all of this alone. She assured me that Dale had never previously so much as raised his voice at her. She knew he wasn't himself, yet she did not understand why any of this had happened.

After finding Dale confused and sitting on the shower floor a year prior, Marian began helping him bathe. When buttons and zippers became too difficult for him, she replaced his jeans and dress shirts with pull-on joggers and pullover tops. She accompanied and helped him through every moment of his day, ensuring he was fed, clean, and clothed. This effort took its toll, with Marian experiencing significant weight loss and back pain over the last year.

Six months earlier, as Dale began losing Physical Function, he began having bowel and bladder accidents throughout their home. Marian recounted sleepless nights and exhausting cleanups until, eventually, she decided to transition Dale into adult diapers despite his fierce resistance.

In the prior three months, Dale had lost interest in eating and dropped 40 pounds, representing 20% of his body weight. He had also begun to cough during mealtime. Carefully attending to his nutrition, Marian fed him extra protein and cut his food into smaller and smaller bites so that he could chew without choking.

When I asked Marian how she was making sense of the changes she had described, she couldn't. She had no idea why any of this was happening. When I asked if there was a diagnosis that she could pin these changes to, she shook her head, "No." When I asked where she thought Dale was in the overall journey with his health, she was unable to say.

As I transitioned the conversation to a discussion of dementia, gently introducing the diagnosis of Alzheimer's disease, I told her that she had been right to seek an answer early on and that the reason a diagnosis likely hadn't been made at that time was that Dale's *cognitive reserve*—his intellectual ability to improvise and find alternative ways to solve problems—had allowed him to avoid detection. If he hadn't had such a high level of education and an intellectually stimulating career, he likely wouldn't have passed the tests so easily. I told her that I was sorry that she had gone through this journey without a diagnosis to help explain what was happening to him.

As I described the major milestones of the Alzheimer's journey, I tied each stage to the specific changes Dale had experienced. When I arrived at the final stage, detailing the physical decline that layers on top of existing cognitive loss, I gently explained my worry that Dale's time was limited. Not surprisingly, Marian was taken aback by this revelation. Although she didn't disagree with my concern, it was too much for her right then to answer any questions about her wishes for him or to make any determination about his care. Respecting her need for time to process our conversation, I wrapped up our discussion for the day.

Before I left her, I took the time to praise her efforts over the years by telling her how fortunate Dale was to have had her looking after him all that time. I emphasized that Dale had done as well as he had, for as long as he had, because of the amazing care she had provided to him at home. Like many caregivers hearing these words for the first time, Marian was grateful for this acknowledgment, her eyes welling with tears.

When I came back to see Marian the following day, she was emotionally ready to move into the next part of our conversation and able to articulate what she thought her husband would want. She felt sure he would want to be comfortable, not to suffer, and to pass peacefully when it was his time.

Hearing Marian articulate these wishes was my queue to transition our conversation into a discussion of hospice care. After asking her to share with me her prior experience (none) and understanding (little) of hospice care, I filled in the gaps for her by painting a picture of what hospice care looks like, describing the hospice philosophy, hospice criteria, and the details of care, cost, and location.

Exhausted from her efforts to care for Dale at home, Marian decided to move him to our community's hospice center, preferring their last chapter together to be that of husband and wife rather than caregiver and patient. Dale lived another month, his wife spending every day with him. When he took his last breath, Marian was there, holding his hand.

~~~

Patients with dementia tend to come in two groups—those with insight into their decline and those without. This dimension adds further complexity and challenge to a caregiver's job, as those with insight range from comfortable to troubled, and those without insight range from apathetic to fiercely defiant.

Ava was early enough in her dementia journey, just starting into Cognitive Function loss, that she was still able to participate in her care planning fully. A warm, friendly, generous woman, she had plenty of insight into her cognitive decline, so much so that she had already given up driving, refused to cook without her husband present, and, because she was afraid of being home alone, wore a medical alert necklace. However, she expressed concern about her ability to remember to wear it or to know what to do with it when needed. Ava was aware that her mind could no longer retain or recall new information, which, she explained, would disappear in the time it took for her to leave one room and cross the threshold into another. Even before I asked, she told me that she didn't want to be a burden to her husband or children and was planning to move into a care facility when it became too difficult for her to live at home.

Tasked with caring for the whole person, palliative care providers cast a wide net of concern for patients and their caregivers. For the reasons indicated throughout this chapter, patients with dementia are particularly vulnerable to the whims of fate that affect their caregivers.

Ava and her husband, Juan, lived alone in a one-story condo into which they had moved two years earlier. Juan looked cachectic and frail when we met, in much poorer health than his wife. As I inquired about his need to assist Ava with IADLs, Juan explained that his poor health made these tasks more difficult. He was working on completing a Medicaid application for Ava, already considering the time when she would need more financial and functional support. When I inquired into Juan's health, he disclosed his stage IV cancer diagnosis.

Concerned, given his appearance, I asked Juan about recent weight loss, changes in appetite, and fatigue. His answers confirmed my hunch that my immediate task in supporting Ava was to begin caring for her husband. I messaged oncology, explaining the situation and my concern that Juan's decline, a poor prognostic indicator, left his wife at significant risk. Any hospitalization Juan might experience would leave Ava home alone, unsafe to make it through her day. Oncology placed a referral to our service for Juan, and when we next met, we focused on his health, how that might impact his wife's journey, and their collective wishes.

As with many cancer patients, Juan lacked insight into the significance of his declining weight, appetite, strength, and wakefulness. He didn't understand the advanced nature of his cancer, that it was incurable, or that it was spreading. He didn't understand that his chemotherapy treatments were palliative in nature, intended to prolong his life, but not intended to cure his disease.

As I gently walked Juan through *The Arc of Conversation*, painting a picture for him of the cancer trajectory and sharing my concern that he had already started down the cliff, he arrived at the decision, within a few weeks, to transition to hospice care at home. He wanted to be present and capable of participating in conversations and care planning for his wife before he passed. He didn't want his ongoing chemotherapy to risk worsening his health to the point that he could not serve her in this way. His primary goal before he died was to ensure that Ava would be safely situated in a care facility after his death. Understanding that he was declining despite his ongoing treatment, he decided to forego further treatment so that he could ensure this final act of love for his wife.

The next time I saw Ava, several months after Juan passed, she was living in her apartment at an assisted living facility. She had accommodated very well to her new surroundings and was thriving. She had made friends who looked out for her, and she very much enjoyed the social setting, where she could connect with others and participate in activities like chair aerobics, bingo, and movie nights.

Ava's insight and lack of psychiatric symptoms make for an ideal situation. I expect she will continue to have a pleasant journey, as she has done well to this point. Our service will help her family transition her to a higher level of care when that time comes and support any needs along the way.

~~~

Like Ava, Anthony has insight into his declining memory and inability to make it through the day without help. However, Anthony experiences significant anxiety, which manifests as agitation in the form of a fixation on his health, which leads to repeated calls to the pharmacy and his provider offices and frequent visits to the ER. A poor historian of his health who cannot recall recent events, Anthony confusedly reports a mixed bag of non-specific symptoms, which have led to extensive workups to rule out various issues. For many months, his hypochondria has led him to report side effects with any new medication, which then get labeled in his chart as allergies, a growing list that is rapidly limiting the medical community's ability to help.

Anthony lives at home with his wife, Sonia, who also has dementia. Both spouses having dementia create a special kind of challenge for caregivers, typically children, who often find themselves navigating this journey with parents with different degrees of insight. This complex dynamic frequently leads to significant conflict, resentment, frustration, and high levels of caregiver strain.

Lacking any insight into her decline, Sonia also fails to recognize the severity of her husband's suffering. Both have lost significant weight as Sonia's ability to plan meals and cook has diminished. Neither are taking their medications reliably, limiting my ability to prescribe antidepressant-type medications to help with Anthony's anxiety. Especially concerning is the fact that Sonia is still driving, adamantly refusing a driving test.

Anthony's anxiety and agitation and the couple's weight loss reflect the fact that they need a higher level of care at home. However, because Sonia steadfastly refuses any form of help, their children, who live out of state, experience significant obstacles in their ability to help.

In situations like this, I encourage children to appreciate the inherent limitations. Barring moving in to oversee a parent's daily life, children can do little aside from continuing to discuss and offer support. That is, until a medical crisis leads to hospitalization, when discharge planning can better investigate the question of a safe return home. This is always a challenging conversation with family members whose hearts are virtually breaking in their frustrated effort to support their loved ones living at home.

For patients like Sonia, who can become very defensive at my mere presence, I often need to avoid in-person visits, which can cause distress and add to the difficult family dynamics. Instead, I offer to meet with spouses and caregivers off-site or by telephone. These, and other forms of *stealth tactics*, a term I learned from Judy Cornish, the developer of the DAWN Method® [88] of support for patients with Alzheimer's disease and other forms of dementia, allow me to continue supporting family members as they help navigate loved ones through this challenging journey.

~~~

As patients with dementia move through their journey and as care needs increase, patients who live alone or whose families are unable to manage them at home will typically require care facility support. The decision to move a loved one from their own home is often fraught, and it can be challenging for families (for financial or other reasons) to match the level of care needed to the acuity of the disease, leading to multiple moves along the way.

Vivian, whose husband died when she was 75, lived independently until she was 80. Her son, Dennis, who lived out of state, didn't initially appreciate the difficulties she was having at home, alone for the first time in her adult life. Realizing that she needed more help when he stayed with her after she experienced a fall and an ER visit, he moved into a house just down the street.

A few weeks before we met, Dennis had moved his mother into a one-bedroom apartment at an independent living facility. This had been a difficult decision as he grappled with the permanence of the move, worried that his mother would suffer from the loss of her personal independence and familiar surroundings. To ease her transition, Dennis decorated her apartment with her personal effects—paintings, photographs, and her collection of dolls.

Without someone to assess where Vivian was in her dementia journey—well into the Personal Care stage at the time of her move—and help anticipate her care needs, Dennis chose to move his mother into an independent living facility, which did not provide the level of care she required. Independent living facilities alleviate the need for adults to manage many of the IADLs, as they often provide transportation, a dining hall, and on-site activities. Patients without dementia can thrive in this setting for many years, as can those with dementia who are early in their journey. But for patients with dementia already in the Personal Care stage, who struggle with ADLs, independent living is typically not an appropriate level of support.

Indeed, Vivian struggled in her new apartment to make it through the day without extra help. She frequently got lost on the way to and from the dining hall, spent much of the day confused about where she was or what she should be doing, and couldn't remember to shower, eat lunch, or change her clothes. Her cognitive decline made it challenging to engage with others in the dining hall, leaving her isolated in her apartment for much of the day. Without understanding why but quickly recognizing the problem, Dennis began piecing together extra support for Vivian across the day.

He arranged for meals to be delivered to her apartment and hired a home health aide for two hours each morning and two hours in the evening to ensure that she took her medications, changed her clothes, had a shower, and ate breakfast and dinner. Dennis spent the lunch hour and afternoon with Vivian, so she was only alone at night. He installed a video camera he could monitor from his phone to keep an eye on her when he wasn't there.

With this level of extra support, Vivian was able to remain in her independent apartment for the better part of a year. However, the need to manage his mother every day eventually took its toll, and Dennis decided to move her to an assisted living facility nearby. There, she would receive round-the-clock nursing support, and when she needed an even higher level of care, she could easily be moved into the facility's memory care wing.

Vivian spent just six weeks in her new assisted living apartment before the staff suggested that she transition to Memory Care, a move that finally matched her care needs with the support she receives. Since moving into Memory Care, Vivian has thrived, making new friends, benefiting from assisted dining support at mealtimes, and living in a space that makes it difficult to get lost.

Other Neurodegenerative Diseases

Patients with neurodegenerative disorders, including Parkinson's disease, progressive supranuclear palsy, amyotrophic lateral sclerosis, multiple sclerosis, myasthenia gravis, muscular dystrophy, and Huntington's disease, can display a varying amount of cognitive decline overlaying a primarily progressive loss of voluntary and involuntary motor function. Families must accommodate declining levels of physical capacity until, eventually, patients become bedbound and dependent on all aspects of personal care. When patients need 24-hour support, family life typically centers around the needs of the patient, which can lead to caregiver and family strain or the need to transition to a care facility, most usually a nursing home, or, like in Vivian's case, a dementia-friendly facility.

In 2023, approximately 1 million Americans were living with a diagnosis of Parkinson's disease, with 60,000 new cases diagnosed each year [89]. More than 35,000 Americans died of Parkinson's disease in 2019 [90]. As with Alzheimer's disease, Parkinson's disease moves through progressive stages characterized by loss of independence and an increasing need for help with IADLs and ADLs. Not every patient with Parkinson's disease will die from this disease. Those who do will exhibit Physical Decline and the metabolic shift evident with Alzheimer's disease, developing issues with swallowing, weight loss, falls, and susceptibility to recurrent infections, including aspiration pneumonia, sepsis, and complications related to poor wound healing, becoming dependent and requiring round-the-clock care.

Patients with amyotrophic lateral sclerosis (ALS) will develop an increasing need for ventilation and feeding support, with many transitioning to a non-invasive ventilator that can support their breathing at home, as well as a feeding tube to support their nutrition. Patients with dysphagia (swallowing dysfunction) who receive feeding tube support are at increased risk of aspiration pneumonia, and respiratory failure is the most common cause of death for patients with ALS [91].[91] With these statistics in mind, discussions ahead of time with patients and families about end-of-life wishes, including the risk of a feeding tube in the setting of dysphagia and the likelihood of needing ventilation support, are critical to aligning patient wishes with end-of-life care. As with patients with heart and lung failure, ALS patients who wish to pass away at home will need to transition to hospice care well before the point in their journey where their inability to wean off invasive ventilation successfully becomes likely.

Palliative care and comprehensive support programs that involve physicians, social workers, chaplains, counselors, and skilled therapists (physical, occupational, and speech and language) are an essential part of helping patients and families navigate the physical, financial, and emotional complexity of these challenging neuro-degenerative journeys.

~~~

The five disease trajectories described in this chapter form the foundation of the technique taught in this book. Discussing wishes for medical care with patients and families requires an accurate and timely assessment of where a patient is in their overall journey with their health. The first step in arriving at such an assessment is the identification of the specific disease trajectory and diagnosis driving a patient's decline. As we will see when learning *The Arc of Conversation* technique, this is the initial step when gathering a patient's history, the goal of asking a patient to *paint a picture of their recent health.*

The ability to appreciate functional and metabolic decline, increasing dependence on others, and to understand healthcare utilization—ER visits, hospital admissions, ICU stays, and trips to rehab—as symptoms of disease progression and decline is necessary for positioning the acute snapshot of a patient's current health condition within the moving picture of their overall journey with their health.

In the next chapter, we will learn the hospice criteria for patients' primary diagnoses at the end of life. Familiarity with hospice criteria, which seems to be largely absent from the medical community's general expertise, is essential for recognizing when a patient has reached the point in their journey when the medical community can no longer be expected to alter the course of their disease, and when our medical interventions may do more harm than good. Medical providers managing patients with serious, chronic, or progressive illnesses should develop familiarity with the hospice criteria.

Patients and families need and deserve accurate, complete, and timely information to make medical decisions that authentically align with their values and priorities. Recognizing the forest for the trees and the elephant lurking therein is essential to providing *truly* patient-centered care.

References

1. Ballentine JM. The five trajectories—supporting patients during serious illness. 2018. https://csupalliativecare.org/wp-content/uploads/Five-Trajectories-eBook-02.21.2018.pdf. Accessed 12 Jun 2022.
2. Glaser BG, Strauss AL. Awareness of death. Chicago: Aldine Publishing Company; 1965.
3. Field MJ, Cassel CK. Approaching death: improving care at the end of life. Washington, DC: National Academies Press; 1997.
4. Glaser B, Strauss AL. Time for dying, vol. 68. Chicago, IL: Aldine Publishing; 1968. p. 2660.
5. Lynn J. Living long in fragile health: the new demographics shape end of life care. Hastings Cent Rep. 2005:S14–S18. PMID: 16468250. https://doi.org/10.1353/hcr.2005.0096.
6. Lunney JR, Lynn J, Hogan C. Profiles of older medicare decedents. J Am Geriatr Soc. 2002;50(6):1108–12. PMID: 12110073. https://doi.org/10.1046/j.1532-5415.2002.50268.x.
7. Murray SA, Kendall M, Boyd K, Sheikh A. Illness trajectories and palliative care. BMJ. 2005;330(7498):1007–11. PMID: 15860843; PMCID: PMC557248. https://doi.org/10.1136/bmj.330.7498.1007.
8. Lunney JR, Lynn J, Foley DJ, Lipson S, Guralnik JM. Patterns of functional decline at the end of life. JAMA. 2003;289(18):2387–92. https://doi.org/10.1001/jama.289.18.2387.
9. Injuries and Violence Are Leading Causes of Death. In: Injury Prevention & Control. 2022. https://www.cdc.gov/injury/wisqars/animated-leading-causes.html. Accessed 2 Jan 2023.
10. Accidents or Unintentional Injuries. In: National Center for Health Statistics. https://www.cdc.gov/nchs/fastats/accidental-injury.htm. Accessed 2 Jan 2023.
11. Kumar A, Avishay DM, Jones CR, Shaikh JD, Kaur R, Aljadah M, Kichloo A, Shiwalkar N, Keshavamurthy S. Sudden cardiac death: epidemiology, pathogenesis and management. Rev Cardiovasc Med. 2021;22(1):147–58. PMID: 33792256. Accessed 2 Jan 2023. https://doi.org/10.31083/j.rcm.2021.01.207.
12. Trzeciak S, Mazzarelli A. Compassionomics. The revolutionary scientific evidence that caring makes a difference. Pensacola, FL: Studer Group; 2019.
13. National Vital Statistics Reports. 2021 Deaths: Final Data 2019. 2021. https://www.cdc.gov/nchs/data/nvsr/nvsr70/nvsr70-08-508.pdf. Accessed 12 Jun 2022.

14. McDermott KW, Roemer M. Most frequent principal diagnoses for inpatient stays in U.S. Hospitals, 2018. 2021. https://www.hcup-us.ahrq.gov/reports/statbriefs/sb277-Top-Reasons-Hospital-Stays-2018.pdf. Accessed 12 Jun 2022.
15. Heart Disease. 2022. https://www.cdc.gov/nchs/fastats/heart-disease.htm. Accessed 15 Jun 2022.
16. Murphy SL, Kochanek KD, Xu J, Arias E. Mortality in the United States, 2020. 2021. https://www.cdc.gov/nchs/products/databriefs/db427.htm. Accessed 12 Jun 2022.
17. Chronic Obstructive Pulmonary Disease (COPD) includes: chronic bronchitis and emphysema. 2022. https://www.cdc.gov/nchs/fastats/copd.htm. Accessed 15 Jun 2022.
18. Chronic Obstructive Pulmonary Disease (COPD). 2022. https://www.who.int/news-room/fact-sheets/detail/chronic-obstructive-pulmonary-disease-(copd). Accessed 15 Jun 2022.
19. Watnick S, Dirkx T. Chronic kidney disease. In: McPhee SJ, Papadakis MA, Rabow MW, editors. 2012 Current medical diagnosis & treatment. New York: McGraw-Hill Medical; 2012. p. 884–92.
20. Kidney Disease. 2022. https://www.cdc.gov/nchs/fastats/kidney-disease.htm. Accessed 15 Jun 2022.
21. Sharma A, Nagalli S. Chronic liver disease. 2022. https://www.ncbi.nlm.nih.gov/books/NBK554597/. Accessed 12 Jun 2022.
22. Chronic Liver Disease and Cirrhosis. 2022. https://www.cdc.gov/nchs/fastats/liver-disease.htm. Accessaed 15 Jun 2022.
23. Alcohol Facts and Statistics. 2022. https://www.niaaa.nih.gov/publications/brochures-and-fact-sheets/alcohol-facts-and-statistics. Accessed 12 Jun 2022.
24. Wei Y, Wang YG, Jia Y, Li L, Yoon J, Zhang S, Wang Z, Zhang Y, Zhu M, Sharma T, Lin YH, Hsieh MH, Albrecht JH, Le PT, Rosen CJ, Wang T, Zhu H. Liver homeostasis is maintained by midlobular zone 2 hepatocytes. Science. 2021;371(6532):eabb1625. Erratum in: Science. 2021 Sep 3;373(6559):eabl8195. PMID: 33632817; PMCID: PMC8496420. https://doi.org/10.1126/science.abb1625.
25. Mailliard ME, Sorrell MF. Alcoholic liver disease. In: Longo DL, Kasper DL, Jameson JL, Fauci AS, Hauser SL, Loscalzo J, editors. Harrison's principles of internal medicine. New York: McGraw-Hill, Health Professions Division; 1998. p. 2589–91.
26. Mitra S, De A, Chowdhury A. Epidemiology of non-alcoholic and alcoholic fatty liver diseases. Transl Gastroenterol Hepatol. 2020;5:16. Published 2020 Apr 5. https://doi.org/10.21037/tgh.2019.09.08.
27. Patel R, Mueller M. Alcoholic liver disease. 2022. https://www.ncbi.nlm.nih.gov/books/NBK546632/. Accessed 12 Jun 2022.
28. Bacon BR. Cirrhosis and its complications. In: Longo DL, Kasper DL, Jameson JL, Fauci AS, Hauser SL, Loscalzo J, editors. Harrison's principles of internal medicine. New York: McGraw-Hill, Health Professions Division; 1998. p. 2592–602.
29. Sanyal AJ. Prediction of variceal hemorrhage in patients with cirrhosis. 2021. https://www.uptodate.com/contents/prediction-of-variceal-hemorrhage-in-patients-with-cirrhosis. Accessed 12 Jun 2022.
30. Fontana RJ. Acute liver failure including acetaminophen overdose. Med Clin North Am. 2008;92(4):761. https://doi.org/10.1016/j.mcna.2008.03.005.
31. Agrawal S, Khazaeni B. Acetaminophen toxicity. 2022. https://www.ncbi.nlm.nih.gov/books/NBK441917/. Accessed 12 Jun 2022.
32. Cancer. 2022. https://www.cdc.gov/nchs/fastats/cancer.htm. Accessed 15 Jun 2022.
33. Ferrell BR, Temel JS, Temin S, Alesi ER, Balboni TA, Basch EM, Firn JI, Paice JA, Peppercorn JM, Phillips T, Stovall EL, Zimmermann C, Smith TJ. Integration of palliative care into standard oncology care: American Society of Clinical Oncology clinical practice guideline update. J Clin Oncol. 2017;35(1):96–112. Epub 2016 Oct 28. PMID: 28034065. https://doi.org/10.1200/JCO.2016.70.1474.
34. Heimburger DC. Malnutrition and nutritional assessment. In: Longo DL, Kasper DL, Jameson JL, Fauci AS, Hauser SL, Loscalzo J, editors. Harrison's principles of internal medicine. New York: McGraw-Hill, Health Professions Division; 1998. p. 605–12.

35. Gannavarapu BS, Lau SKM, Carter K, Cannon NA, Gao A, Ahn C, Meyer JJ, Sher DJ, Jatoi A, Infante R, Iyengar P. Prevalence and survival impact of pretreatment cancer-associated weight loss: a tool for guiding early palliative care. J Oncol Pract. 2018;14(4):e238–50. Epub 2018 Feb 21. PMID: 29466074; PMCID: PMC5951294. https://doi.org/10.1200/JOP.2017.025221.

36. Madeddu C, Gramignano G, Astara G, Demontis R, Sanna E, Atzeni V, Macciò A. Pathogenesis and treatment options of cancer related anemia: perspective for a targeted mechanism-based approach. Front Physiol. 2018;9:1294. PMID: 30294279; PMCID: PMC6159745. https://doi.org/10.3389/fphys.2018.01294.

37. Bailey CH, Jameson G, Sima C, Fleck S, White E, Von Hoff DD, Weiss GJ. Progression-free survival decreases with each subsequent therapy in patients presenting for phase I clinical trials. J Cancer. 2012;3:7–13. Epub 2011 Nov 28. PMID: 22211140; PMCID: PMC3245603. https://doi.org/10.7150/jca.3.7.

38. Stone JB, DeAngelis LM. Cancer-treatment-induced neurotoxicity—focus on newer treatments. Nat Rev Clin Oncol. 2016;13(2):92–105. Epub 2015 Sep 22. PMID: 26391778; PMCID: PMC4979320. https://doi.org/10.1038/nrclinonc.2015.152.

39. Finn L, Markovic SN, Joseph RW. Therapy for metastatic melanoma: the past, present, and future. BMC Med. 2012;10:23. https://doi.org/10.1186/1741-7015-10-23.

40. Baron RB. Protein-energy malnutrition. In: McPhee SJ, Papadakis MA, Rabow MW, editors. 2012 Current medical diagnosis & treatment. New York: McGraw-Hill Medical; 2012. p. 1225–6.

41. Bruera E. In: Smith T, Givens J, Savarese D, editors. Assessment and management of anorexia and cachexia in palliative care. Waltham, MA: UpToDate; 2022. https://www.uptodate.com/contents/assessment-and-management-of-anorexia-and-cachexia-in-palliative-care. Accessed 10 May 2022.

42. Yoshida T, Delafontaine P. Mechanisms of cachexia in chronic disease states. Am J Med Sci. 2015;350(4):250–6. https://doi.org/10.1097/MAJ.0000000000000511.

43. von Haehling S, Anker SD. Cachexia as a major underestimated and unmet medical need: facts and numbers. J Cachexia Sarcopenia Muscle. 2010;1(1):1–5. Epub 2010 Oct 26. PMID: 21475699; PMCID: PMC3060651. https://doi.org/10.1007/s13539-010-0002-6.

44. Gom I, Fukushima H, Shiraki M, Miwa Y, Ando T, Takai K, Moriwaki H. Relationship between serum albumin level and aging in community-dwelling self-supported elderly population. J Nutr Sci Vitaminol (Tokyo). 2007;53(1):37–42. PMID: 17484377. https://doi.org/10.3177/jnsv.53.37.

45. Ritchie C, Yukawa M. In: Schmader K, Seres D, editors. Geriatric nutrition: nutritional issues in older adults. Waltham, MA: UpToDate; 2022. https://www.uptodate.com/contents/geriatric-nutrition-nutritional-issues-in-older-adults. Accessed 10 May 2022.

46. Wong CJ. Involuntary weight loss. Med Clin North Am. 2014;98(3):625–43. Epub 2014 Mar 21. PMID: 24758965. https://doi.org/10.1016/j.mcna.2014.01.012.

47. Gaddey HL, Holder KK. Unintentional weight loss in older adults. Am Fam Physician. 2021;104(1):34–40. PMID: 34264616.

48. Evans WJ, Morley JE, Argilés J, Bales C, Baracos V, Guttridge D, Jatoi A, Kalantar-Zadeh K, Lochs H, Mantovani G, Marks D, Mitch WE, Muscaritoli M, Najand A, Ponikowski P, Rossi Fanelli F, Schambelan M, Schols A, Schuster M, Thomas D, Wolfe R, Anker SD. Cachexia: a new definition. Clin Nutr. 2008;27(6):793–9. Epub 2008 Aug 21. PMID: 18718696. https://doi.org/10.1016/j.clnu.2008.06.013.

49. Medical guidelines for determining appropriateness of hospice referral: disease-specific guidelines. https://www.uptodate.com/contents/image?imageKey=ONC%2F61282. Accessed 12 May 2022.

50. Medical guidelines for determining appropriateness of hospice referral: non-disease-specific baseline guidelines plus comorbidities. https://www.uptodate.com/contents/image?imageKey=PALC%2F87321. Accessed 12 May 2022.

51. Alzheimer's Association. Alzheimer's disease facts and figures. Alzheimers Dement. 2022;2022:18. https://www.alz.org/media/documents/alzheimers-facts-and-figures.pdf. Accessed 15 May 2022.

52. Schulz R, Beach SR. Caregiving as a risk factor for mortality: the caregiver health effects study. JAMA. 1999;282(23):2215–9. PMID: 10605972. https://doi.org/10.1001/jama.282.23.2215.
53. National Alliance for Caregiving & Evercare. Evercare® Study of Caregivers in decline: a close-up look at the health risks of caring for a loved one. Bethesda, MD and Minnetonka, MN: National Alliance for Caregiving and Evercare; 2006. https://www.caregiving.org/wp-content/uploads/2020/05/Caregivers-in-Decline-Study-FINAL-lowres.pdf. Accessed 12 Jun 2022.
54. Shaw WS, Patterson TL, Semple SJ, Ho S, Irwin MR, Hauger RL, Grant I. Longitudinal analysis of multiple indicators of health decline among spousal caregivers. Ann Behav Med. 1997;19(2):101–9. PMID: 9603684. https://doi.org/10.1007/BF02883326.
55. AAOS Updates clinical practice guideline for Management of hip Fractures in older adults. 2021. https://www.aaos.org/aaos-home/newsroom/press-releases/aaos-updates-clinical-practice-guideline-for-management-of-hip-fractures-in-older-adults/. Accessed 12 Jun 2022.
56. Kazaure H, Roman S, Sosa JA. High mortality in surgical patients with do-not-resuscitate orders: analysis of 8256 patients. Arch Surg. 2011;146(8):922–8. https://doi.org/10.1001/archsurg.2011.69.
57. Schnell S, Friedman SM, Mendelson DA, Bingham KW, Kates SL. The 1-year mortality of patients treated in a hip fracture program for elders. Geriatr Orthop Surg Rehabil. 2010;1(1):6–14. https://doi.org/10.1177/2151458510378105.
58. Morri M, Ambrosi E, Chiari P, Orlandi Magli A, Gazineo D, D'Alessandro F, Forni C. One-year mortality after hip fracture surgery and prognostic factors: a prospective cohort study. Sci Rep. 2019;9(1):18718. PMID: 31822743; PMCID: PMC6904473. https://doi.org/10.1038/s41598-019-55196-6.
59. Downey C, Kelly M, Quinlan JF. Changing trends in the mortality rate at 1-year post hip fracture—a systematic review. World J Orthop. 2019;10(3):166–75. PMID: 30918799; PMCID: PMC6428998. https://doi.org/10.5312/wjo.v10.i3.166.
60. Dimet-Wiley A, Golovko G, Watowich SJ. One-year Postfracture mortality rate in older adults with hip fractures relative to other lower extremity fractures: retrospective cohort study. JMIR Aging. 2022;5(1):e32683. PMID: 35293865; PMCID: PMC8968577. https://doi.org/10.2196/32683.
61. Scarano KA, Philp FH, Westrick ER, Altman GT, Altman DT. Evaluating postoperative complications and outcomes of orthopedic fracture repair in nonagenarian patients. Geriatr Orthop Surg Rehabil. 2018;9:2151459318758106. PMID: 29619274; PMCID: PMC5871047. https://doi.org/10.1177/2151459318758106.
62. Vaillant-Molina M, Bahrick LE, Flom R. Young infants match facial and vocal emotional expressions of other infants. Infancy. 2013;18. https://doi.org/10.1111/infa.12017.
63. Winfrey O, Perry BD. What happened to you? Conversations on trauma, resilience, and healing. New York: Flatiron Books; 2021.
64. Reisberg B, Franssen EH, Souren LE, Auer SR, Akram I, Kenowsky S. Evidence and mechanisms of retrogenesis in Alzheimer's and other dementias: management and treatment import. Am J Alzheimers Dis Other Dement. 2002;17(4):202–12. PMID: 12184509. https://doi.org/10.1177/153331750201700411.
65. Lum JA, Conti-Ramsden G, Page D, Ullman MT. Working, declarative and procedural memory in specific language impairment. Cortex. 2012;48(9):1138–54. https://doi.org/10.1016/j.cortex.2011.06.001.
66. Camina E, Güell F. The neuroanatomical, neurophysiological and psychological basis of memory: current models and their origins. Front Pharmacol. 2017;8:438. https://doi.org/10.3389/fphar.2017.00438.
67. Blumenfeld H. Neuroanatomy overview and basic definitions. In: Neuroanatomy through clinical cases. 2nd ed. Sunderland, MA: Sinauer Associates; 2010. p. 13–46.
68. Rogers SL, Friedman RB. The underlying mechanisms of semantic memory loss in Alzheimer's disease and semantic dementia. Neuropsychologia. 2008;46(1):12–21. https://doi.org/10.1016/j.neuropsychologia.2007.08.010.

69. Petersson KM, Hagoort P. The neurobiology of syntax: beyond string sets. Philos Trans R Soc Lond Ser B Biol Sci. 2012;367(1598):1971–83. https://doi.org/10.1098/rstb.2012.0101.

70. Braun CM, Dumont M, Duval J, Hamel-Hébert I, Godbout L. Brain modules of hallucination: an analysis of multiple patients with brain lesions. J Psychiatry Neurosci. 2003;28(6):432–49. PMID: 14631455; PMCID: PMC257791.

71. Johnston B, Harper M, Landefeld CS. Geriatric disorders. In: McPhee SJ, Papadakis MA, Rabow MW, editors. 2012 Current medical diagnosis & treatment. New York: McGraw-Hill Medical; 2012. p. 58–73.

72. Blumenfeld H. Somatosensory pathways. In: Neuroanatomy through clinical cases. 2nd ed. Sunderland, MA: Sinauer Associates; 2010. p. 276–316.

73. Goodman C, Rycroft Malone J, Norton C, Harari D, Harwood R, Roe B, Russell B, Fader M, Buswell M, Drennan VM, Bunn F. Reducing and managing faecal incontinence in people with advanced dementia who are resident in care homes: protocol for a realist synthesis. BMJ Open. 2015;5(7):e007728. PMID: 26163032; PMCID: PMC4499729. https://doi.org/10.1136/bmjopen-2015-007728.

74. Na HR, Cho ST. Relationship between lower urinary tract dysfunction and dementia. Dement Neurocogn Disord. 2020;19(3):77–85. PMID: 32985147; PMCID: PMC7521953. https://doi.org/10.12779/dnd.2020.19.3.77.

75. Kalia M. Dysphagia and aspiration pneumonia in patients with Alzheimer's disease. Metabolism. 2003;52(10 Suppl 2):36–8. PMID: 14577062. https://doi.org/10.1016/s0026-0495(03)00300-7.

76. Blumenfeld H. Brainstem I: surface anatomy and cranial nerves. In: Neuroanatomy through clinical cases. 2nd. ed. Sunderland, MA: Sinauer Associates; 2010. p. 494–563.

77. Alzheimer's Disease. 2022. https://www.cdc.gov/nchs/fastats/alzheimers.htm. Accessed 15 Jun 2022.

78. Melkas S, Jokinen H, Hietanen M, Erkinjuntti T. Poststroke cognitive impairment and dementia: prevalence, diagnosis, and treatment. Degener Neurol Neuromuscul Dis. 2014;5(4):21–7. PMID: 32669898; PMCID: PMC7337160. https://doi.org/10.2147/DNND.S37353.

79. What is Vascular Dementia? 2014. https://www.jpaget.nhs.uk/media/275007/What-is-vascular-dementia.pdf. Accessed 10 Jun 2022.

80. Sakakibara R. Overactive bladder as a brain Disease. J Neurol Disord Stroke. 2013;1(2):1002.

81. Rabinovici GD, Miller BL. Frontotemporal lobar degeneration: epidemiology, pathophysiology, diagnosis and management. CNS Drugs. 2010;24(5):375–98. https://doi.org/10.2165/11533100-000000000-00000.

82. Byers AL, Yaffe K. Depression and risk of developing dementia. Nat Rev Neurol. 2011;7(6):323–31. PMID: 21537355; PMCID: PMC3327554. https://doi.org/10.1038/nrneurol.2011.60.

83. Reisberg B, Franssen E, Souren LEM, Kenowsky S, Janjua KS, Veigne SW, Guillo-Benarous F, Singh S, Khizar A, Shah U, Shah RG, Bhandal A, Auer S. Alzheimer's disease. In: Moroz A, Flanagan SR, Zaretsky H, editors. Medical aspects of disability for the rehabilitation professional. New York: Springer Publishing Company, LLC; 2017. p. 31–90.

84. Maslow AH. A theory of human motivation. Psychol Rev. 1943;50(4):370–96. https://doi.org/10.1037/h0054346.

85. What is cognitive reserve? 2020. https://www.health.harvard.edu/mind-and-mood/what-is-cognitive-reserve. Accessed 11 Jun 2022.

86. Jennings LA, Hollands S, Keeler E, Wenger NS, Reuben DB. The effects of dementia care co-management on acute care, hospice, and long-term care utilization. J Am Geriatr Soc. 2020;68(11):2500–7. Epub 2020 Jun 23. PMID: 32573765. https://doi.org/10.1111/jgs.16667.

87. Jennings LA, Turner M, Keebler C, Burton CH, Romero T, Wenger NS, Reuben DB. The effect of a comprehensive dementia care management program on end-of-life care. J Am Geriatr Soc. 2019;67(3):443–8. Epub 2019 Jan 24. PMID: 30675898; PMCID: PMC9859712. https://doi.org/10.1111/jgs.15769.

88. Cornish J. Dementia with dignity, living well with Alzheimer's or dementia using the DAWN method®. 2019.
89. Statistics. https://www.parkinson.org/Understanding-Parkinsons/Statistics.
90. Rong S, Xu G, Liu B, et al. Trends in mortality from Parkinson disease in the United States, 1999-2019. Neurology. 2021;97:e1986. https://doi.org/10.1212/WNL.0000000000012826.
91. Wolf J, Safer A, Wöhrle JC, Palm F, Nix WA, Maschke M, Grau AJ. Todesursachen bei amyotropher Lateralsklerose : Ergebnisse aus dem ALS-Register Rheinland-Pfalz [Causes of death in amyotrophic lateral sclerosis : results from the Rhineland-Palatinate ALS registry]. Nervenarzt. 2017;88(8):911–8. German. PMID: 28184974. https://doi.org/10.1007/s00115-017-0293-3.

Hospice Criteria: Determining That Time Is Limited

5

When we survey Americans about where they want to be at the end of their lives, 70% say they want to pass away at home [1]. Just 1 in 10 says they would prefer to die in a hospital [1]. When we ask Americans what the priority should be at the end of life, 70% say, "helping people die without pain, discomfort, and stress" [1]. Less than 20% express an end-of-life priority for "preventing death and extending life as long as possible" [1].

In my experience, the actual numbers are closer to 99% in favor of passing away at home and 1% in the hospital. I rarely encounter a patient at the end of life who prefers to continue to seek inpatient medical care when they know that their time is very limited.

I lead with these statistics when training new providers in our service and the doctors in our local family medicine residency program, emphasizing how easy it is to give people what they want at the end of their lives.

When I worked as a wedding photographer, I knew that customer service was the heart and soul of my business. My personal mandate was to say "Yes" as often as possible to increase the joy and quality my clients experienced. I understood that weddings are more than a single moment in time. Rather, they are a collective family experience that extends well before and beyond the wedding day itself.

A wedding is a journey that starts in the hearts and minds of two people in love long before they share vows, a kiss, and a slice of cake. The months of preparation, decision making, and planning are characterized by ebbs and flows, hiccups, hurdles, and occasionally, the momentary forced exhale. Not uncommonly, emotional, physical, and spiritual strain impacts friendships and family dynamics, reflected in seating arrangements and wedding attendant configurations.

The weaving together of two lives shares much in common with the unraveling that occurs at the end of a human existence. Weddings and disease are motion pictures that involve myriad sets, cast members, and often, multiple directors. Just as it was with my wedding photography, my work in palliative care centers the primary participants but also involves family, friends, and other professionals. My entire purpose is to improve the quality and experience of people's lives. Many days, my

© The Author(s), under exclusive license to Springer Nature Switzerland AG 2024
A. Shaw, PA, *The Arc of Conversation*,
https://doi.org/10.1007/978-3-031-70495-6_5

job feels like going to church, for honoring a patient and family's experience and personal wishes is nothing short of a spiritual endeavor. Being able to say "Yes" at the end of someone's life is the ultimate act of customer service.

If you walk into a patient's room, you can be nearly guaranteed that they will want to spend their final days, weeks, or months in the comfort of their own homes or wherever they live, surrounded by their family, friends, and pets. They will want to wrap up their affairs, say their goodbyes, and be allowed to focus on what matters most to people—expressing and experiencing love. Hospice care will enable your patients to achieve this.

Honoring patient choice by talking about and helping transition patients to hospice care, the ultimate alignment of patient personal values and wishes, is one of the easiest ways to serve patients and families with our medical care. It is one of the most beautiful and rewarding efforts in our work to support patient autonomy and provide high-quality, patient-centered care.

One thing is certain: *If patients are not asked about end-of-life preferences ahead of time, providers cannot align their wishes with their care when that time comes.*

The Surprise Question and Trends in End-of-Life Care

To be able to talk about and transition patients to hospice care, we must first recognize that a patient is experiencing a terminal trajectory, the focus of the previous chapter. Next, we must evaluate the patient's disease status with respect to hospice criteria to determine whether their time is limited.

Knowledge of hospice criteria has traditionally fallen under the purview of hospice care teams. Hospice eligibility guidelines are not widely understood, taught, learned, or utilized by the medical community, even those working with patients with predictably terminal diagnoses. Despite working in cardiology for three years, I never once heard the phrase *hospice criteria*, nor did I observe any of the cardiologists I worked with using or discussing the hospice criteria for heart disease to evaluate where a patient was in their overall health journey or to inform the physicians' decisions about the treatment options they offered and discussed with patients.

Recently, a cardiology colleague asked me what the hospice criteria are for heart failure. As mentioned previously, heart failure was the leading cause of death for Americans in 2020 and, in 2018, the second leading cause of hospital admissions [2–4]. That a cardiologist can make it through four years of medical school, three years of internal medicine residency training, and an additional three years of a cardiology residency without encountering or learning the hospice criteria for heart failure signifies a breathtaking misalignment of focus between our medical training and the reality and impact of disease, particularly with respect to what matters most to people in the end.

Cardiologists are not alone in their ignorance of hospice criteria. I have yet to meet a single medical provider outside of hospice care who has learned and regularly uses hospice criteria to better understand the health status of their patients.

From a training standpoint, the problem is a matter of focus. Throughout my two years of didactic and clinical training in PA school, the entire focus remained on diagnosis and treatment—recognizing the presence of disease where it did not formerly exist and learning to "fix" the underlying pathology and its attendant symptoms. The end of life was entirely ignored, and I left PA school in 2014 without a robust understanding of disease as a progressive and often terminal process of decline, with no training in palliative or hospice medicine. In speaking with my physician colleagues, they report a similar experience in medical school and residency training.

Likewise, medical textbooks focus almost entirely on diagnosis and treatment, ignoring the end of life. Harrison's *Principles of Internal Medicine*, a two-volume, 3600-page opus, dedicates just 18 pages to palliative and hospice care [5], most of which focus on symptom management. Just one sentence devoted to the determination of hospice eligibility, "Two physicians must certify that the patient has a prognosis of ≤ 6 months if the disease runs its natural course," gives the impression that recognition of the end of life is so formidable as to require not just one, but two medical degrees. Yet, nowhere is the reader taught how to determine when a disease has reached the end of its course, with *hospice criteria* absent from the chapters relating to the major diagnoses of terminal decline and the index.

Rather than being taught hospice criteria, which is an objective set of medical and functional standards, providers are taught, if we are taught at all, to use an ambiguous and equivocal approach called the "surprise question", in which the provider asks themselves some variation of the question:

> *Is this person sick enough that it would be no surprise for the person to die within the next six months, or a year?* [6].

Joanne Lynn, a palliative care thought leader, introduced this question in 2005 in a powerful article commenting on and challenging the medical system's approach to end-of-life care. She pointed out the underlying goal of this question is to determine whether a patient has reached a point in their disease where any change in health status could mean the end [6]. Lynn was not recommending that the "surprise question" be used to determine this point, but rather, was acknowledging that palliative care teams were already using this question to do so.

The "surprise question" has become an element of informal training and can also be found in medical textbooks [7], guidelines [8, 9], and approaches to care for the frail and elderly in the hospital [10, 11], even though physicians remain notoriously poor prognosticators [12, 13], and that the question has been found to be confusing and difficult to use [10]. Not surprisingly, recent systematic reviews of studies utilizing the "surprise question" to predict the prognosis of patients at the end of life found wide variation in its accuracy and consistency, ranging from poor to (just) adequate [14, 15].

Appealing in its simplicity, providers typically use this question as the threshold for when to involve palliative care. Because physicians tend to significantly overestimate prognosis [12], more so the longer they've known the patient, utilizing the "surprise question" carries the risk of waiting too long to involve care teams trained to align patient wishes with care and to improve quality of life, delaying even beyond the point for many patients where they are still able to experience what matters most.

Additionally, many providers erroneously believe that hospice care is appropriate and available for just the final days or weeks of life, when in truth, hospice care is available to patients and families for *at least six months*, but possibly longer, should the patient continue to qualify, and without a limit of total time for enrollment. The underlying assumptions are that hospice care is only appropriate when no other treatment options are available, or for patients who are in the throes of death—*actively dying*—and have only a few days or hours left. Basing the timing of a referral to palliative or hospice care on the "surprise question" almost guarantees the misalignment of patient wishes and their end-of-life care.

It is unfathomable that instead of mastering the hospice criteria for the major terminal trajectories, our medical system, which is virtually obsessed with evidence-based medical care and objective algorithms, has chosen instead to rely on such an absurdly subjective and inexact approach to identifying such a critically important moment of patients' lives.

I want to take a moment here to pause for a thought experiment. Imagine, if you will, how you would feel if, instead of relying on a stereotactic biopsy, a highly sophisticated, precise, and objective test to determine whether you have breast cancer, decisions about your diagnosis and treatment were based entirely on the radiologist's hunch?

I know what you're thinking. That would be ridiculous, unimaginable, and absurd.

I have experienced palliative care referrals so late that one of my patients died while I was in their home performing my initial consultation. It is not uncommon for patients to pass within hours of being enrolled in hospice care, either at home or shortly after arriving at our hospice center. I have seen oncology patients die on the same or the following day as the recommendation for chemotherapy treatment. Our palliative care service has received more referrals than we can count for patients who have passed before they could be seen.

Healthcare utilization trends at the end of life in the United States bear out these observations, painting a picture of a system that predominantly focuses on extending life instead of providing comfort at the end.

Consistently, over the past several decades, one-quarter of all Medicare spending has been for care to beneficiaries during the last year of their lives, despite just 5% of Medicare decedents dying each year [16–18]. Much of this care is hospital-based, focusing on cure rather than comfort. Although a study of Medicare spending during the last year of beneficiary life from 1978 to 2006 showed a downward trend in spending on hospital care from a whopping 76.3% in 1978 to a still significant 50.2% in 2006, hospice care, which got its start in 1983 as a Medicare benefit, accounted for just 0.6% of Medicare spending in 1988, with an increase to just 9.7% by 2006 [19].

During that same time, various studies have shown an upward trend in the use of aggressive care toward the end of life, including ICU care and multiple hospitalizations [19–21]. A 2009 study showed that nearly one-third of Medicare patients experienced an ICU stay in the last few months of life [20]. A study looking at end-of-life care for patients with heart failure between 2000 and 2007 showed that 80% of patients experienced a hospitalization in the last six months of life, that ICU length of stay increased from 3.5 to 4.6 days, and that while fewer patients died in the hospital over time (40.2% in 2000, 35.2% in 2007), more patients died in the ICU (42.4% in 2000, 50.2% in 2007) [19].

In the last two decades, Medicare Advantage (MA) and Accountable Care Organizations (ACOs) have been introduced to impact healthcare outcomes while reducing Medicare spending. At the time of this writing, investigations of the impact of MA and ACOs on end-of-life care and spending were limited. However, a 2019 study found that ACOs had no meaningful effect on end-of-life spending [22]. A 2022 study investigating ICU utilization from 2007 to 2017 for Medicare beneficiaries showed that although non-ICU hospitalizations declined by 20.3% over that period, ICU admissions increased by 29.2% [23].

Notably, a systematic review published in 2016 looking at care to hospitalized patients during the last six months of life showed that 33% to 38% of patients experienced aggressive and costly interventions, which the authors labeled *nonbeneficial treatment* [21]. This care was defined as "aggressive management such as invasive procedures, operations, complex medications and costly actions commencing or occurring in the last six months to the last days of life, a period that qualified 'terminal illness,'" and included

> chemotherapy in the last two weeks, parenteral hydration, artificial nutrition, dialysis, intensive care admission in the last few days of life, mechanical ventilation (MV) in the last days, cardiopulmonary resuscitation (CPR) in terminal patients, intravenous (IV) antibiotics in terminal care, transfusion and any invasive non-palliative treatments which were either administered against patient wishes, delivered due to clinician's uncertainty of prognosis, personal beliefs, sense of duty to cure or moral obligation, or considered unwarranted by treating staff but were administered due to family demands or health system accountability pressures [21].

Much can and should be said about care that goes against patients' wishes or is delivered for any of the unfortunate reasons listed above. Suffice it to say that care that does not align with patient or family wishes or is offered simply because providers do not know how to evaluate prognosis does not support the medical ethic of respect for patient autonomy and presents an important opportunity for improving end-of-life care.

A 2018 study by leading economists looking at end-of-life Medicare spending suggests that it can be challenging to predict which hospitalized patients are likely to die and because low-intensity end-of-life hospitalizations do not always lead to death, targeting spending at the end of life is problematic [24]. Rather than utilizing hospice criteria, researchers used predictive machine learning algorithms to attempt to predict which patients were likely to pass. Commenting on the low accuracy of their computer-generated predictions, the authors wrongly suggest that better predictions are unlikely to be had either from physicians or the electronic medical record.[1]

In the current system, where providers use the "surprise question" to determine whether a patient is likely to die, subjective physician prediction is unreliable and unlikely to be accurate. However, it is possible to determine whether a patient meets hospice criteria from a chart review. Palliative care teams do this every day. This requires training in using the objective hospice criteria and knowing where to look in the patient's chart. I would disagree that because low-intensity, end-of-life hospitalizations do not always lead to death, targeting end-of-life spending is problematic. Instead, this is precisely where the opportunity best lies to improve end-of-life quality and comfort for patients and families.

End-of-life spending is simply a stand-in for the medical community's approach to end-of-life care, reflecting our philosophy, training, and orientation toward helping patients and families at this stage of disease. Given our discussion in the last chapter of the predictable approaches to the end of life, and the expected need for increasingly invasive care in the setting of metabolic, organ system, and functional decline, it is easy to understand why nonbeneficial treatment, including care delivered during low-intensity, end-of-life hospitalizations, occurs.

Sepsis at the end of life is an excellent case in point. In the United States, sepsis is the leading cause of hospital deaths [27], making it the focus of significant prevention efforts. Taking into account patient health status, including functional decline, comorbidities, and severity of acute illness at presentation, a 2019 study looking at terminal admissions found that most cases of sepsis (88%) were not preventable [27]. Moreover, using hospice criteria, researchers found that 40% of patients who died with sepsis met hospice criteria at the time of admission due to advanced cancer, organ failure (heart or lung), dementia, or stroke. Sepsis is very much a natural part of disease progression and, as we shall see, a component of hospice criteria for various terminal trajectories.

If patients reaching the end of life are not offered an alternative approach to care that enables them to remain comfortably at home, then hospitalizations for events like sepsis will continue to be an expected part of their journeys. Training providers to recognize the signs of disease progression and decline, to acknowledge when a patient meets hospice criteria, and to be comfortable with having earlier and more

---

[1] Machine learning and artificial intelligence (AI) have evolved rapidly since 2018, irrevocably changing the human landscape since I began writing this book in late 2021. The arrival of ChatGPT in November of 2022 signaled the beginning of a new era, placing AI-powered tools in the hands of every Internet-connected human on Earth. AI-powered tools are already being deployed across the healthcare system to assist providers' clinical decision making, such as in skilled nursing facilities (SNFs), to improve chronic disease management and reduce hospital admissions [25]. In 2023, a study was published in the journal *Nature*, which assessed the efficacy of NYUTron, a large language model (LLM) driven by AI, in predicting in-hospital mortality and 30-day readmissions, among other things [26]. The results showed that NYUTron had an area under the curve (AUC) of $94.9\% \pm 0.168\%$ on in-hospital mortality prediction. The potential for AI-powered tools to enhance clinician capabilities and improve patient outcomes is game-changing.

frequent collaborative goals of care conversations with patients, and, most importantly, to confidently offer hospice care as a viable option for treatment, is precisely
how we can improve quality of life at the end of life, and reduce end-of-life
spending.

Awareness and utilization of hospice care have improved over the decades since
hospice care became a guaranteed Medicare benefit in 1983. In 2019, nearly 50% of
Medicare decedents experienced hospice care at the end of their lives, ranging from
just under 30% of those younger than 64 to just over 60% of those age 85 or older
[28]. However, half of those patients experienced just 18 or fewer days of hospice
care, a number (the median) that has barely budged over the last 15 years [28, 29].
One in four patients experienced just five or fewer days of hospice care, and despite
being available for *at least six months* at the end of their lives, in 2019, the vast
majority (75%) of Medicare decedents experienced less than just three months of
hospice care [28]. Referrals to palliative and hospice care, many relying on physician hunch instead of objective criteria, are still being made far too late into patients'
journeys.

Patients and families deserve better. They deserve the respect and consideration
that we would want for one of our own loved ones, including an accurate and timely
assessment of their medical trajectory and decline, so that their decisions can align
with their internal compasses, enabling their journeys to end in a manner that provides dignity, comfort, and peace. Competence with objective disease evaluation is
as important at the end of a journey as at the start. The medical education and
healthcare system has a responsibility to correct this gross neglect of one of the
most important aspects of our training.

Hospice Mindedness and Hospice Criteria

Hospice criteria, as currently defined, reflect natural disease progression and establish the point in a patient's journey where it is reasonable to expect that curative
medical care can no longer alter the course of a patient's disease or significantly
prolong a patient's life. To enroll in hospice care, patients must be *hospice minded*
and meet *hospice criteria.*

Being ***hospice minded*** means that patients and families have arrived at the stage
of life where they are ready to allow nature to take its course. This is the language I
use when asking people about their preparedness for hospice, asking them directly,
"Are you ready to allow nature to take its course when the time comes?" Asking the
question in this manner allows patients to think about their experience of disease
and determine whether they are ready to pass without further medical interventions
intended to prolong their lives.

Almost everyone, including those with the most tenacious grip on living, eventually gets to the point where the quality of life matters more than its quantity. The
experience of being hospitalized time and time again is distressing to patients and

families. For many patients, time spent in the hospital and away from their homes in rehabilitation facilities will eventually surpass the amount of time they experience feeling well at home. When this happens, the internal quality-of-life scale tips, and patients decide to stop seeking care in the hospital. This is especially true when we explain that future hospitalizations—an expected part of their journey—can be avoided with the intervention that we call hospice care.

For this reason, it is so vital for the medical community to learn to recognize that a patient is declining. Collaborative conversations across a disease trajectory should explain the disease course, put hospital and rehab admissions and functional and physical decline into context, and paint a picture of the expected journey ahead so that patients and families can become hospice minded naturally and at a time that is right for them.

Aside from recognizing disease progression and decline, the other critical component to supporting patient and family hospice mindedness is accurately representing hospice care as an appropriate treatment option in a manner that communicates its purpose and practical application. Knowledge of hospice care is something every medical professional should possess, for two very important reasons.

First and foremost, medical professionals must understand the treatment options available to patients. Death is not a surprise at the end of a human life but rather the expected outcome for every one of us. Hospice care is the appropriate treatment for the final leg of everyone's journey, providing the soft landing everyone seeks and allowing patients to pass peacefully and with dignity.

Second, hospice care is the treatment option that allows the medical community to give patients and families what they want during the final leg of their journey. Hospice care, especially when it is offered and engaged early enough during end-stage decline, enables patients to avoid the distressing and nonbeneficial hospitalizations that are an expected part of each terminal trajectory, instead allowing patients to experience what matters most at the end of life—experiencing and expressing love.

Hospice mindedness is the most crucial component of hospice eligibility, for until patients and families are ready to allow nature to take its course, they cannot enroll in hospice care. To empower and support the emotional and spiritual labor of deciding to engage hospice care, patients and families need accurate and timely communication about their disease and what is ahead, as well as accurate information about hospice care.

Because the end of life happens to every patient, all medical professionals, regardless of their level of training, should be able to explain and discuss hospice care and address the typical hospice-related fears and concerns that patients and families share. To this end, a primer on hospice care, with template language that can be used to explain this treatment option, is included in Chap. 17.

In addition to being hospice minded, patients must meet *hospice criteria*, either for the single disease predominantly driving their decline or via a compelling picture that accounts for multiple interrelated disorders impacting the patient's long-term physical and functional prognosis and which the medical community is no longer able to manage well.

Patients may have multiple diagnoses, but every disorder will likely not play a critical role in their end-of-life decline. When assessing a patient's overall disease progression, clinicians must identify the diagnosis (or multiple diagnoses) primarily responsible for the patient's decline while recognizing how their other complicating diagnoses impact the patient's overall health. The diagnoses covered in the previous chapter are the most common primary disease trajectories patients follow as they approach the end of life.

Limitations of Hospice Criteria

Hospice criteria are intended to help identify the point in a terminal trajectory where the patient's prognosis is expected to be six months or less. Although the purpose of this timeframe is to ensure that patients are not offered end-of-life care prematurely during a time when medical interventions might yet extend patients' lives, the hospice criteria, as currently defined, have several limitations.

It can be the case that patients become hospice minded well before meeting hospice criteria. This is especially true for patients with dementia, whose families recognize that admission to the hospital and rehab are distressing and, at some point, of diminishing benefit. Hospice mindedness in the setting of a terminal diagnosis in which the patient or family is willing to forego hospital admissions and other forms of life-prolonging or curative care should satisfy eligibility for hospice care, regardless of prognosis.

Hospice care improves the quality of life and comfort for patients and families alike [30–34] and allows patients to avoid distressing, costly, and non-beneficial hospital and rehab care at the end of life [35]. When patients and families are ready to focus on quality of life over quantity, our medical system should support that choice. A 2023 study of the Medicare Care Choices Model (MCCM), which provided concurrent hospice care to patients receiving curative treatment for terminal disease, showed a 13% reduction in Medicare expenditures, a 26% reduction in hospital admissions, a 12% reduction in ER visits, and an 18% increase in hospice utilization [36]. At this time, concurrent hospice care is unavailable to patients in the United States.

Families of loved ones who voice the preference of avoiding hospitalizations or further curative treatment long before patients meet hospice criteria can be supported by palliative care teams that can work closely with families to manage symptoms, and through continual assessment of patient decline, to transition patients to hospice care the minute they meet hospice criteria. Although not always successful, this approach can help patients avoid distressing and unwanted end-of-life hospitalizations.

As we shall see, for many of the terminal trajectories, hospital admissions and escalations of care are supporting and, in some cases, a required component of hospice eligibility. This reflects a poor appreciation for disease progression and decline and risks missing the six-month prognosis point. Several studies investigating dementia have shown that the hospice criteria for dementia fail to serve as a reliable marker for the six-month point [37–39].

By now, we understand that hospital admissions and escalations of care are an expected part of end-stage disease and will occur if patients are not offered the high level of care that hospice affords. Rather than requiring patients to advance so far into the terminal phase of disease that they experience frequent end-stage hospitalizations, the hospice criteria should be refined to enable patients and families who wish to avoid end-of-life hospitalizations and escalations of care, especially in the last six months of life, to do so.

Relatedly, the different disease trajectories follow different patterns of terminal decline, some with terminal phases that are potentially far longer than six months. This is the case for many patients with COPD and heart failure, as well as for those with dementia and many other neurodegenerative diseases. Our service supported a patient with progressive supranuclear palsy (PSP), a rare neurodegenerative disease, for nearly four years at the end of his life. His disease had wreaked such havoc on his physical body that he was essentially *locked in*, able only to blink his eyes and grunt to express his needs. Although an extreme example, lengthy terminal phases are not at all uncommon.

Recall Evelyn, from the previous chapter, who met hospice criteria with COPD at our initial visit, a full two years before her death. Over the years that I knew Evelyn, she suffered from a significant symptom burden of shortness of breath and anxiety, each exacerbating the other. She also experienced multiple hospital admissions, including an ICU stay during which she was intubated one month before her death. Evelyn was the perfect candidate to benefit from the high level of support that hospice provides, which would have better managed her symptoms and helped her avoid the distressing hospital visits and escalations of care that she experienced.

Although I broached the topic of hospice care with Evelyn early on in our visits, she remained reluctant to enroll for two primary reasons. First, her pulmonologist, in whom she placed a great deal of trust, had reassured her, after my initial discussion of hospice care with her, that she still had "many good years left." This carrot of hope, though well intended, effectively nullified Evelyn's willingness to consider hospice care a viable option until the very end.

Second, like many patients and providers, Evelyn believed that hospice care was intended for people with only a very short amount of time left. This misconception likely derives from the six-month prognosis cutoff imposed by the hospice criteria, as well as from the medical community's failure to refer patients to hospice until their time is limited to weeks or days rather than months. Having seen other people die in hospice care after just a few days, patients frequently associate hospice care with imminent death and come to fear hospice. Because the medical community does not dissuade them from this misconception, patients fail to appreciate the power of hospice care to provide comfort for a prolonged period at the end of life.

In Evelyn's case, because her trusted pulmonologist did not broach the topic of hospice care with her earlier in her journey but rather offered her an optimistic picture of longevity, my efforts to educate her about the benefits of hospice care remained stymied. It is natural for patients to put a great deal of faith in the judgment of their physicians, but for this reason, many of us working in palliative care often feel as though we are swimming upstream.

It would be far better for patients like Evelyn if the specialist and the palliative care provider were on the same page—the page where the patient is asked what she wants for herself in whatever time she has left and where the providers work together to make that happen—rather than avoiding the question altogether, by providing an inaccurate or misleading assessment, or by failing to discuss and offer hospice care as a viable treatment option until it is nearly too late.

Patients like Evelyn, who can experience many months in the terminal phase, would benefit from a medical community better trained to recognize the moment hospice care would become appropriate and to discuss and offer hospice care as an appropriate treatment option, as well as hospice eligibility criteria that lengthen the time patients can benefit from this high level of care.

Regarding the length of time a patient can remain on hospice care, while it is true that patients who survive beyond six months with the support of hospice care may continue to receive hospice care, they must show some observable measure of decline to continue to remain eligible. Patients are periodically evaluated for hospice eligibility—after the first 90 days and at 60-day intervals thereafter—and decline from one certification period to the next must be documented for CMS to continue reimbursing for hospice care. Those who do not show continued decline must be discharged from hospice [40], which is frequently problematic.

A patient who previously met hospice criteria carries a significant risk of meeting hospice criteria again soon. As mentioned earlier, trends tend to persist. Organ failure, dementia, many neurodegenerative diseases, age-related decline, and cancer follow predictably terminal trajectories. When patients are discharged from hospice care because of improvement or stabilization in symptoms, weight, or function, the most critical question remains, "Does the patient want to once again return to the hospital for care?" If the answer is "No," then unless the patient has moved entirely off the current trajectory with a definitive cure, which typically only occurs with cancer, following discharge from hospice, patients often experience additional hospital admissions (expected), escalations of care (often unwanted), rebounding readmission to hospice care or, as my team often sees, death within a short amount of time (frequently unsupported by hospice care).

Rather, patients with an expected terminal diagnosis who have willingly decided to forego curative and hospital care should be allowed to remain in hospice until death without the necessity of showing an objective decline. The combination of their qualifying diagnosis and hospice mindedness should sufficiently satisfy hospice eligibility. Until CMS hospice eligibility criteria and policies are retooled to address these concerns, it is important to keep these limitations in mind.

Functional Assessment

A core element of a hospice evaluation is an assessment of a patient's functional status—their ability to make it through the day without help. As reviewed in the previous chapter, a patient's functional status represents what I consider to be *the most important vital sign*, informing a patient's sense of purpose, well-being, and *joie de vivre.* It is a patient's functional status that eventually flickers out as the light wanes at the end of the tunnel, with all terminal trajectories following a course of progressive and permanent functional loss, leaving patients entirely dependent on others before their death.

Hospice teams assess functional status using the Palliative Performance Scale (PPS), which evaluates five domains of a patient's capacity including ambulation, activity level, evidence of disease, ability to perform self-care, oral intake, and wakefulness [41]. Patients are given a percentage score, called the PPS score, which ranges from 0%, representing a dead person, to 100%, representing someone without limitations (Table 5.1). A PPS score is part of the inclusion criteria for many hospice trajectories defined by CMS [42, 43].

In addition to the Palliative Performance Scale, the Karnofsky Performance Scale (KPS), which evaluates patient functional status in a similar range from 0 (dead) to 100 (fully functional), can be substituted for the PPS and is also referenced

Table 5.1 Palliative Performance Scale (PPS)

Palliative Performance Scale (PPS)					
%	Ambulation	Activity and evidence of disease	Self-care	Intake	Conscious level
100	Full	Normal activity No evidence of disease	Full	Normal	Full
90	Full	Normal activity Some evidence of disease	Full	Normal	Full
80	Full	Normal activity with effort Some evidence of disease	Full	Normal or reduced	Full
70	Reduced	Unable to do normal job/work Some evidence of disease	Full	Normal or reduced	Full
60	Reduced	Unable to do hobby/house work Significant disease	Occasional assistance necessary	Normal or reduced	Full or confusion
50	Mainly sit/lie	Unable to do any work Extensive disease	Considerable assistance required	Normal or reduced	Full or confusion
40	Mainly in bed	As above	Mainly assistance	Normal or reduced	Full or drowsy or confusion
30	Totally bed bound	As above	Total care	Reduced	Full or drowsy or confusion
20	As above	As above	Total care	Minimal sips	Full or drowsy or confusion
10	As above	As above	Total care	Mouth care	Drowsy or coma
0	Death	–	–	–	–

Anderson F, Downing GM, Hill J, Casorso L, Lerch N. Palliative performance scale (PPS): a new tool. J Palliat Care. 1996 Spring;12(1):5–11. PMID: 8857241. Reprinted with permission [41]

in some of the hospice criteria [44]. With its five separate assessment domains, the PPS system is more useful across the patient population. Although I refer exclusively to the PPS in this volume, note that a KPS score can be used instead of a PPS score.

The Palliative Performance Scale has been shown to have both good intra- and interrater reliability [45, 46] and, in my experience, takes little time to master. A patient's PPS score provides a snapshot of a patient's functional status at a given moment. PPS scores can evolve, shifting from day to day or month to month. Thus, PPS scores provide a way of tracking improvement or decline and contextualizing acute health status changes within overall disease progression. Very conveniently, the PPS maps directly to the y-axis of the disease trajectory diagrams described by Lunney et al. [18] and Ballentine [47], as in Fig. 5.1, which illustrates this relationship using the Organ Failure trajectory.

Patients without many limitations, symptoms, or other evidence of disease, who can care for themselves, and who experience a normal level of wakefulness, appetite, and ability to eat will have a PPS score of 80% to 100%. These are adults with overall good health or a disease that is well- or mostly well-controlled and does not overwhelmingly impact their ability to get through or experience their day-to-day life. These patients would be expected to survive for several years, barring any unfortunate event that might dramatically impact their prognosis. Rarely do I encounter patients with this level of function in palliative care, and almost no patients admitted to the hospital, to a rehab center, or an acute or long-term care facility score in this range.

Patients with a PPS score of 60% to 70% are beginning to show signs of disease or decline, with less available energy for a job, housework, or hobbies, or for being up and around like they once were. They may need occasional assistance, have a

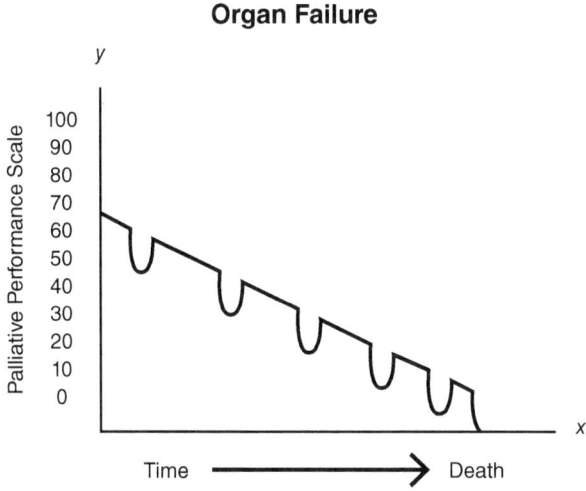

Fig. 5.1 Organ failure. (Adapted with permission from Lunney et al. (2002). *Profiles of Older Medicare Decedents.* Journal of the American Geriatrics Society [18])

reduced appetite, and find themselves napping more frequently. Many older adults who acknowledge that they are *slowing down* and whose families are beginning to step in to help, as well as those with a disease that is starting to impact their daily lives, score in this range. Patients here may be transitioning along a disease trajectory that will eventually impact their longevity, and patients with a downward trend in PPS score may sooner than later require a transition toward a facility that provides additional support, such as an independent or assisted living facility. Most stable patients with chronic disease exist in this range from month to month, shifting at times to a lower status when they experience an exacerbation or acute crisis. Trends that do not correct relatively quickly (within weeks to a few months) are always concerning and represent an opportunity to revisit patient wishes and care needs.

Arrival at the PPS 50% point indicates an important milestone of disease progression and decline. Patients at this range have significant evidence of disease that impacts their ability to make it through the day, limiting their energy and capacity to perform housework, a job, and hobbies. Patients here require considerable assistance and spend much of their day sitting or lying down. They may experience a reduced appetite and level of wakefulness, with many reporting that they *nod off* throughout the day. Many patients receiving palliative care have a baseline PPS score of 50%, and it is at this point that a patient with a progressive and terminal illness may enter the end stage with the expectation of reduced longevity. Hospice care may be appropriate, and a PPS score equal to or less than 50% is part of the inclusion criteria for many hospice trajectories defined by CMS [42, 43].

A patient's PPS score should indicate their *actual* effort, ability, and energy level throughout the day, not their *potential* effort, ability, and energy level. Patients with dementia, whose disease has robbed them of the mental capacity and awareness of the need for much work but who might still technically be physically capable of doing more, should be scored in a manner that reflects their *actual* effort and energy level. By the time patients with dementia have arrived at the Personal Care stage, in which they need assistance with all activities of daily living (ADLs), they typically have a PPS score of 50% or less, like patients whose advanced heart failure or COPD has rendered them equally, though primarily *physically*, incapable of much activity.

While it is undoubtedly true that patients may recover from acute decline with the help of modern medical interventions, patients with advanced or progressing disease or a background of baseline decline often have too little reserve to recover from any subsequent illness or injury. It is helpful to know the patient's baseline level of functional status so that any acute shift can be contextualized appropriately. Knowing that a patient's PPS score can shift from daily, during an acute crisis, or at the end of life, it is important to understand the significance of a drop in PPS to 40% or below.

At a PPS of 40%, patients are primarily bedbound, exhibiting extensive symptomatology and functional dependence, requiring assistance for almost all aspects of living, including the instrumental activities of daily living (IADLs) and ADLs. Patients at this level may be able to feed themselves. Still, they will likely have a reduced appetite and may sleep more throughout the day, with little available energy for visiting or participating in conversations. Patients with this level of PPS decline have an expected prognosis in the range of weeks to month(s) [48–50], and hospice care is appropriate for most patients at this level.

Below a PPS of 40%, patients carry a significantly increased risk of mortality, with studies showing survival times limited on the order of weeks, days to week(s), and days and for those with a PPS of 30%, 20%, and 10%, respectively [48–50]. The descriptions of the following PPS levels are intended to serve as a *sliding scale* for mortality recognition as patients approach the end of their lives.

At 30% PPS, patients are fully bedbound, unable to perform any act of personal care, exhibit a significantly reduced oral intake and level of wakefulness, and have an expected prognosis in the range of weeks. Patients may still be able to visit occasionally with family, but eating and engaging in conversation may exhaust what little energy they still have available.

Families often worry at this point that their loved one will *starve* to death. It is important to explain that a person's body making the metabolic transition at the end of life can no longer utilize nutrition as it once did and that the introduction of food or liquid can overwhelm organs that can no longer manage that nutrient or volume source. Extra fluid, for instance, IV hydration, can easily overwhelm a failing heart or kidneys, whose job is to maintain the body's volume level in the blood vessels. Patients receiving extra fluid at the end of life can experience extremity or pulmonary edema, ascites, and skin breakdown as a result, and additional nutrition can contribute to constipation, all of which can add to a patient's discomfort. Loved ones also benefit from the knowledge that when a patient's body arrives at the final leg of the journey, they do not experience hunger and thirst as they once did. Because most people's concerns relate to patient comfort, education about these considerations becomes essential support at this challenging time.

At 20% PPS, patients are fully bedbound, require total care, take only sips of liquid by mouth, and are much less responsive, spending nearly the entire day asleep. At this point, patients are said to be *actively transitioning* toward death, with an expected prognosis of days to week(s).

From this point on, patients may experience *terminal restlessness*, which can be alleviated by antianxiety medications, and the *death rattle*—the sound of secretions collecting toward the upper airway—may be audible. This sound tends to be more discomforting to families than the patient and can be addressed by applying atropine eye drops or a scopolamine patch behind the ear. Skin changes, including mottling (a lacy venous pattern evident on otherwise pale skin) and coldness, indicate that the body is limiting resources to the extremities to preserve the function of the vital organs of the interior.

At 10% PPS, a patient's death is said to be *imminent*—expected within the next few hours to day(s). At this point, patients sleep throughout the day, require 24-hour support, and do not drink or eat at all. To ensure the patient's comfort, oral care consists of wet swabs and lip balm. As organs shut down, urine production becomes scant, if at all, and no energy remains available for communication. However, families are encouraged to continue to speak to their loved ones and provide physical comfort through touch.

Patients in the final hours to days of life may experience terminal fevers, which can be alleviated with acetaminophen to ensure patient comfort. Additionally, following a period of nonresponsiveness, patients may experience a brief period of clarity and energy called *terminal lucidity*, which can be confusing to families, who may believe that their loved one has turned the corner with signs of recovery. As the vital organs begin to shut down, breathing may become disorganized, with long pauses called *apnea*, indicating that a patient's time on Earth has nearly run out. As patients experience and exhibit these physical changes, families are best supported by hospice teams well-versed in what to expect.

Prognostication (A Note of Advice)

Providing prognostic information to patients and families can be a delicate endeavor. It is important to keep in mind the following clinical pearls.

First, as we will learn in the next section of this book when discussing the *Ground Rules for Communication*, it is never appropriate to march in and forcefully confront or undo someone's belief systems. This applies to spiritual beliefs—beliefs about God and the afterlife—and to medical beliefs—beliefs about healing, prognosis, and when the medical end of a journey might occur. Our job as medical practitioners is to *meet people where they are*, respect their beliefs, and refrain from forcing our medical opinions down anyone's throat.

For this reason, prognostic information should only ever be delivered once you have received some indication from the patient and family that they are emotionally and spiritually ready to receive that information. Providing a prognosis without a patient or family's readiness risks offending their beliefs, which is inappropriate. Believe me when I report that patients and families remember precisely what they were told and by whom whenever a prognosis is mentioned. It can be emotionally devastating for patients and families to be told how long they have left without first positioning that information within the landscape of their understanding of the disease, their decline, and their beliefs about who or what is in charge of the end of their lives.

Save yourself the near-guaranteed margin of error and refrain from prognosticating with any amount of specificity or authority beyond a range like *hours to days*, *days to weeks*, *weeks to months*, or *months to years*. I learned this vital advice from Dr. Faryal Michaud, whose podcast *Write Your Last Chapter* contains clinical wisdom and guidance about end-of-life care [51]. As Dr. Michaud suggests, when providing prognostic information, always hedge your bets by offering a humble disclaimer, such as, "While we cannot know for sure, I worry that your prognosis is on the scale of X. Some patients will live longer, and some will not live that long." Whatever you do, remember to never provide prognostic information before receiving some indication from the patient and family that they, too, worry that the patient's time is limited, that they believe the end is near, or that they are ready and willing to receive that information.

In the coming chapters, we will discuss ways of detecting that the patient and family are ready to receive prognostic information and specific approaches to delivering that information.

Determining Hospice Eligibility

To qualify a patient for the Medicare hospice benefit, the hospice care team must convey a compelling clinical picture demonstrating that the patient is terminally ill [52, 53]. This is called a *certificate of terminal illness (CTI)*. To furnish a CTI, CMS defines two types of qualifying criteria, allowing for two approaches to supporting hospice eligibility.

First, a patient can meet hospice criteria with a single *disease-specific indication*, reflecting a situation in which one primary diagnosis is responsible for their decline. This can occur with organ failure, cancer, dementia, or any of the other neurodegenerative diseases, HIV (human immunodeficiency virus), or with a catastrophic event that leaves the patient in critical functional and physical decline, for example, a stroke or traumatic brain injury.

Alternatively, a patient can meet hospice criteria with a *decline in clinical status*, which CMS defines as the single *non-disease-specific indication*. In this case, a patient must have experienced a dramatic and recent drop in functional status and show evidence of physical decline, with at least one comorbidity impacting their symptomatology and overall prognosis. This path for meeting hospice criteria allows for a situation where one specific diagnosis is not driving the patient's decline; instead, multiple factors contribute.

Despite these two mechanisms for certifying patients for hospice care, there remains a glaring omission in the hospice criteria as currently defined. CMS does not allow for patients to meet hospice criteria specifically and solely on the merits of *age-related decline*. There are no specifically defined criteria for patients without comorbidities who are reaching the end of their lives, like my grandmother, who *died of old age*. It is not enough to qualify a patient for hospice care with only *debility* or *adult failure to thrive* [52]. This is unfortunate and puts hospice centers in a bind because many patients approach the end of life with nothing other than *age-related decline*.

The following narrative provides an example of the documentation CMS requires to support a patient's suitability for hospice care. As you will see, this narrative paints a clear picture of ongoing functional and physical decline, detailing the patient's symptom burden and need for assistance throughout the day, as well as specifying the required elements of hospice criteria for heart failure—in this case, a reduced ejection fraction (EF) and symptoms at rest.

> The patient meets hospice criteria with a diagnosis of end-stage heart failure with a reduced EF of 15% and NYHA Class IV symptoms, including shortness of breath and difficult-to-control chest pain at rest. The patient has a long-standing history of coronary artery disease, with three-vessel disease repaired by coronary artery bypass graft (CABG) 25 years ago. In the last five years, the patient has been hospitalized seven times for various heart-related

events, including an ST-elevation myocardial infarction (STEMI), which was treated with percutaneous coronary intervention (PCI), during which the patient received a stent to a failed graft. Despite optimal medical therapy, including dual-antiplatelet medications, the stent subsequently reoccluded, leading to a second STEMI and a reduced EF that has not recovered. In the last six months, the patient has experienced three hospitalizations for heart failure exacerbations, requiring IV diuretics. The patient's volume status remains difficult to control, with the patient experiencing ongoing edema, weeping skin, and lower extremity tissue breakdown. The patient's difficult-to-control volume status and low baseline blood pressure make his angina challenging to control as well, as the anti-anginal medications further reduce the patient's blood pressure, leading to ongoing symptoms of light-headedness, dizziness, and fatigue.

At this point, the patient prefers to avoid life-prolonging interventions, including the placement of an implantable cardioverter-defibrillator (ICD), which is the standard of care for patients with a chronically reduced EF. His quality of life is severely limited by his worsening and significant symptoms at rest, which limit his ability to exert himself beyond short distances (bed to chair, bed to bathroom). The patient's PPS is 50%; he requires assistance with all IADLs and most ADLs. The patient is ready to allow nature to take its course, has a DNR order, is hospice minded, and prefers to avoid future hospitalizations. He wishes to remain at home in whatever time he has left, where he continues to be well-supported by his wife of 45 years. This patient has an expected prognosis of less than six months and will be enrolled in home-based hospice care.

Although intentionally wordy, to make my point, this documentation adequately constitutes a CTI.

The hospice criteria below reference the local coverage determination (LCD), available online at the Medicare Coverage Database [42, 43, 54]. As the hospice criteria are continually updated, it is advisable to use this chapter as a guide, but it is important to refer to the current hospice criteria guidelines [42, 43, 54].

Disease-Specific Hospice Criteria

Catastrophic Event Trajectory (Fig. 5.2)

Coma
Responsiveness and arousal inhabit a continuum that ranges from the fully intact and normally functioning healthy brain to *brain death*—the complete and irreversible loss of brain function. At the healthy extreme, among other things, patients can respond to conversation, follow commands, breathe independently, swallow normally, and exhibit a healthy arousal system with a sleep-wake cycle easily disturbed by noxious stimuli. At the other end of the continuum, brain death represents the absence of these functions due to widespread damage to the brainstem, cerebellum, and cerebral cortex. Between these two endpoints exists a host of disordered expressions of consciousness and responsiveness, including concussion, dementia, delirium, akinetic mutism, abulia, catatonia, minimally responsive state, vegetative state, and coma, reflecting wide variation and severity of brain injury [55].

Impaired consciousness is evaluated and monitored using a clinical scale called the Glasgow Coma Scale (GCS), which assesses brainstem, cerebellum, and

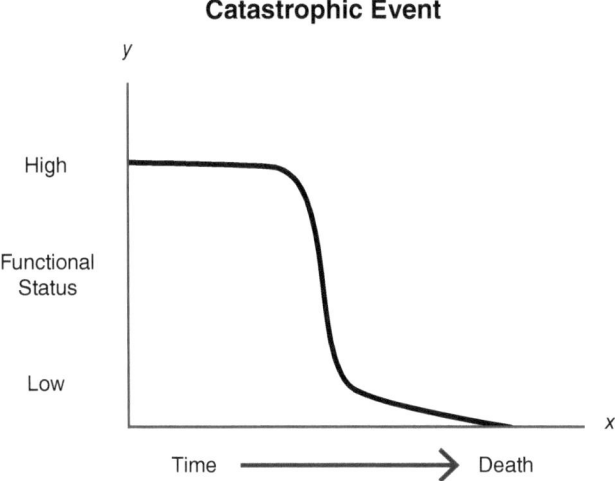

Fig. 5.2 Catastrophic event. (Adapted with permission from Ballentine, J. M. (2018). *The Five Trajectories: Supporting Patients During Serious Illness.* CSU Shiley Haynes Institute for Palliative Care. Copyright © Jennifer Moore Ballentine. All rights reserved [47])

cortical function by evaluating eye-opening and verbal and motor response to stimuli (pain, sound, and command). The GCS exam provides a rapid evaluation of head injury in the ER as well as continual monitoring of patient response to therapy in the ICU and on the medical floor. Patients are given a score between 3 (low) and 15 (high), with 3 representing the absence of all responses and 15 representing an oriented patient who can follow commands and open their eyes spontaneously [56]. Scores in the range of 3 to 8 signify severe head injury with profoundly impaired consciousness, with patients generally requiring endotracheal intubation and mechanical ventilation [57]. Scores of less than 5 are associated with an 80% risk of mortality or persistent vegetative state [58].

Brain death can result from any number of physical or metabolic causes, including seizure, stroke, hemorrhage, infection, trauma, tumor, or anoxia. Brain death is a clinical diagnosis that reflects the irreversible loss of brain function in which patients remain unconscious, exhibit absent brainstem reflexes, are unable to breathe on their own, and do not follow commands, verbalize, or respond to pain or sound. Cerebral, cerebellar, and brainstem blood flow and metabolism are absent as a result of catastrophic brain cell death [59].

A diagnosis of brain death is determined by hospital policy, which dictates who may diagnose and what specific clinical evidence is required. To evaluate the respiratory reflex, patients undergo an *apnea test*, during which ventilator support is turned off for a short period (8–10 minutes at my hospital) to observe whether the brainstem can spontaneously resume control of breathing. Other tests providing evidence of catastrophic brain injury, such as a cerebral blood flow study confirming the absence of perfusion,[2] can be used to support a diagnosis of brain death but are not required.

All patients experiencing brain death require ICU-level care and mechanical ventilation. When families decide to withdraw treatment, patients are terminally extubated in the ICU and typically pass within a few minutes to hours. Because patients diagnosed with brain death cannot survive long without breathing machine support, these patients are typically not enrolled in hospice care, and brain death is not included as a separate, specific hospice criterion.

Unlike brain death, *coma* is not a specific clinical diagnosis or etiology but rather an umbrella term representing cerebrocortical-brainstem dysfunction, one step removed from brain death. A patient in a coma will exhibit upper brainstem and cerebral injury, remaining unconscious and without willful verbal or motor response, but will show abnormal brainstem reflexes and may retain the ability to breathe on their own [55]. Brain metabolism is typically reduced in a coma, and electroencephalogram (EEG) activity is usually abnormal [55]. Coma typically resolves in one way or another within two to four weeks, as patients either improve—moving into a vegetative state, minimally conscious state, or recovering more fully—or deteriorate further, with many going on to a diagnosis of brain death [55].

In speaking with my ICU and hospitalist colleagues, the concept of *coma* represents a gray area of diagnosis in which prognosis can be challenging. Because brain function, including the respiratory and swallow reflexes, cannot be fully assessed while patients are sedated, the direction in which a coma is resolving is often masked while patients are intubated. This was the case with a patient cared for at my hospital with severe COVID-19, who required a significant amount of sedative while being ventilated. Although the medical team was successful in recovering this patient from the virus, the patient had experienced profound brain injury and brain death while sedated, due to an embolic stroke that went undiscovered until extubation. Hopeful for the patient's complete recovery, the family and medical team alike were caught unawares by this devastating actuality.

In truth, *coma* is more lay language than medical terminology, used to describe a state of unconscious unresponsiveness rather than serving as a specific diagnosis. My grandmother, who arrived at the ER in a *coma* following the worst headache of her life, was found to have suffered a *cerebral artery aneurysm* and *massive brain hemorrhage*. After confirmation of *brain death*, she passed away in the hospital following the withdrawal of ventilation support in the ICU. Rather than identifying coma as the diagnosis, physicians name the etiology responsible for the patient's profound decline in clinical status—in my grandmother's case, an aneurysm causing a hemorrhage.

---

[2] The definition, and therefore acknowledgment of brain death, is an evolving and even controversial topic in neurology.

To meet hospice criteria with a coma, any 3 of the following on day 3 of the coma must be documented [42]:

- Abnormal brainstem response
- Absent verbal response
- Absent withdrawal response to pain
- Serum creatinine >1.5 mg/dL

An elevated creatinine level reflects the finding that acute kidney injury occurs early and often with traumatic brain injury and denotes a poor prognosis [60, 61].

To support a picture of a patient meeting hospice criteria with coma, evidence portending poor prognosis, including end-stage metabolic decline sequelae, large volume stroke or hemorrhage, or stroke or hemorrhage involving the brainstem, should be documented [42].

Evidence of end-stage metabolic decline sequelae can include any of the following medical complications occurring in the previous 12 months in the setting of ongoing decline [42]. As described in the previous chapter in the section on the General Decline trajectory, these findings indicate that a patient's metabolism has shifted into a state of hypercatabolism, leaving the patient susceptible to recurrent infections and poor wound healing.

- Aspiration pneumonia
- Upper urinary tract infections (pyelonephritis)
- Refractory (resistant to healing) and advanced stage (3–4) decubitus ulcers
- Recurrent fever after antibiotics

Note that the current CMS criteria for coma, as listed above, do not fully capture the range of manifestations of profound brain injury that patients can experience, and that carries a poor prognosis.

An illustrative case is a patient of mine who experienced a rapidly progressing and devastating form of dementia with profound cognitive decline over six months. Just six months after his original diagnosis, this patient was found unresponsive and unconscious at home. Arriving at the ER with a GCS score of 3, he was found to be severely hypertensive, bradycardic, and apneic, for which he required emergent intubation, mechanical ventilation, and ICU-level care. An early extubation attempt revealed a loss of respiratory reflex, leading to urgent re-intubation. Despite recovering his ability to open his eyes to stimulation with light and to follow simple commands, he remained unconscious unless stimulated and unable to breathe without support. Given his recent and rapid cognitive decline and loss of independent respiratory drive, the patient's family decided to withdraw care, and he passed in our ICU within the hour of being terminally extubated.

This is an example of a patient who was neither brain dead nor in a coma, as presently defined by hospice criteria, yet whose brain injury, the etiology for which was never precisely determined, resulted in such profound dysfunction that he required life support to remain alive. Vegetative state and minimally conscious state, two other profoundly diminished conditions on the arousal and responsiveness continuum, would also not meet hospice criteria for coma.

In the vegetative state, patients regain their sleep-wake cycle but remain unconscious, with a PPS of 30% or lower, exhibiting brainstem-mediated reflexes but no purposeful movement, remaining bowel and bladder incontinent, and requiring a feeding tube [55]. In the minimally conscious state, patients experience minimal ability to follow commands, have some verbal response, and some sense of self-awareness, but also remain bowel and bladder incontinent and require a feeding tube. Patients in the minimally conscious state will have a PPS score of 40% or lower. In both conditions, patients require around-the-clock care [55]. Neither condition meets the present definition of hospice criteria for coma. Patients with these conditions can be qualified for hospice with the Non-disease-specific guidelines, described below.

Perhaps more than any other condition, the continuum of profound brain injury provides a compelling illustration of the importance of positioning the patient's acute condition within their overall clinical picture because long-term prognosis, intensity of care need, and symptomatology intersect with quality of life to impact family decisions in these situations. This was certainly the case with my uncle, whose family chose to withdraw his life support and allow him to pass in the ICU as a way of honoring his identity and sense of purpose as an avid outdoorsman who would not have wanted his family to be burdened with his high level of required care.

Finally, although a clinical diagnosis of brain death or coma may seem like a hard medical stop due to the patient's negligible chance of recovery, it is important to keep in mind that surrogate decision-makers bring to the table a variety of personal beliefs about who or what is ultimately in charge of the end of life, and also do not always have the benefit of medical or biology-based education. Faith-based hope for recovery, beliefs about miracles, and limitations in medical literacy must be respected, even when such perspectives directly oppose what the medical community may consider biologically possible or medically reasonable.

Consider the example of Frank, from the previous chapter in the section on Catastrophic Event, who declined to a minimally conscious state following his catastrophic stroke and cerebral hemorrhage. Frank lived for many months with a feeding tube and urinary catheter, requiring a high level of around-the-clock care and experiencing recurrent infections and other complications. Families like Frank's often need plenty of time to arrive at a point where their medical understanding of recovery more evenly matches the medical community's. As families navigate these complex and challenging considerations, doing the emotional and spiritual work of making sense of their loved one's new reality, they are best supported by palliative care teams and providers trained to sensitively assist this fraught labor.

Stroke

Following a stroke, patients can experience a profound functional and nutritional decline. For those with an intact arousal system who can follow commands and breathe independently, a swallow study will be completed to evaluate their ability to swallow safely without aspiration. Patients unable to swallow safely will first be offered a nasogastric (NG) feeding tube, which can provide nutrition while protecting their lungs from aspirating while working with speech and language therapy to recover their swallow function. An NG tube can be left in place for a short time-frame, typically no longer than four to six weeks. After this time, patients unable to recover their swallow function will be offered a permanent feeding tube, which will be inserted into the abdomen. As discussed previously, a permanent feeding tube carries the risk of aspiration pneumonia, particularly for patients with a degraded swallow function.

There are two elements to meeting hospice criteria with a stroke [42]:

1. The patient's functional status must be declined to a PPS of 40% or lower, meaning that the patient is mostly or totally bedbound, unable to ambulate independently, and requires assistance with most aspects of living [42].
2. The patient's nutritional status must be impacted so they cannot adequately maintain their nutrition orally. Any of the following situations would satisfy this component of the hospice criteria [42]:

   - A clinically significant amount of weight loss (10% of total body weight in the prior six months or >7.5% of total body weight in the prior three months)
   - A serum albumin of 2.5 g/dL or less (normal range 3.5–5.5 g/dL)
   - A calorie count showing insufficient caloric intake
   - Post-stroke aspiration pneumonia in the setting of dysphagia that is not improving despite speech and language therapy interventions
   - Dysphagia preventing adequate nutritional intake in which the patient refuses or chooses to discontinue artificial nutrition and hydration by tube

Evidence of end-stage metabolic decline sequelae can include any of the following medical complications occurring in the previous 12 months in the setting of ongoing decline [42]. As described in the previous chapter in the section on the General Decline trajectory, these findings indicate that a patient's metabolism has shifted into hypercatabolism, leaving the patient susceptible to recurrent infections and poor wound healing.

- Aspiration pneumonia
- Upper urinary tract infections (pyelonephritis)
- Refractory (resistant to healing) and advanced stage (3–4) decubitus ulcers
- Recurrent fever after antibiotics

In stroke patients, imaging studies of findings associated with very poor prognosis should be documented [42].

In the case of a hemorrhagic stroke, this can include any of the following [42]:

- Large volume hemorrhage identified on CT scan:
  - Infratentorial (cerebellum and brainstem) $\geq$ 20 mL
  - Supratentorial (cerebral cortex) $\geq$ 50 mL

- Extension of the hemorrhage into the ventricles
- Involvement of 30% or more of the surface area of the cerebrum
- Midline shift $\geq$1.5 cm

Blockage of the cerebrospinal fluid, called obstructive hydrocephalus, in which the patient declines or is not a candidate for therapy with a ventriculoperitoneal (VP) shunt.

In the case of a thrombotic or embolic stroke, diagnostic imaging findings can include any of the following [42]:

- Large anterior stroke affecting both the cortex/subcortical structures
- Large strokes affecting both hemispheres
- Strokes involving arteries that supply the brainstem:
    - Basilar artery
    - Bilateral vertebral arteries

Recall Walter and Frank, patients we encountered in the previous chapter in the section on Catastrophic Event. Both suffered strokes and were unable to recover their swallow function. Both received a feeding tube, and both ended up in the hospital with aspiration pneumonia. Both patients would have met the qualification for hospice criteria following their strokes had their families chosen not to pursue a permanent feeding tube.

Following Frank's stroke, his PPS score remained in the 40% to 30% range. During the time that I followed him, Frank exhibited signs of metabolic decline despite his feeding tube. He lost a clinically significant amount of weight, his albumin declined, and he experienced poor wound healing and recurrent infections, including aspiration pneumonia, UTIs, and sepsis. Frank would have met hospice criteria at the point where his weight loss and declining album met the thresholds listed above.

Finally, when Frank and Walter's feeding tubes were discontinued, each patient met hospice criteria.

These cases illustrate how a single disease trajectory can meet hospice criteria at different points along the way and in different ways. In this instance, the hospice criteria appropriately provide flexibility in qualifying patients, allowing for variation in disease expression and patient and family preference.

Organ Failure Trajectory (Fig. 5.3)

Heart Disease

Cardiologists evaluate the severity of heart disease using an assessment tool called the New York Heart Association (NYHA) Classification, which describes the impact of heart disease on a patient's functional status [62]. As heart disease worsens and the heart slowly loses its ability to keep up with the body's demands, patients experience an increasing symptom burden and intolerance for exertion, eventually experiencing *angina* (chest pain) or *dyspnea* (shortness of breath) at rest. The NYHA Classification ranks heart disease progression from Class I (early stage) to Class IV (end-stage) as follows [62] (Table 5.2).

As with the PPS, the NYHA Classification maps directly to the *y*-axis of the Heart Disease trajectory diagram (Fig. 5.4).

Just like with other forms of organ failure, patients with heart failure will experience progressive worsening of their disease, with periodic *exacerbations*, in which symptoms of their increasing dysfunction require medical intervention for management. Symptoms will depend on the underlying structural or functional defect.

Table 5.2 NYHA
Classification— The Stages
of Heart Failure

NYHA Class I	No symptoms, no limits to ordinary activity
NYHA Class II	Mild symptoms, slight limits to ordinary activities
NYHA Class III	Marked symptoms and limitations. Comfortable only at rest
NYHA Class IV	Symptoms at rest, severe limitations

Bashore TM, Granger CB, Hranitzky P, Patel MR. Heart Disease. In: McPhee S J, Papadakis MA, Rabow MW, editors. 2012 Current Medical Diagnosis & Treatment. New York: McGraw-Hill Medical; 2012. p. 317–419. Reprinted with permission [62]

Organ Failure

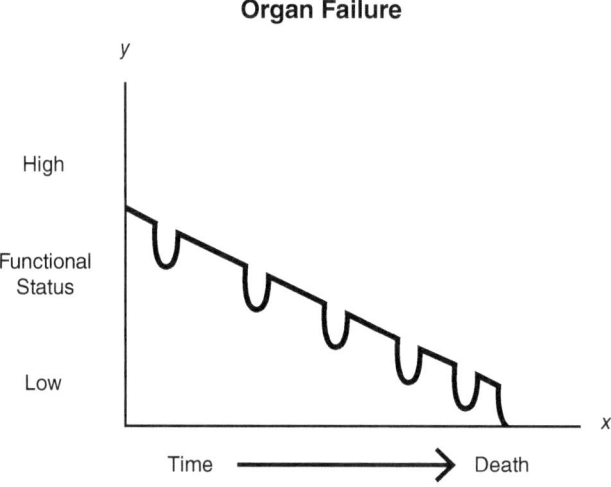

Fig. 5.3 Organ failure. (Adapted with permission from Lunney et al. (2002). *Profiles of Older Medicare Decedents. Journal of the American Geriatrics Society* [18])

Patients with electrical issues, such as atrial fibrillation, may experience palpitations, light-headedness, and syncope, which can lead to symptoms of pump failure—shortness of breath, weight gain, and edema. Patients with plumbing issues—*atherosclerosis*, or coronary artery disease (CAD)—may experience chest pain, shortness of breath, fatigue, and symptoms of pump failure. Those with valvular disease or pump failure can experience any of the symptoms listed here.

Depending on the patient's particular history, a patient may progress through each of the NYHA stages, or, following a significant event such as a silent, evolving, and major heart attack, a patient may begin their heart failure journey at a more advanced, symptom-burdensome baseline. As heart disease progresses toward end-stage, the lungs and kidneys also often fail, leaving patients at risk of increasingly invasive forms of support in the hospital, including pressors (drugs that force the heart to pump), BiPAP, mechanical ventilation, and hemodialysis.

Heart Disease

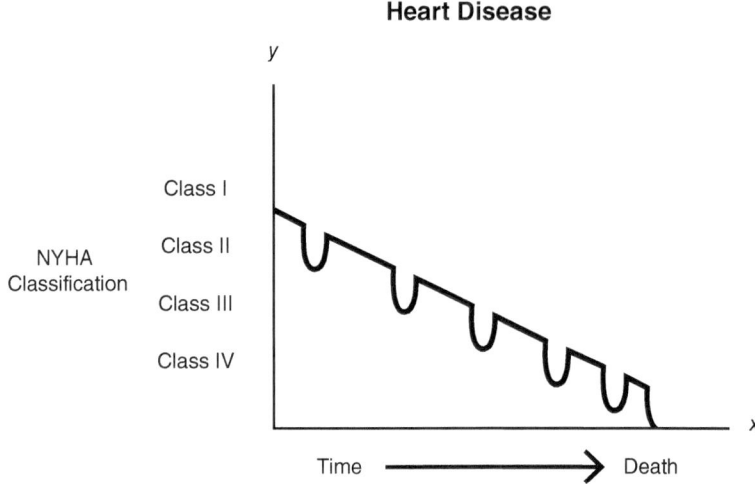

Fig. 5.4 Heart disease. (Adapted with permission from Lunney et al. (2002). *Profiles of Older Medicare Decedents.* Journal of the American Geriatrics Society [18])

Patients with NYHA Class II symptoms will show some indication of functional decline, with a typical PPS in the range of 90% to 60%. Those with NYHA Class III symptoms, who are comfortable only at rest, will have a typical PPS in the range of 60% to 40% as they gravitate toward spending more of their day seated or lying down. Those with NYHA Class IV symptoms, who are not comfortable even at rest, will have a typical PPS in the range of 50% to 40% or less, exhibiting a bed-to-chair existence in which their disease dramatically limits their ability to move about their homes.

Over time, as patient symptoms increase and functional status declines, caregiver demand increases, with NYHA Class IV patients requiring assistance with all aspects of daily living.

There are two elements to meeting hospice criteria with heart disease [42]:

1. Patients must exhibit NYHA Class IV symptoms at rest [42].
2. Patients must either be optimally treated or intolerant of optimal treatment, or they must not be candidates for surgical procedures or have declined those procedures [42].

This second element of the heart disease criteria provides incredible flexibility for qualifying any heart disease that causes patients to experience symptoms at rest. Together, these two elements create a robust set of criteria, enabling patients with heart disease to experience a long terminal phase supported by hospice care teams.

To support a picture of a patient meeting hospice criteria with heart disease, evidence portending poor prognosis, including end-stage or treatment-resistant disease, should be documented. This can include any of the following, though none of these items are required [42]:

- An EF of $\leq 20\%$
- Treatment-resistant symptomatic supraventricular or ventricular arrhythmias

- History of cardiac arrest or resuscitation
- History of unexplained syncope (loss of consciousness)
- Brain embolism of cardiac origin
- Concomitant HIV disease

Recall Derrick, from the previous chapter, who experienced progressive and eventually terminal heart failure caused by a constellation of electrical, plumbing, and structural problems with his heart, including atrial fibrillation, CAD, and pump failure. Despite numerous interventions, Derrick's EF remained chronically reduced, at 40%, leading to constant edema that was difficult to control because of chronically low blood pressure (*hypotension*). His chronic edema led to weeping skin and long-standing wounds that became increasingly resistant to healing despite close follow-up by wound care. By his final hospital admission, Derrick could not tolerate walking more than ten steps from his hospital bed to the adjoining bathroom, and as we visited, he remained short of breath with the effort of speaking. Derrick met hospice criteria with NYHA Class IV symptoms, including shortness of breath and edema that were not amenable to treatment because of his blood pressure.

Lung Disease

Pulmonologists evaluate lung function using a noninvasive breathing assessment called the pulmonary function test (PFT), which measures various lung volumes, capacities, and airflow as patients forcibly exhale. The PFT is instrumental in staging and monitoring the development of COPD and other forms of progressive lung disease. Although the specifics of PFT testing are beyond the scope of this text, what is important to understand is that COPD and other forms of obstructive lung disease lead to air trapping within the lungs, making it difficult for patients to exhale the expected volume with expiration. To help force the air from their lungs, patients often purse their lips and actively engage their chest muscles as they exhale.

Measured during a PFT, the air a patient can forcibly exhale over one second is called the forced expiratory volume (FEV1). Healthy lungs can exhale 65% to 70% of the lung volume during the first second of an exhalation. This volume progressively declines with COPD until, per the *GOLD criteria* [63]—the staging system used to monitor COPD and obstructive lung disease progression—FEV1 declines to 30% or less. At this point, patients are said to have very severe or end-stage disease.

Over time, patients with lung failure expend more and more of their daily energy in the effort to breathe, leaving them with less energy for eating, talking, exerting themselves, or participating in the activities they once enjoyed. Patients often exhibit *pulmonary cachexia*, which shows up as early satiety and weight loss (as described in the previous chapter). Eventually, patients with COPD will get to the point where they spend their days in their chairs or beds. The journeys of heart and lung failure are very similar in this regard, and the NYHA classification perfectly describes the progression of lung disease symptoms and functional decline as patients move from Class I (early stage) to Class IV (end-stage) disease. At the end of their journey, a patient with lung failure will also not be comfortable even at rest and will exhibit a typical PPS in the range of 50% to 40% or less.

Depending on the patient's particular lung history, a patient may progress from early to late-stage disease progressively, or, following a significant event such as scarring pneumonia, a patient may begin their lung failure journey at a more advanced, symptom-burdensome baseline.

Like all organ failure patients, patients with lung disease will experience periodic *exacerbations*, in which symptoms of their increasing lung dysfunction require medical intervention for management of shortness of breath, cough, wheezing, and congestion. Patients with COPD, who are very susceptible to viral infections, can very quickly develop bacterial pneumonia, making early treatment (on day one or two of an exacerbation) with steroids and antibiotics an essential part of their ongoing care.

As lung disease approaches its end stage, the heart also often fails, leaving patients at risk of increasingly invasive forms of support in the hospital, including BiPAP, mechanical ventilation, and pressors. As is the case with all of the terminal trajectories, patients with lung disease will get to the point where any subsequent hospitalization may be their last, as their chance of passing away in the hospital increases with each exacerbation.

As patient symptoms increase and their functional status declines, caregiver demand increases, with patients with end-stage lung failure requiring assistance with all aspects of daily living.

Currently, there are three elements to meeting hospice criteria for lung disease [42]:

1. Disabling dyspnea at rest, poorly responsive or unresponsive to bronchodilators, resulting in decreased functional capacity, e.g., bed-to-chair existence, fatigue, and cough [42]

   Documentation of forced expiratory volume in 1 second (FEV1), < 30% predicted value after bronchodilator, is objective evidence for disabling dyspnea but is not necessary to obtain.

2. Progression of end-stage disease, as shown by increasing visits to the emergency department or hospitalizations for pulmonary infections and/or respiratory failure or increasing clinician home visits prior to initial certification [42]

   Documentation of serial decrease of FEV1 > 40 mL/year is objective evidence for disease progression but is not necessary to obtain.

3. Hypoxemia at rest on room air, as evidenced by $pO_2 \leq 55$ mmHg or oxygen saturation $\leq 88\%$, determined either by arterial blood gases or oxygen saturation monitors (these values may be obtained from recent hospital records), or hypercapnia, as evidenced by $pCO_2 \geq 50$ mmHg (this value may be obtained from recent (within 3 months) hospital records) [42].

To support a picture of a patient meeting hospice criteria with lung disease, evidence portending poor prognosis, including end-stage or treatment-resistant disease, should also be documented. This can include any of the following, although none of these items are required [42]:

- Right-sided heart failure secondary to pulmonary disease (*Cor pulmonale*, not secondary to left heart failure or valvulopathy)

- Unintentional progressive weight loss >10% of total body weight in the preceding 6 months
- Resting tachycardia >100/minute

Recall Evelyn, from the previous chapter, who experienced a long terminal phase—at least two full years—with her COPD. When we met, Evelyn exhibited a baseline that easily met hospice criteria for lung disease. She was short of breath at rest, spent most of her day seated at her dining room table, had lost more than 10 pounds (>10% of her total body weight) in the previous 12 months, and had experienced four recent hospital admissions for COPD exacerbations. Her O_2 saturation level would drop into the high 60% to low 70% range when she removed her supplemental oxygen, and her PFT showed no response to bronchodilators and an FEV1 of 41%.

Evelyn's air hunger, shortness of breath, and resulting anxiety could have been managed by the hospice care team, who, visiting weekly, could have also treated her COPD exacerbations, preventing the hospital admissions that she experienced during her last two years.

Because her pulmonologist did not broach the topic of hospice care or discuss that treatment option as a viable, appropriate, and timely intervention, Evelyn remained resistant to the idea until she experienced intubation and mechanical ventilation, the expected escalation of care for terminal lung failure patients. It is incumbent on physicians to learn the hospice criteria for their specialties and to appropriately represent and offer hospice care as a viable treatment option so that patients can make decisions that reflect their values.

Although we will never know how long Evelyn would have survived with the support of hospice care had she chosen that type of treatment option earlier in her journey, hospice care would have certainly allowed her to avoid the distressing, nonbeneficial, and taxing admissions, trips to rehab, and escalations of care that she experienced, and her final months would have been much more comfortable, given the higher level of symptom management that the hospice team would have provided.

Kidney Disease

Kidney function is evaluated by a calculated value called the *glomerular filtration rate* (GFR), which approximates the rate at which the kidneys filter the blood. The GFR can be determined by measuring the amount of creatinine cleared by the kidneys in 24 hours, a lab value called *creatinine clearance* (CrCl), or by a calculation that utilizes the *serum creatinine* level that arrives at an *estimated glomerular filtration rate* (eGFR) [64].

The normal range for serum creatinine is 0.8 to 1.4 mg/dL; the normal range for creatinine clearance is 88 to 128 mL/minute/1.73 m^2 in females and 97 to 137 mL/minute/1.73 m^2 in males [64]; and the normal range for eGFR is > 90 mL/minute/1.73 m^2.

GFR is used to stage chronic kidney disease, with patients at end stage (stage 5) exhibiting a decline in GFR to < 15 mL/minute/1.73 m^2 [65] (Table 5.3).

Table 5.3 Stages of chronic
kidney disease

CKD stage	GFR (mL/minute/1.73 m^2)
I	> 90
II	60–89
III	30–59
IV	15–29
V	< 15 (or dialysis)

Watnick S, Dirkx T. Kidney Disease. In: McPhee S J, Papadakis MA, Rabow MW, editors. 2012 Current Medical Diagnosis & Treatment. New York: McGraw-Hill Medical; 2012. p. 874–911. Reprinted with permission [65]

Chronic Kidney Disease

Patients with chronic kidney disease experience a decline in their GFR over several months to years, often without signs or symptoms until stage 5, when they can show evidence of the *uremic syndrome*, which results from a build-up of nitrogenous waste products, including urea. A host of non-specific symptoms and signs, including fatigue, weakness, poor appetite, easy bruising, metallic taste, shortness of breath, nausea, weight loss, erectile dysfunction, neuropathy, pallor, edema, rales, pleural effusion, high blood pressure, enlarged heart, confusion, and stupor characterizes the uremic syndrome [65].

The recommendation to start dialysis is based on a combination of uremic symptoms and low GFR. Typically, patients are started on dialysis therapy with a GFR of 5 to 10 mL/minute/1.73 m^2. Patients who require but decline dialysis treatment can be expected to die within one to two weeks [65].

By the time CKD patients start dialysis treatment, most have already reached the terminal phase of their lives, with a yearly mortality rate of nearly 20% [66] and just 1 in 3 surviving beyond five years [67]. Despite their high risk of mortality, less than 40% of dialysis patients have completed advanced care planning directives, and few understand that their journey will be characterized by aggressive and invasive healthcare utilization until the very end of their lives [67].

As compared to patients with heart failure and cancer, patients on dialysis experience higher rates of ICU admissions and hospitalizations in the last month of life [67]. They are much more likely than patients with other terminal trajectories to pass away in the hospital setting, with rates of hospice use much lower for dialysis patients (20%) than for cancer (55%) and heart failure (39%) patients [67]. Because the hospice criteria for kidney failure require that patients discontinue dialysis, with CKD patients having a mean survival time of just 8.2 days from discontinuation of dialysis [68], dialysis patients experience much shorter stays in hospice at the end of their lives [67]. These statistics represent the poor alignment of dialysis patient end-of-life care with what we know most people want at the end of their lives. However, this is not surprising in the context of a medical system that focuses almost entirely on the prolongation of life and is ill-trained to recognize when the end is near [67].

Painting this picture of end-stage CKD patient care, Grubbs et al. make three solid recommendations for improving end-of-life dialysis care in the United States: (1) nephrologists should be better trained to recognize the end of the kidney failure patient's journey and to usher patients through goals of care conversations more expertly; (2) a standardized approach to **palliative dialysis** should be developed; and, (3) the fiscal impact of palliative dialysis should be investigated, with the implication that to support end-of-life wishes for CKD patients, an effort should be made to alter hospice policy to allow for palliative dialysis to be reimbursed [67].

Established in several European countries, palliative dialysis (often in the form of RN-supported home dialysis) differs from maintenance dialysis in that it focuses entirely on supporting the quality of life and comfort of the patient, with adjustments made to timing, frequency, and intensity of dialysis according strictly to patient symptoms and comfort, rather than CMS-determined quality metrics [67]. Currently, palliative dialysis while patients are receiving hospice care is not covered by Medicare in the United States.

Currently, there are two major elements to meeting hospice criteria with chronic kidney disease [42]:

1. The patient is not seeking dialysis or kidney transplant or is discontinuing dialysis [42].

   To this element, CMS adds [42]:

   - As with any other condition, an individual with kidney disease is eligible for the hospice benefit if that individual has a prognosis of 6 months or less if the illness runs its normal course. There is no regulation precluding patients on dialysis from electing hospice care. However, the continuation of dialysis will significantly alter a patient's prognosis and thus potentially impact that individual's eligibility.
   - When an individual elects hospice care for ESKD [end-stage kidney disease] or for a condition related to the need for dialysis, the hospice agency is financially responsible for the dialysis. There is no additional reimbursement beyond the per diem rate. The only situation in which a beneficiary may access both the hospice benefit and the ESKD benefit is when the need for dialysis is not related to the patient's terminal illness.

2. One of the following two lab values must be present, indicating end-stage disease [42]:

   - Creatinine clearance

     - < 10 mL/minute in a non-diabetic patient without chronic heart failure (CHF)
     - < 15 mL/minute in a diabetic patient without CHF
     - < 15 mL/minute in a non-diabetic patient with CHF
     - < 20 mL/minute in a diabetic patient with CHF

   - Serum creatinine

     - > 8.0 mg/dL in a non-diabetic patient
     - > 6.0 mg/dL in a diabetic patient

To support a picture of a patient meeting hospice criteria with chronic kidney disease, evidence portending poor prognosis, including end-stage or treatment-resistant disease, should also be documented. This can include any of the following, although none of these items are required [42]:

- Uremia (high levels of urea in the blood)
- Oliguria (low urine output) (< 400 cc/24 hours)
- Intractable hyperkalemia (high potassium) (> 7.0 mEq/L), not responsive to treatment
- Uremic pericarditis (inflammation of the lining of the heart)
- Hepatorenal syndrome (liver and kidney involvement)
- Intractable fluid overload, not responsive to treatment

Recall Isaac and Hank from the previous chapter in the section on Kidney Failure. Although both patients probably met hospice criteria earlier in their journeys, given their declining metabolic and functional status, neither patient would have qualified for hospice care until their families decided to discontinue dialysis treatments.

Acute Kidney Disease

Acute kidney injury (AKI), previously termed acute kidney failure, occurs when an insult leads to a sudden and dramatic decline in GFR. Very common in hospitalized patients, AKI is seen in up to 7% of overall admissions and up to 67% of ICU admissions [69]. Most commonly caused by decreased renal perfusion, if not reversed, AKI can lead to renal ischemia, resulting in permanent loss of kidney tissue and function [65].

AKI is a common occurrence in advanced cancer, age-related decline, and heart, lung, and liver failure, with nearly half of the in-hospital cases of AKI occurring in the presence of sepsis [69], which by now we have come to understand is an expected part of all terminal trajectories. Not surprisingly, sepsis-associated AKI (SA-AKI) is very common in elderly patients, who are at increased risk of experiencing invasive interventions such as mechanical ventilation and pressor drugs [69]. SA-AKI also carries a higher mortality rate in the hospital and ICU than AKI without sepsis (29.7% in-hospital mortality rate versus 21.6%; 19.8% ICU mortality rate versus 13.4%) [69]. Providers caring for patients with SA-AKI should be well-versed in the disease trajectories and hospice criteria and should understand SA-AKI as a significant marker of terminal decline.

Because treatment for severe AKI often involves intermittent dialysis, the hospice criteria for AKI are very similar to that of CKD.

There are two major elements to meeting hospice criteria with acute kidney disease [42]:

1. The patient is not seeking dialysis or kidney transplant or is discontinuing dialysis [42].

   To this element, CMS adds [42]:

   - As with any other condition, an individual with kidney disease is eligible for the hospice benefit if that individual has a prognosis of 6 months or less if the illness runs its normal course. There is no regulation precluding patients on dialysis from electing hospice care. However, the continuation of dialysis will significantly alter a patient's prognosis and thus potentially impact that individual's eligibility.

- When an individual elects hospice care for ESKD or for a condition related to the need for dialysis, the hospice agency is financially responsible for the dialysis. There is no additional reimbursement beyond the per diem rate. The only situation in which a beneficiary may access both the hospice benefit and the ESKD benefit is when the need for dialysis is not related to the patient's terminal illness.

2. One of the following three lab values must be present, indicating end-stage disease [42].

- Estimated glomerular filtration rate (eGFR) < 10 mL/minute/1.73 m^2
- Creatinine clearance
  - < 10 mL/minute in a non-diabetic patient without CHF
  - < 15 mL/minute in a diabetic patient without CHF
  - < 15 mL/minute in a non-diabetic patient with CHF
  - < 20 mL/minute in a diabetic patient with CHF
- Serum creatinine
  - > 8.0 mg/dL in a non-diabetic patient
  - > 6.0 mg/dL in a diabetic patient

To support a picture of a patient meeting hospice criteria with acute kidney failure, evidence portending poor prognosis, including escalations of care and advanced-stage comorbidities, should also be documented. This can include any of the following, although none of these items are required [42]:

- Mechanical ventilation
- Malignancy (other organ system)
- Chronic lung disease
- Advanced cardiac disease
- Advanced liver disease
- Immunosuppression/AIDS
- Albumin < 3.5 g/dL
- Platelet count < 25,000/μL
- Disseminated intravascular coagulation
- Gastrointestinal bleeding

Liver Disease

Liver function can be monitored by a variety of laboratory values, including alanine aminotransferase (ALT), aspartate aminotransferase (AST), alkaline phosphatase (ALP), gamma-glutamyltransferase (GGT), albumin, total bilirubin (TBIL), prothrombin time (PT), the international normalized ratio (INR), and platelet count. A diagnosis of cirrhosis is considered in patients with abnormal liver function for longer than six months who have risk factors for liver disease, such as metabolic syndrome, alcohol abuse, or hepatitis B or C [70]. A liver biopsy can establish a definitive diagnosis of cirrhosis but is not required; symptomatic patients can be diagnosed clinically.

Cirrhosis is staged according to the absence or presence of symptoms of advanced disease, which include esophageal hemorrhage, ascites, jaundice, and hepatic encephalopathy [71]. Early on, when the liver can maintain homeostasis and symptoms are absent, disease is considered *compensated*, with patients experiencing a median survival time of greater than 12 years [71]. The arrival of symptoms, typically during an exacerbating event that requires hospitalization, marks the transition into the terminal, or *decompensated*, phase of disease. Overall, patients with decompensated liver failure have a median survival time of two years [71], with an acute decompensation carrying a 14% risk of 90-day mortality [72].

Ascites (fluid buildup in the abdomen) is often the earliest symptom of decompensated liver failure, its presence carrying a 50% risk of two-year mortality [73]. By the time ascites becomes refractory to treatment and repeat US paracentesis is required, either on a scheduled basis or during admissions for exacerbations, patients have a median survival time of just six months [73]. Severe or refractory encephalopathy carries a mean survival time of 12 months. *Hepatorenal syndrome* (HRS), in which the kidneys fail in the setting of liver disease, is an ominous sign, with a median survival time of less than two weeks [74], with 90% of patients passing by 10 weeks [74]. Infections carry a very high risk (30%) of 30-day mortality [73].

Patients at any stage of liver disease, including those yet undiagnosed, can experience an acute decline in liver function that leads within a few short weeks to multiple organ failure. This presentation is labeled *acute on chronic liver failure* (ACLF) [72]. Thirty percent of patients with acutely decompensated liver failure will go on to develop ACLF, with 50% of patients with ACLF passing within 90 days [75].

In the absence of long-standing liver failure, *acute liver failure* portends a very poor prognosis, with a mortality rate as high as 85% [76].

Fortunately, transplantation provides a hopeful escape from the liver failure trajectory for many thousands of patients each year. Just over 9000 Americans received a liver transplant in 2021 [77]. At the time of this writing, in 2022, 11,000 patients were awaiting a liver transplant in the United States [78].

Orchestrated by the United Network for Organ Sharing (UNOS), eligibility and priority for liver transplantation in the United States is determined by a scoring system called the Model for End-Stage Liver Disease (MELD), which predicts three-month mortality based on serum levels of creatinine, bilirubin, and the international normalized ratio (INR). Accounting for the fact that hyponatremia worsens with worsening liver failure and is an independent risk factor for mortality in advanced disease, serum sodium level was added to the scoring system (MELD-Na) in 2016 [79].

With the MELD-Na calculation, patients are scored between 6 and 40, with 3-month mortality risk increasing with an increasing score, as follows: 9 or less (1.9% 3-month mortality); 10–19 (6.0% 3-month mortality); 20–29 (19.6% 3-month mortality); 30–39 (52.6% 3-month mortality); 40 (71.3% 3-month mortality) [80].

Evaluation for liver transplant is typically begun at a MELD score of 10, with patients included on the transplant list when their MELD score reaches 15 or higher [81]. Given the mortality risk, patients with acute liver failure are given top priority for a donor organ, followed by patients with decompensated liver failure, particularly those with hepatorenal syndrome.

Numerous contraindications to liver transplant exist, such as advanced heart or lung disease, AIDS, non-hepatic cancer, hepatic cancer with metastasis, non-compliance with treatment, and lack of social support [81]. Patients with a history of alcohol abuse are typically required to participate in an abstinence program, show a minimum of six months of sobriety, and have appropriate social support to maintain ongoing abstinence [81]. Although many eligible patients will receive a liver transplant, many patients will become too sick to remain on the transplant list, while others will die waiting for an organ.

There are two major elements to meeting hospice criteria with liver disease [42]:

1. Two of the three following lab values must be severely deranged [42]:

   - Serum albumin < 2.5 g/dL, **and**
   - Either:

     - PT greater than 5 s over control, meaning 5 s longer than the high limit of normal, or
     - International Normalized Ratio (INR) > 1.5.

   The serum albumin level requirement can be disregarded for patients receiving periodic infusions of albumin.

2. One of the following sequelae must be present, indicating end-stage disease [42]:

   - Ascites, refractory to treatment, or patient non-compliant
   - Spontaneous bacterial peritonitis (SBP)
   - Hepatorenal syndrome (elevated creatinine and BUN with oliguria (< 400 mL/day) and urine sodium concentration < 10 mEq/L)
   - Hepatic encephalopathy, refractory to treatment, or patient non-compliant
   - Recurrent variceal bleeding, despite intensive therapy

To support a picture of a patient meeting hospice criteria with liver failure, evidence portending poor prognosis, including liver-damaging or life-limiting comorbidities, should also be documented. This can include any of the following, although none of these items are required [42]:

- Progressive malnutrition
- Muscle wasting with reduced strength and endurance
- Continued active alcoholism (> 80 g ethanol/day)
- Hepatocellular carcinoma
- Chronic hepatitis B virus infection (HBsAg-positive)
- Hepatitis C infection, refractory to interferon treatment

Of note, patients who are awaiting liver transplant are eligible for hospice enrollment and can be discharged from hospice should a donor organ become available.

Enrolling those waiting for a liver transplant in hospice care is an excellent way of supporting patients with two possible futures—the one in which they receive the good news that a donor's liver is available and the other, where their life is cut short while waiting. Understanding that concurrent hospice enrollment is a possible option for those on the liver transplant list is an important means of ensuring that patients reaching the end of the liver failure journey can be well-supported at that time [73].

Recall Darryl from the previous chapter in the section on Liver Failure. Darryl met hospice criteria seven weeks before I met him, during his first admission for liver decompensation, with PT, INR, and album levels of 19 s, 1.8, and 2.3 g/dL, respectively. Like many liver failure patients I have cared for, Darryl experienced a number of hospital admissions in a short amount of time, leading to death shortly after admission to hospice care.

Cancer Trajectory (Fig. 5.5)

Cancer

In the United States, most cancer deaths are caused by solid tumor cancers, most commonly lung, colon, pancreas, breast, prostate, and liver, followed by the hematopoietic cancers, leukemia, and non-Hodgkin lymphoma [82].

Imaging studies, surgical results, tumor markers, and genetic features of a tumor are used by oncologists, surgeons, and pathologists to evaluate the extent of oncologic disease, with various staging systems in use. Solid tumor cancers are most commonly staged using the tumor-node-metastasis (TNM) system, which accounts for the primary tumor size (T), involvement of lymph nodes (N), and the presence of metastasis (M) [83] (Table 5.4).

Tracking cancer progression from its primary organ of origin to distant metastatic spread, the TNM system maps onto a staging convention familiar to most

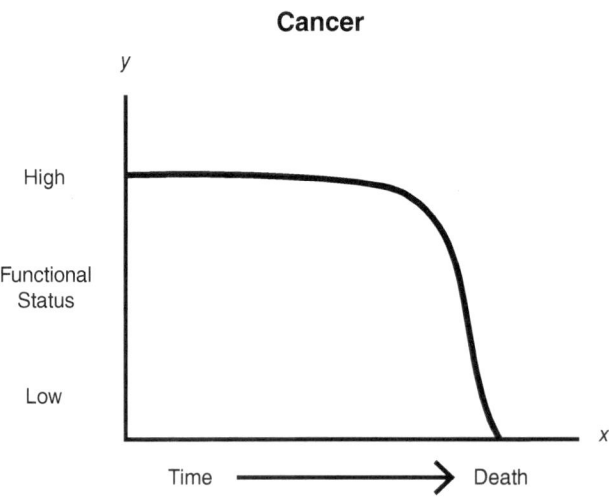

Fig. 5.5 Cancer. (Adapted with permission from Lunney et al. (2002). *Profiles of Older Medicare Decedents.* Journal of the American Geriatrics Society [18])

Table 5.4 TNM classification

TNM classification	
The **T category** describes the original (primary) tumor	
TX	Primary tumor cannot be evaluated
T0	No evidence of primary tumor
Tis	Carcinoma in situ
T1–4	Increasing size and/or local extent of the primary tumor
The **N category** describes whether or not the cancer has reached nearby lymph nodes	
NX	Regional lymph nodes cannot be assessed
N0	No regional lymph node metastasis
N1-N3	Increasing involvement of regional lymph nodes
The **M category** tells whether there are distant metastases (spread of cancer to other parts of the body)	
M0	No distant metastasis
M1	Distant metastasis

Brierley J, Gospodarowicz MK, Wittekind C, Union for International Cancer Control. TNM Classification of Malignant Tumours. Eighth ed. Chichester, West Sussex, UK: Wiley Blackwell; 2017. Reprinted with permission [83]

Table 5.5 Cancer staging and TNM classification

Stage	Description	TNM classification
Stage 0	Abnormal cells are present but have not spread to nearby tissue. Also called carcinoma in situ, or CIS. CIS is not cancer, but it may become cancer	T1, N0, M0
Stage I, Stage II, and Stage III	Cancer is present. The higher the number, the larger the cancer tumor and the more it has spread into nearby tissue	T1–T4, N0–N3, M0
Stage IV	The cancer has spread to distant parts of the body (metastatic)	T1–T4, N1–N3, M1

Cancer staging was originally published by the National Cancer Institute [84]

patients (stages 0 to IV) [84, 85], reflecting increasing tumor burden and declining curability, as shown in Table 5.5.

The hematopoietic cancers (myeloma, leukemia, lymphoma) are each staged differently, according to their unique patterns of progression and spread. These staging systems, which are beyond the scope of this text, can be referenced in the U.S. National Cancer Institute's Surveillance, Epidemiology, and End Results (SEER) Training Modules [86].

Oncologists always refer to a patient's cancer by its stage at diagnosis, even if the cancer progresses. In their notes, oncologists will detail new information about treatment choices and response and any progression of disease in a narrative tied to the original diagnosis.

In addition to staging disease, oncologists monitor patient functional status using the Eastern Cooperative Oncology (ECOG) Performance Scale, which rates patient capacity to make it through the day without assistance on a scale of 0 to 5, with disability increasing with increasing number [44] (Table 5.6).

Table 5.6 Eastern Cooperative Oncology Group (ECOG) Performance Scale

Grade	ECOG performance status
0	Fully active, able to carry on all pre-disease performance without restriction
1	Restricted in physically strenuous activity but ambulatory and able to carry out work of a light or sedentary nature, e.g., light housework, office work
2	Ambulatory and capable of all self-care but unable to carry out any work activities. Up and about more than 50% of waking hours
3	Capable of only limited self-care, confined to bed or chair more than 50% of waking hours
4	Completely disabled, cannot carry on any self-care, totally confined to bed or chair
5	Dead

Longo DL. Approach to the Patient With Cancer. In: Longo DL, Kasper DL, Jameson JL, Fauci AS, Hauser SL, Loscalzo J, editors. Harrison's Principles of Internal Medicine. New York:McGraw-Hill, Health Professions Division, 1998. p. 646–654. Reprinted with permission [44]

Table 5.7 ECOG performance status and PPS score [87, 88]

ECOG grade	PPS score
0	100, 90
1	80, 70
2	60, 50
3	40, 30
4	20, 10
5	0

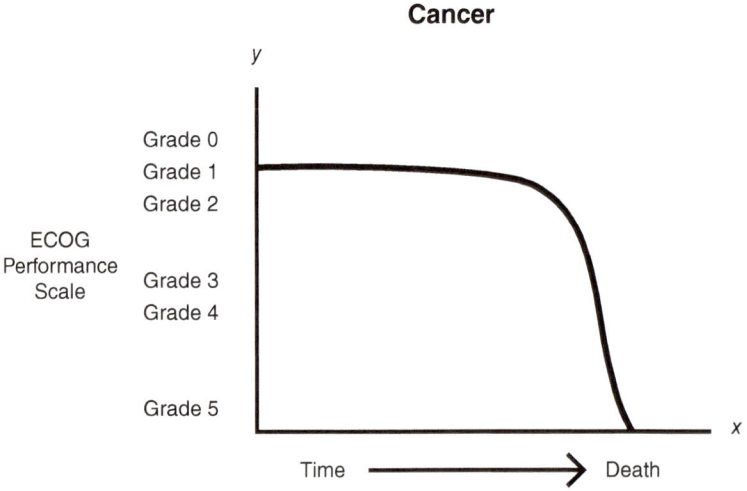

Cancer

Fig. 5.6 Cancer. (Adapted with permission from Lunney et al. (2002). *Profiles of Older Medicare Decedents*. Journal of the American Geriatrics Society [18])

The relationship between the ECOG scoring system and the PPS system is shown in Table 5.7 [87, 88].

As with the PPS and NYHA Classification, the ECOG scoring system maps directly to the *y*-axis of the Cancer trajectory diagram, as shown in Fig. 5.6. The ECOG scale provides less nuance than the PPS in evaluating the functional status of patients with a PPS score of 50% or lower.

Many patients with cancer do not understand how their functional and metabolic decline relates to their disease. This is unfortunate because patients cannot make medical decisions that reflect their personal values and priorities without an accurate understanding of their particular journey. Because patients with cancer are at risk of dramatic decline in a short amount of time, accurate functional and metabolic assessment and ongoing discussions that contextualize any decline are critical to supporting patient autonomy.

There are three paths to meeting hospice criteria with cancer, including *metastasis at presentation*, *progression to metastatic disease*, and *cancer with poor prognosis* [42].

Metastasis at Presentation   To meet criteria in this manner, the patient will exhibit metastatic disease at presentation [42].

Progression to Metastatic Disease   To meet criteria in this manner, the patient will exhibit disease that has progressed from an earlier stage of disease to metastatic disease with either [42]

- Continued decline despite therapy, or
- Patient declines further disease-directed therapy.

As stated earlier, decline due to cancer typically occurs either because the cancer outpaces the treatment or the treatment makes the patient too sick to pursue further treatment. Evidence of decline might include metabolic changes (declining serum albumin, weight loss), functional loss (declining PPS or increasing ECOG score), hospital admissions and escalations of care, or treatment-related complications that impact the patient's quality of life or treatment options, such as myelosuppression.

Cancer with Poor Prognosis   To meet criteria in this manner, the patient will have a diagnosis of cancer with poor prognosis, such as small cell lung cancer, brain cancer, or pancreatic cancer. In this case, the patient need not show progression or metastasis to be qualified for hospice [42].

Recall Richard, Yasmin, and Rita from the previous chapter in the section on Cancer. Richard qualified for hospice care with his diagnosis of pancreatic cancer. Aligning with his wish to avoid aggressive or extensive medical care, the five sessions of palliative radiation Richard underwent proved beneficial for several months. Having previously discussed end-of-life treatment options, when his pain worsened, Richard was well-prepared to transition to hospice care.

Yasmin also qualified for hospice care with pancreatic cancer. Found to have advanced and metastatic disease, Yasmin's PPS score (40%) was much lower than Richard's (60%) at diagnosis. Recall that her functional ability declined precipitously following just two chemotherapy treatments to a bed-bound status of 10%, at which point her family chose to transition her to hospice care. Yasmin's story illustrates the intersection between functional decline and the cancer trajectory, as well as the challenge oncologists face when discussing and offering treatments to patients.

A fighter, Yasmin immediately adopted the warrior role our culture has endorsed for patients with cancer. Willing to try anything to survive, she eagerly accepted the risk of chemotherapy, and despite hearing from the oncologist that it would be merely *palliative*, believed she would not only survive but return to her former status as an athlete and world traveler, neither of which was likely to happen in her case. Reluctant to displace patient hope, it is understandable why oncologists offer aggressive therapy to patients like Yasmin, particularly those as young as she was. However, the medical ethical principle of *nonmaleficence*, in which providers are obligated not to inflict harm intentionally, would seem to question whether chemotherapy in a patient like Yasmin is an appropriate offering.

Rita was also offered successive options for chemotherapy despite ongoing functional decline, to the point that she became entirely dependent for all personal care. Rita met hospice criteria when her cancer continued to progress despite ongoing therapy, at which point she was offered salvage chemotherapy. As with other specialists, patients put great faith in their oncologists. In Rita's case, the oncologist did not discuss end-of-life and hospice care, leaving the question central to this book: Is a decision for treatment made without an accurate understanding of one's medical reality truly adherent to the ethical principle of respect for patient autonomy?

HIV

It is estimated that 40 million people have died from an AIDS-related illness since the beginning of the HIV pandemic in the early 1980s [89]. Currently, an estimated 35 million people are infected with HIV worldwide, most (25 million) living in sub-Saharan Africa [90]. In 2021, 1.5 million people became infected with HIV worldwide, and 650,000 people died from an AIDS-related illness. In the United States, 35,000 people become infected with HIV each year, and in 2019, 5000 Americans died of AIDS [91].

An HIV infection proceeds through three stages [92]. Following initial exposure to the virus, an acute phase (*acute HIV*) occurs when the virus rapidly multiples and attacks the CD4 T lymphocytes, the immune system's primary defense against infections [93]. Until antibody levels become sufficient to control viral replication, during a process called *seroconversion*, patients may experience several weeks of flu-like symptoms and non-life-threatening infections, including shingles, pneumonia, and thrush [93, 94].

Following the acute phase, untreated patients can experience a long, asymptomatic period (*chronic HIV*). As the virus slowly multiplies [92, 93] and their CD4 count gradually declines at a rate of approximately 50 cells/μL per year [90, 94] from a normal range of 500 to 1000 cells/μL [95], patients become susceptible to an evolving variety of opportunistic infections and other conditions not commonly seen in the immunocompetent population [94].

At a CD4 count of 500 cells/μL, patients can experience bacterial infections, tuberculosis (TB), herpes simplex and herpes zoster, vaginal candidiasis, hairy leukoplakia, and Kaposi sarcoma [96]. At a CD4 count of 200 cells/μL, patients can experience *Pneumocystis jiroveci* pneumonia, TB, cryptococcal meningitis, toxoplasmosis, coccidioidomycosis, and cryptosporidiosis [96]. Below a CD4 count of 50 cells/μL, patients frequently experience disseminated *Mycobacterium avium* complex (MAC), histoplasmosis, cytomegalovirus (CMV) retinitis, and lymphoma [96]. The most life-threatening conditions for HIV patients, those occurring at or below a CD4 count of less than 200 cells/μL, and which historically served as hallmarks of end-stage disease, are referred to as *AIDS-defining illnesses* [94].

In addition to these opportunistic conditions, patients with HIV can develop heart disease, kidney disease, hepatobiliary disease, endocrine or rheumatologic disease, blood disorders, and dermatologic conditions [94]. Patients can experience dementia, seizures, and encephalopathy, as well as exhibit cachexia (loss of > 10% of total body weight) in the setting of prolonged (>1 month) diarrhea, a condition known as *wasting syndrome* [96]. Patients also frequently suffer from a host of symptoms, including but not limited to fever, nausea, night sweats, chronic sinusitis, myopathy, and gastroenteritis [96].

Acquired immune deficiency syndrome (AIDS), the terminal phase of an HIV infection, can be diagnosed at a CD4 count of 200 cells/μL or less, or when a patient exhibits an AIDS-defining illness. In the untreated population, the median time for the development of an AIDS-defining illness after the initial infection is 10 years [94], and the median time for the development of an AIDS-defining illness upon reaching a CD4 count of 200 cells/μL is 12 to 18 months [97]. Most untreated patients with AIDS will die within two years [98].

The development of antiretroviral therapy (ART) significantly altered the natural course of an HIV infection [92]. Whereas before ART, all patients with HIV developed AIDS and died from an AIDS-defining illness within a shortened window of time, today, by keeping a patient's viral load at essentially undetectable levels, ART can delay the onset of AIDS by several decades, conferring an average lifespan when started at a CD4 count over 500 cells/μL [99]. Even when started at a CD4 count of 200 cells/μL, ART can bring a patient with AIDS back from the brink, extending their life by 10 years or more [90].

Presently, the course of an individual patient's HIV journey depends on early diagnosis and treatment, which depend on myriad socio-economic factors that, in the end, determine the disease's geographic and demographic distribution [100]. In sub-Saharan Africa, where most of the world's HIV population resides and where 1 in 3 people are infected with tuberculosis [101], AIDS-related illnesses, particularly TB and other opportunistic infections, remain the leading cause of death for patients with HIV [102, 103]. In this area of the world, a co-infection of TB carries a significant risk of mortality, with up to 30% of patients passing away during the initial TB treatment regimen and another 25% of patients passing away during the following year [101].

By contrast, in resource-rich settings, most HIV patients (2 out of 3) no longer die from AIDS but rather from a non-AIDS-related illness, most commonly a non-AIDS-related malignancy, followed by heart disease and liver disease [94, 104].

Today, just 1 in 3 patients with HIV in resource-rich settings die from an AIDS-related illness [105], most commonly non-Hodgkin lymphoma [106]. In resource-rich settings, HIV patients with good adherence to ART can expect a lifespan similar to that of the non-HIV population. However, they will experience fewer healthy years and will develop common comorbidities (heart disease, lung disease, liver disease, and kidney disease) at an earlier age [99].

The HIV hospice criteria is placed here, alongside the Cancer trajectory, because the leading causes of death for patients with a diagnosis of AIDS in both resource-rich and resource-poor settings (AIDS-related malignancies and TB with high risk of mortality, respectively) follow a pattern of significant decline in a short amount of time.

The decline in patients with HIV driven by a non-AIDS-defining comorbidity can be evaluated either with the hospice criteria for the disease driving decline, such as heart failure, or by the hospice criteria for frailty, which will be discussed below.

There are three elements to meeting hospice criteria with HIV [42]:

1. At least one of the following lab values must be severely deranged [42]:

    - CD4 T lymphocyte count < 25 cells/μL
    - Persistent (2 or more assays at least 1 month apart) viral load > 100,000 copies/mL

2. One of the following sequelae must be present, indicating end-stage disease [42]:

    - Central nervous system (CNS) lymphoma, untreated or persistent despite treatment
    - Wasting (loss of at least 10% lean body mass)
    - *Mycobacterium avium* complex (MAC) bacteremia, untreated, unresponsive to treatment, or treatment refused
    - Progressive multifocal leukoencephalopathy
    - Systemic lymphoma with advanced HIV disease and partial response to chemotherapy
    - Visceral Kaposi sarcoma, unresponsive to therapy
    - Kidney failure in the absence of dialysis
    - *Cryptosporidium* infection
    - Toxoplasmosis, unresponsive to therapy

3. The patient's functional status must be declined to a PPS of 50% or lower [42].

To support a picture of a patient meeting hospice criteria with HIV, evidence portending poor prognosis, including life-limiting comorbidities or comorbidities that put patients at risk of poor treatment compliance, should also be documented. This can include any of the following, although none of these items are required [40]:

- Chronic persistent diarrhea for 1 year
- Persistent serum albumin < 2.5 g/dL
- Concomitant, active substance abuse
- Age > 50 years
- Absence of or resistance to effective antiretroviral, chemotherapeutic, or prophylactic drug therapy specifically for HIV disease

- Advanced AIDS dementia complex
- Toxoplasmosis
- Heart failure, NYHA Class IV, symptomatic at rest
- Advanced liver disease

Because patients at an advanced stage of HIV can benefit from initiation of ART, it is recommended that every effort should be made to start all patients on ART, regardless of viral load, CD4 count, or symptomatology. Effective response to ART is monitored by CD4 count recovery: within one to two months following initiation of ART, the CD4 count should increase by at least 50 cells/µL; within one year, the CD4 count should increase by between 100 and 150 cells/µL; and after that, the CD4 count should increase by 50 to 100 cells/µL per year [107].

With little available literature helping to identify patients unlikely to respond to antiretroviral therapy, or detailing prognosis following the development of various AIDS-associated illnesses, clinicians understandably struggle with knowing when to initiate conversations about hospice care [108], with one study indicating very poor alignment of what we know patients want at the end of life and end-of-life care for HIV patients in an urban US setting [109].

Looking at outcomes of 367 HIV patients being cared for in a hospital in Parkland, Texas, researchers found that 28% of patients died while being hospitalized, with just 6% having received a palliative care consultation, less than 10% having documentation of code status, and just 6% experiencing hospice care at the end of their lives. Of those who received hospice care, the average time to death was just 11 days [109], a whole week shorter than the national U.S. median time on hospice care (18 days) [28].

Again, one thing is certain: *if patients are not asked about end-of-life preferences ahead of time, providers cannot align their wishes with their care when that time comes.* Until physicians are better trained to assess disease progression and to have effective goals of care conversations in which they offer hospice care as an appropriate option for patients with advanced disease, earlier and more consistent use of palliative care consultations and follow-up should be a standard part of care for HIV patients.

It seems reasonable to postulate that patients experiencing clinically significant cachexia with a declining or chronically low albumin level, functional decline, advanced interventions (such as tube feeding, dialysis, or mechanical ventilation), treatment resistance disease or sequelae, or advanced comorbidities like heart failure or liver disease—in other words, those who have already made the transition far down the disease trajectory cliff—would be far less likely to benefit from treatment with antiretroviral therapy and therefore, recover from end-stage disease. Further research into the clinical picture of HIV/AIDS patients with a prognosis of less than one year is warranted.

Dementia/Frailty Trajectory (Fig. 5.7)

Dementia

Neurologists and hospice teams evaluate the severity of Alzheimer's dementia using the Functional Assessment Staging of Dementia (FAST) [110], which was introduced in 1988 by Dr. Barry Reisberg, whose long and influential career in dementia research has contributed significantly to our foundational understanding of the

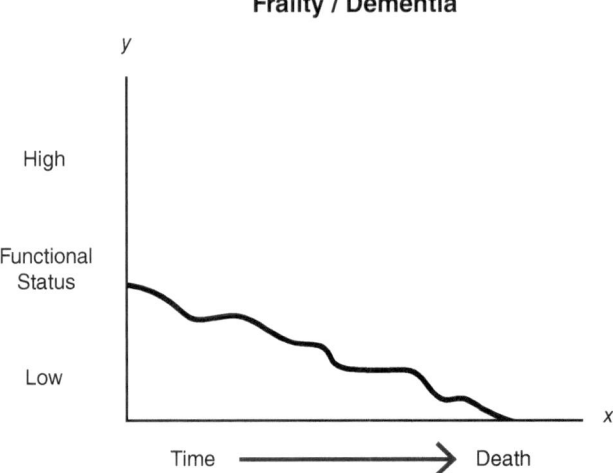

Fig. 5.7 Frailty/Dementia. (Adapted with permission from Lunney et al. (2002). *Profiles of Older Medicare Decedents*. Journal of the American Geriatrics Society [18])

course of Alzheimer's disease and was instrumental in the development of the major approaches and medications used in its treatment [111] (Table 5.8).

The FAST system details the *retrogenesis* [112] process that occurs in Alzheimer's disease, first described by Dr. Reisberg, in which patients *go from infancy to adulthood, in reverse*, losing the skills they gained during development, in roughly the reverse order of acquisition. By asking caregivers whether patients need help with the tasks described at each stage, the FAST scale can be used to clinically assess where a patient is in their dementia journey.

It is important to understand that neither Dr. Reisberg nor I am suggesting that patients *become children* during their dementia journey. Rather, their cognitive processing power declines over the course of their journey, affecting their ability to problem-solve the tasks adults need to navigate successfully to make it through the day on their own. As the stakes become increasingly high for mistakes patients can make along the way, for instance, in handling their finances or medications, caregivers will need to step in to manage patient affairs to keep patients safe, as well as understand that at some point, patients should not be left home alone. By the end of their journey, when patients need assistance with all aspects of living, having lost the ability to walk, talk, smile, and eat, their processing power will decline to that of a dependent infant.

Despite this loss of processing power, each patient brings unique life experiences, life skills, and memories into their journey. As patients lose access to their memories and skills, some even losing the ability to recognize or recall their spouses, they will retain the capacity to read social cues and experience joy, and all patients will maintain an inherent need to experience dignity, as well as a sense of competence, capability, and control over their own lives to an evolving extent. Being armed with the knowledge that dementia is a progressive loss of processing power that

Table 5.8 Functional Assessment Staging (FAST) of Alzheimer's disease

Functional Assessment Staging (FAST)	
Stage	Functional impact
1	No difficulties, either subjectively or objectively
2	Complains of forgetting location of objects. Subjective work difficulties
3	Decreased job functioning evident to co-workers; difficulty in traveling to new locations. Decreased organizational capacity
4	Decreased ability to perform complex tasks (e.g., planning dinner for guests), handling personal finances (forgetting to pay bills), difficulty shopping, etc.
5	Requires assistance in choosing the proper clothing to wear for the day, season, or occasion; patient may wear the same clothing repeatedly, unless supervised
6	A—Difficulty putting clothing on properly without assistance B—Unable to bathe property (e.g., difficulty adjusting bath water temperature) C—Inability to handle mechanics of toileting (e.g., forgets to flush the toilet, does not wipe properly or properly dispose of toilet tissue) D—Urinary incontinence, occasional or more frequent E—Fecal incontinence, occasional or more frequent
7	A—Ability to speak limited to approximately a half dozen different words or fewer, in the course of an average day or in the course of an intensive interview B—Speech ability limited to the use of a single intelligible word in an average day or in the course of an interview (the person may repeat the word over and over) C—Ambulatory ability lost (cannot walk without personal assistance) D—Ability to sit up without assistance lost (e.g., the individual will fall over if there are no lateral rests (arms) on the chair) E—Loss of the ability to smile

Reisberg B, Franssen E, Souren L EM, Kenowsky S, Janjua KS, Veigne SW, Guillo-Benarous F, Singh S, Khizar A, Shah U, Shah RG, Bhandal A, Auer S. Alzheimer's Disease. In: Moroz A, Flanagan SR, Zaretsky H, editors. Medical Aspects of Disability for the Rehabilitation Professional. New York: Springer Publishing Company, LLC; 2017. P. 31–90. Reprinted with permission [113]

robs patients of their ability to manage themselves through their day successfully empowers families to adjust their expectations of their loved ones' capacity and adapt the patients' environments to keep them safe.

Because it can feel cumbersome to discuss seven different stages when describing the dementia journey to patients and families, I have begun instead to describe *four stages of cognitive (clinical) impact*, detailed in the previous chapter (Recent Memory, Cognitive Function, Personal Care, and Physical Function). This descriptive framework can be mapped onto the FAST scale, as shown in Table 5.9.

Research published by Dr. Reisberg and colleagues in 2021 investigating the pattern, severity, and rate of neurodegenerative loss across the Alzheimer's trajectory similarly clumps the FAST stages into the three most important stages of neuronal loss, beginning with FAST 3–4, in which neuronal loss is most severe; FAST 5–6, in which neuronal loss is most rapid; and FAST 7, in which neuronal loss reaches floor level [114].

I have found this simple framework useful when speaking with families. Providing details about the type of memory and specific brain regions impacted as the disease progresses transforms a confusing jumble of experiences into an understandable and ongoing process of loss. Referencing four major stages of cognitive decline allows for individual variation in the timing of specific capacity loss at each

Table 5.9 Four stages of dementia

Cognitive/ clinical impact	Impact on patient capacity, recommendations for caregivers, and appropriate level of care facility support	FAST stage
	No difficulties	1
Recent Memory (mild disease)	Hippocampus impacted	2
	Loss of "short-term memory" (i.e., recent memory, which encodes new pieces of information about personal experience and environment)	
	Patients become poor historians about their own lives; patients should be accompanied by a close family member during appointments	
	Questioning patients about recent events (e.g., what did you eat for breakfast? Who visited last week? When is your dentist appointment?) can force a confrontation with the patient's cognitive deficits, which can leave them feeling incompetent, incapable, and like things are not in their control; understand that when questions are asked, patient responses may not be accurate or reliable	
	Manage tone of voice and facial expression when interacting with patients to support their sense of competence, capability and control, as well as their sense of dignity	
	Many patients can participate in their own advanced care planning at this stage	
Cognitive Function (moderate/ advanced disease)	Cerebral cortex impacted	3
	Loss of logic, reason, abstract thinking, computation, anticipation, planning, judgment, impulse control, self-awareness, etc.	4
	Problems with IADLs (cooking, cleaning, driving, shopping; managing finances, appointments, medications, mealtime, the home, and pets)	
	Ongoing loss of semantic memory and conceptual inventory (words, ideas, language)	
	Efforts to "convince" or "reorient" patients to reality can undermine their sense of competence, capability and control; rather move into the patient's reality, provide reassurance, redirect, and help manage the patient's mood	
	The **Just Do It** stage; because the stakes are high for mistakes at this stage, family members will need to just step in to manage IADLs to keep patients safe	
	Patients will lose their capacity to make complicated medical decisions, including advanced care planning during this stage	
	Independent living can be appropriate if the patient has family or other support to manage IADLs, including medications; however, assisted living with RN support for medication management is the appropriate level of care for patients at this stage who cannot be managed at home	
	At this stage and earlier, discussion of the dementia journey and caregiver needs with the patient present can force a confrontation with the patient's sense of competence, capability, and control, as well as undermine their dignity; support can be provided by meeting with the family without the patient present	

(continued)

Table 5.9 (continued)

Cognitive/ clinical impact	Impact on patient capacity, recommendations for caregivers, and appropriate level of care facility support	FAST stage
Personal Care (severe disease)	Loss of procedural knowledge (e.g., motor-related tasks such as making a sandwich, taking a shower)	5
		6A
	Problems with ADLs (dressing, feeding, bathing, and toileting)	6B
	Problems learning new skills	6C
	Ongoing loss of semantic memory and conceptual inventory (words, ideas, language)	
	Patients should not be left home alone	
	Narrate the present and keep options and instructions simple and concrete (e.g., "Let's get dressed," "Let's have a snack")	
	Although many patients with family support can remain at home throughout their journey, the Personal Care stage can be very taxing on spouses, particularly elderly spouses with limited mobility or other health conditions; memory care, in which patients are kept safe from wandering and have around-the-clock RN support, is appropriate at this stage for patients who cannot be managed at home	
	Hospital-to-rehab cycle often begins at this stage, which can be very distressing to patients and families	
	Many families become hospice minded for their loved ones during this stage	
Physical Function (end-stage disease)	Incontinence (bladder and bowel)	6D
	Cachexia (weight loss)	6E
	Dysphagia leading to aspiration pneumonia	7A
	Falls and fractures	7B
	Recurrent infections (UTIs, aspiration pneumonia, sepsis)	7C
	Escalations of care are increasingly likely at this stage; family are very likely to be hospice minded at this stage	7D
		7E
	Hospice care is appropriate at this stage	

Four stages of cognitive/clinical impact of dementia as related to the Functional Assessment Staging (FAST) of Alzheimer's disease

stage, avoiding the incorrect assumption implied by the FAST scale that patients make a linear progression through the dementia journey [115]. Tying the required cognitive capacities to their corresponding real-world skills prepares families to recognize and intervene as capacity is lost, providing a focus for caregiver support where the stakes are highest and empowering families to better appreciate the appropriate level of care that a patient might need at a care facility. Finally, because patient symptoms can be so taxing on caregivers, recommendations for supportive and loving interactions are strengthened when caregivers understand the *why* behind the patient's difficulties, transforming caregiver expectations, and as a result, alleviating their stress and strain. Ultimately, this framework provides a very clear picture of dementia progression, allowing families to anticipate care needs, adapt to changing circumstances, and prevent avoidable crises. Language for explaining this framework to family members is provided in Chap. 15.

Patients with dementia typically experience a disease course lasting 8 to 10 years, with a median survival time following a diagnosis of Alzheimer's disease of 4 to 5 years and a median survival time following a diagnosis of Lewy body and frontotemporal dementia of 2.9 to 3.9 years [116]. Patient prognosis varies according to age at diagnosis [117], how far into the dementia journey a patient is diagnosed, and the presence of significant comorbidities such as heart failure and COPD. Diagnosis is often missed until well into the journey because the disease masks itself so well, and the medical community is not well-trained to understand, recognize, or evaluate its presence and severity.

There are two elements to meeting hospice criteria with Alzheimer's disease [42]:

1. Patients must be FAST Stage 7 or beyond [42]

   To this element, CMS adds that patients must show all of the following characteristics [42]:

   - Unable to walk without assistance
   - Unable to dress without assistance
   - Unable to bathe without assistance
   - Urinary and fecal incontinence, intermittent or constant
   - No consistently meaningful verbal communication; stereotypical phrases only or the ability to speak is limited to 6 or fewer intelligible words

   Of note, a patient meeting these criteria would technically be FAST 7C, unable to ambulate without assistance.

2. At least one of the following medical complications must be documented within the past 12 months, indicating end-stage disease [42]:

   - Aspiration pneumonia
   - Pyelonephritis
   - Septicemia
   - Multiple stage 3 to 4 decubitus ulcers
   - Recurrent fever after antibiotics
   - Inability to maintain sufficient fluid and calorie intake

     ▪ $\geq 10\%$ weight loss over the previous 6 months, or
     ▪ Serum album < 2.5 g/dL.

As currently written, the hospice criteria for dementia require that a patient experiences disease progression to the point of needing assistance with ambulation *as well as* clinically significant weight loss or some other significant sequelae of metabolic decline, including infections typically identified only during a hospitalization (aspiration pneumonia, sepsis, and pyelonephritis). For many patients, this will be far too late into their journey to benefit from the entire six months of hospice care allowed by CMS. Indeed, studies show that requiring patients to advance in their journey to FAST 7C misses the 6-month prognosis mark [115, 118].

Many patients with dementia will show a metabolic shift with clinically significant weight loss, portending poor prognosis *before* losing their ambulatory ability. This metabolic shift puts patients at risk of life-limiting complications, like sepsis and hip fractures, *independently* of complications from ongoing neuronal loss (e.g., brainstem degradation leading to loss of the swallow reflex leading to aspiration pneumonia).

Families of patients with dementia, when appropriately educated about disease progression, including the end-stage sequelae and accompanying risk of hospitalizations, often become hospice minded for their loved ones well before FAST 7, preferring to avoid hospital admissions or rehab stays and keep their loved ones at home or in their familiar care facility setting. Noting how the disease so dramatically limits the patient's quality of life, families who are well-educated about disease course readily sign DNR orders and specify that they are *ready to allow nature to take its course when the time comes*, not wanting advanced interventions intended only to prolong the patient's life, usually long before the patient meets hospice criteria. When families become hospice minded in their loved one's dementia journey, the medical community should be empowered to support them with hospice care.

Furthermore, because the dementia journey toward the end so dramatically diminishes patients' quality of life, leading caregivers and families to become hospice minded for patients long before they meet hospice criteria by current guidelines, CMS policy for hospice reimbursement should be retooled to cover hospice care for patients with dementia whose families become hospice minded for them, regardless of prognosis.

More than any other disease, dementia highlights the importance of the medical community shifting its focus from acute stabilization to broader recognition and assessment of disease progression and patient decline. When it is understood that dementia is an ongoing and progressive loss of capacity to make it through the day without help, it becomes much easier to recognize the disease and stage its baseline and recent progression during a hospital admission. Whereas it has been suggested that it can be challenging to differentiate between delirium (an altered state of consciousness characterized by confusion and disorientation that is often associated with acute illness) and dementia and that sepsis increases the risk of dementia [119], I would suggest that these and similar problems are a matter of perspective that can be resolved with a better understanding of the dementia journey.

By appropriately staging a patient's dementia baseline clinically, that is, through a conversation investigating patient capacity and need for assistance at home, we can make sense of a patient's confusion during a hospitalization, either understanding it as consistent with the patient's baseline (dementia) or identifying when it is not (delirium). Likewise, recognizing a patient's dementia baseline and any recent progression allows for better contextualization of expected sequelae, such as sepsis, a hip fracture, aspiration pneumonia, weight and appetite loss, or poor wound healing. Recognizing these events as an expected part of end-stage dementia should prompt the medical community to evaluate the patient's cognitive baseline and recent decline and evaluate the patient's status against dementia hospice criteria to position the patient's disease along its trajectory accurately.

Recall John, age 93, from Chaps. 2 and 3, whose pneumonia was relatively easy to recognize as a sign of end-stage dementia, given his bowel and bladder incontinence, limited speech, need for assistance with all ADLs, and 20% total body weight loss in the preceding 12 months. Although John met hospice criteria at admission and likely had for several months, the hospitalist, missing the forest for the trees, had intended to discharge John to a rehabilitation center, a distressing and likely nonbeneficial event. Once John's son appropriately understood what his father had been experiencing and where in the dementia journey John was, John's son readily expressed hospice mindedness for his dad and we were able to discharge John home with hospice care.

Recall Dale from the previous chapter in the section on Dementia. On admission, Dale exhibited end-stage metabolic sequelae, including UTI-related sepsis, frequent falls, and a diminished functional status with a PPS of 40%. Dale had likely met hospice criteria for several months, given his significant weight loss (20% of his total body weight) in the previous three months, bowel and bladder incontinence (which had started six months prior), and albumin of 2.2 g/dL. As with John's son, helping Dale's wife to understand the progressive nature of the disease she had witnessed so closely over the previous 10 years empowered her to choose hospice care, aligning her wishes for her husband's quality of life with his medical care.

ALS

Amyotrophic lateral sclerosis (ALS) is a progressive and eventually terminal motor neuron disease (MND) caused by the destruction of upper and lower motor neurons. Resulting skeletal muscle denervation affects the upper and lower limbs, diaphragm, and oral apparatus, leading to functional loss across four domains: respiratory (breathing), bulbar (speech, salivation, and swallowing), fine motor (e.g., handwriting), and gross motor (e.g., walking) [120]. Although patients retain control of their bowel and bladder, progressive weakness, muscle atrophy, and wasting lead to increasing dependence for all aspects of daily living until, eventually, most patients succumb to respiratory failure [121]. Cognitive impairment affects up to 50% of patients with ALS, with up to 15% of patients exhibiting frontotemporal dementia [122].

Whereas a minority of cases (10%) are inherited, most (90%) are sporadic, with familial disease tending to present at an earlier age (47–52 years) than sporadic disease (58–63 years) [123]. Overall, ALS patients exhibit a median survival time of 30 months, with prognosis decreasing with older age of onset [123]. Approximately 30,000 Americans are living with ALS, with approximately 5000 Americans newly diagnosed each year [124].

A diagnosis of ALS is made using the El Escorial World Federation of Neurology criteria, adopted in 1990, which requires the presence of both upper and lower motor neuron symptoms, progression from one body region to another, and the absence of evidence of an alternative diagnosis [125].

Although not yet adopted by the neurology community, a staging system proposed by Roche and colleagues in 2012 reveals valuable information about ALS progression and prognosis [120] (Table 5.10).

Looking at the timing of important milestones across the ALS journey, Roche and colleagues found that regardless of the total time from symptom onset to death, patients exhibited predictable intervals of progression across the journey. Approximately one-third of total disease course (35%) was experienced before diagnosis, with symptoms initially constrained to one body region (bulbar, respiratory, upper limbs, or lower limbs). At approximately 38% into disease course,

Table 5.10 ALS staging system proposed by Roche et al. 2012

Proposed staging system for ALS	
ALS stage	Description
1	Symptom onset (involvement of first region)
2A	Diagnosis
2B	Involvement of a second region
3	Involvement of a third region
4A	Need for gastrostomy
4B	Need for respiratory support (non-invasive ventilation)

Roche JC, Rojas-Garcia R, Scott KM, Scotton W, Ellis CE, Burman R, Wijesekera L, Turner MR, Leigh PN, Shaw CE, Al-Chalabi A. A proposed staging system for amyotrophic lateral sclerosis. Brain. 2012 Mar;135(Pt 3):847–52. doi: 10.1093/brain/awr351. Epub 2012 Jan 23. PMID: 22271664; PMCID: PMC3286327. Reprinted with permission [120]

patients developed symptoms in a second region, followed by a third region at approximately 61% of disease course. The need for feeding tube and ventilator support occurred close together, at approximately 77% and 80% into disease course, respectively. Most patients (75%) exhibited limb symptoms at presentation, with a minority (25%) exhibiting bulbar symptoms at onset [120]. No patients in the Roche study exhibited respiratory symptoms at onset, a rare presentation with a very poor prognosis [121].

Although researchers found that the need for feeding tube or ventilator support occurred close together in time and indicated very advanced disease, variability in the timing of these supports depended on the pattern of symptom onset. Whereas patients with bulbar onset were found to need feeding tube support before ventilator support, those with limb onset were found to need ventilator support before a feeding tube [120].

In addition to the difficulties with oral intake created by bulbar dysfunction, patients with ALS have been found to exhibit a hypermetabolic state at rest, which increases weight loss and skeletal muscle wasting [126]. As with other disease trajectories, significant weight loss in the setting of ALS increases mortality risk [127, 128]. Nutritional support, including placement of a feeding tube, should occur before lung capacity declines to a forced vital capacity (FVC) level of 50% or less, a level of lung dysfunction that independently increases mortality risk in patients with ALS [128].

The need for ventilation support is determined by symptoms (dyspnea and orthopnea) and evidence of worsening lung function as determined by pulmonary function testing or bloodwork (arterial blood gas) [123]. With declining respiratory function, patients are initially offered non-invasive ventilation support with NIPPV (non-invasive positive pressure ventilation), which has been found to prolong survival time by a median of 205 days and to increase patient quality of life [129]. As respiratory muscles continue to weaken, or for those unable to tolerate non-invasive ventilation due to excessive salivation in the setting of impaired swallowing, invasive ventilation with tracheostomy can be offered. Although tracheostomy has also been shown to prolong survival, this option reduces patient quality of life [123] and increases demand on caregivers.

Functional status can be monitored using the Revised Amyotrophic Lateral Sclerosis Functional Rating Scale (ALSFRS-R), which evaluates function across the primary skeletal muscle domains impacted by ALS (bulbar, respiratory, fine motor, gross motor) [130]. Because faster progression is associated with increased mortality risk, awareness of a patient's rate of functional loss is critical to anticipating both patient and caregiver needs [129].

There are two paths to meeting hospice criteria with ALS, including *critically impaired breathing capacity* and *severe nutritional insufficiency* [42].

Critically Impaired Breathing Capacity   To meet criteria in this manner, patients who do not elect tracheostomy and invasive ventilation must exhibit critically impaired respiratory function (with or without noninvasive positive pressure ventilation (NIPPV)), defined by [42]

- Forced vital capacity (FVC) < 40% predicted (seated or supine), along with 2 or more of the following symptoms and/or signs:
    - Dyspnea (shortness of breath) at rest
    - Orthopnea (shortness of breath when lying down that is relieved by sitting or standing)
    - Use of accessory respiratory musculature
    - Paradoxical abdominal motion
    - Respiratory rate > 20/minute
    - Reduced speech/vocal volume
    - Weakened cough
    - Symptoms of sleep-disordered breathing
    - Frequent awakening
    - Daytime somnolence/excessive daytime sleepiness
    - Unexplained headaches
    - Unexplained confusion
    - Unexplained anxiety
    - Unexplained nausea

Patients who are unable to perform vital capacity tests meet the criteria if they manifest three or more of the above symptoms/signs.

To this element, CMS adds:

These revised criteria rely less on the measured FVC and, as such, reflect the reality that not all patients with ALS can or will undergo routine pulmonary function testing [42].

Severe Nutritional Insufficiency   To meet criteria in this manner, patients must exhibit [42]:

- Dysphagia (difficulty swallowing) with progressive weight loss of at least 5% of body weight
- With or without election for gastrostomy tube insertion

The hospice criteria for ALS are quite elegant, simple, and easy to remember. Insofar as they do not restrict patients from receiving tube feeding or ventilator support and require minimal weight loss (5% as opposed to 10% of total body weight) but without the end-stage sequelae of metabolic decline (e.g., sepsis, aspiration pneumonia, or stage 3 or 4 decubitus ulcers), these criteria appropriately identify the point at which the terminal phase of the ALS journey begins—at the need for extracorporeal respiratory or nutritional support.

No part of the hospice criteria for ALS prevents patients from receiving tube feeding or ventilator support while also receiving hospice care. However, such services and supplies will likely exhaust the daily hospice reimbursement amount CMS provides, and for this reason, hospice services may be unable to provide these services for patients in their care. Although patients who wish to continue with tube feeds or ventilator support while enrolled in hospice care have the option of paying for the services and supplies on their own, this is usually cost-prohibitive for families.

Frailty

In line with its linguistic definition, medically speaking, frailty is a condition of weakness and physiologic dysfunction that leaves patients vulnerable to internal and external stressors. When we talk about patients having or not having *reserve* to withstand or recover from an illness or insult, we are talking about whether their bodies have shifted into a state of frailty [131].

Per the 2012 Frailty Consensus Conference, frailty is defined as [132]:

> A medical syndrome with multiple causes and contributors that is characterized by diminished strength, endurance, and reduced physiologic function that increases an individual's vulnerability for developing increased dependency and/or death.

Frailty results from the aging process, wherein accumulated cellular and molecular damage that outpaces the body's ability to self-repair leads to organ and system decline, resulting in the inability to compensate in the face of physical or psychosocial challenges. Affecting the brain, endocrine system, immune system, and skeletal muscle [131], frailty leads to weight loss, loss of strength and speed, and decline in energy level and physical activity [132]. As stated earlier, it is in the context of frailty that patients often fall and break a hip (femur) or humerus. In addition to increasing the risk of falls, frailty increases patient risk of hospitalizations, trips to rehab, and death [131].

At a metabolic level, patients with frailty can experience sarcopenia (loss of muscle mass associated with aging) and cachexia (loss of weight in the setting of a chronic illness), both of which are complex metabolic changes associated with chronic disease [133], and which are not easily differentiated in a single patient. Both conditions can lead to muscle loss, weakness, anorexia, and functional limitations. In patients able to tolerate physical exertion, sarcopenia can be treated with resistance exercise and physical therapy [134], whereas currently, there is no effective treatment for cachexia [133]. As stated earlier, cachexia is seen in every terminal disease trajectory and is an indication that disease is advanced, serving as an indicator of poor prognosis.

As a clinical syndrome, frailty can sometimes improve with physical therapy and nutritional support [132]. Where things get complicated, and I believe why frailty in the elderly population can be so difficult for physicians to navigate, is that it can be challenging to know whose metabolic dysfunction is yet amenable to intervention—that is, whose muscle mass, weight loss, and functional decline are being caused by sarcopenia versus cachexia.

Not surprisingly, while various definitions and tools have been developed to assess patient frailty [132], the medical community has yet to adopt a single diagnostic criterion or instrument, and importantly, no diagnostic criteria exist to acknowledge a state of frailty that cannot be reversed. In clinical practice, frailty, like functional decline, is often ignored in a medical system ill-prepared to recognize disease progression and decline.

This is unfortunate because, as an approach to the end of life, Frailty is incredibly common. In their research revealing the patterns of terminal decline, in which they looked at 0.1% of all Medicare decedents between the years 1993 and 1998, researchers Lunney, Lynn, and Hogan found that Frailty was the most common end-of-life trajectory, experienced by 47% of decedents, followed by Cancer (22%), Organ Failure (16%), and Sudden Death (7%) [18]. As the world's population of those over 65 increases from nearly half a billion to an expected 2 billion by 2050 [131], I cannot emphasize enough how important it is that the medical community be trained to acknowledge, assess, and contextualize this prevalent end-of-life approach.

In my personal practice, I refer to this trajectory as *age-related decline*, something that readily resonates with patients and families who often answer my inquiry, "How are you making sense of the changes you've been experiencing?" by stating the obvious, "I'm old."

Although some research suggests that the term *frailty of old age* is ageist and that, for this reason, the terms *old age* or *debility of old age* should not be listed as causes of death on death certificates [135], I believe such research, based on opinions of medical providers likely not well-trained in the end-of-life trajectories, misses the mark of acknowledging that a patient without another apparent cause of terminal decline will, at some biological point, reach their own shelf life. The fact remains that frailty *is* associated with increasing age, practically speaking, by definition. Frailty is not a condition of the young.

While it is undoubtedly true that specific age is not a determinant of frailty, each of us, in the absence of another progressive and terminal condition, would reach a point *eventually* where our metabolism would shift, we would begin to wither away, and we would pass away naturally. Merely because this metabolic shift would occur at a different age for each of us does not mean that labeling it as a condition associated with advanced age is erroneous or discriminatory. The medical community must come to terms with the fact that all of our patients, at some point, will follow their body's plan, not ours, declining despite our most optimistic interventions. This is natural and expected and should be embraced.

Qualifying patients on the Frailty trajectory for hospice care can be challenging. As stated earlier, there are no specific hospice criteria for patients without comorbidities who are reaching the end of their lives, like my grandmother did, by simply *dying of old age*. CMS has repeatedly rejected my hospice center's claims for patients being qualified for hospice with a diagnosis of *severe protein-calorie malnutrition*, an ICD-10 code that serves as a stand-in for cachexia, *unless we specify that this condition is occurring in the setting of an advanced comorbidity*, such as COPD, heart failure, diabetes, cancer, or dementia.

For patients without comorbidities, meeting hospice criteria requires that they progress so far into terminal decline that they become imminently terminal, most usually by becoming bedbound with minimal oral intake or by suffering a catastrophic event like a fall and hip fracture, from which they are unable to recover. With minimal time remaining, such patients will have long since passed the six-month prognosis mark by the time a referral to hospice is made, missing their opportunity to benefit fully from the high level of care and comfort that hospice services can provide at the end of their lives.

Recall my grandmother and patients Charles, Bernice, and Virginia, whom we encountered in the previous chapter in the section on Frailty. Each patient likely began their terminal phase of life months before their deaths, around the time that their weight loss reached 5% to 10% of total body weight. Earlier referrals to palliative care for symptom assessment and conversations about medical wishes could potentially have led to earlier transitions to hospice care, helping them avoid the crisis-level hospital admissions that they each experienced in the final days to weeks of life.

Non-Disease-Specific Hospice Guidelines Plus Comorbidities

Patients on the Frailty trajectory with at least one impactful comorbidity can be qualified for hospice using the *non-disease-specific* criteria [43]. This set of criteria can be used for patients whose metabolic dysfunction and resulting frailty is the predominant driver of their decline but who are also showing signs, symptoms, or laboratory evidence of advanced comorbid conditions such as heart failure, peripheral vascular disease, liver or kidney failure, metastatic cancer, neurodegenerative disease, dementia, or severe autoimmune disease. Of note, CMS does not specify how many of the components of this criteria are required for qualification in this manner [43].

This criteria set is split into Part I. Decline in Clinical Status Guidelines and Part II. Non-disease-Specific Baseline Guidelines [43].

Part I. Decline in Clinical Status Guidelines [43]

Functional status decline:

- Decline in PPS due to progression of disease
- Progression to dependence on assistance with 2 or more activities of daily living (feeding, ambulation, continence, transfer, bathing, dressing)

Metabolic status decline:

Progressive inanition (fatigue due to lack of nutritional intake) as documented by:

- Weight loss of at least 10% of body weight in the prior 6 months, not due to reversible causes (e.g., depression or use of diuretics)
- Decreasing anthropomorphic measurements (mid-arm circumference, abdominal girth), not due to reversible causes (e.g., depression or use of diuretics)
- Observation of ill-fitting clothes, decrease in skin turgor, increasing skin folds, or other observation of weight loss in a patient without a documented weight
- Decreasing serum albumin or cholesterol
- Dysphagia leading to recurrent aspiration and/or inadequate oral intake documented by decreasing food portion consumption

Evidence of end-stage sequelae of metabolic decline:

- Recurrent or intractable serious infections, such as pneumonia, sepsis, or pyelonephritis
- Progressive stage 3 or 4 pressure ulcers despite optimal care
- History of increasing emergency department visits, hospitalizations, or clinician visits related to the hospice primary diagnosis prior to election of the hospice benefit

Symptoms:

- Dyspnea with increasing respiratory rate
- Cough, intractable
- Nausea or vomiting poorly responsive to treatment
- Diarrhea, intractable
- Pain requiring increasing doses of narcotic pain medications more than briefly

Signs:

- Decline in systolic blood pressure to below 90 or progressive postural hypotension
- Ascites
- Venous, arterial, or lymphatic obstruction due to local progression or metastatic disease
- Edema
- Pleural or pericardial effusion
- Weakness
- Change in level of consciousness

Laboratory evidence of disease progression (when available; lab testing is not required to establish hospice eligibility):

- Increasing pCO_2 or decreasing pO_2 or decreasing SaO_2

- Increasing calcium, creatinine, or liver function studies
- Increasing tumor markers (e.g., CEA, PSA)
- Progressively decreasing or increasing serum sodium or increasing serum potassium

Dementia progression:

- Progressive decline in FAST for dementia (worsening from 7A on the FAST)

Part II. Non-Disease-Specific Baseline Guidelines [43]

Patients must exhibit both:

- Decline in PPS to < 70%
- Dependence on assistance for 2 or more activities of daily living (feeding, ambulation, continence, transfer, bathing, dressing)

Patients must exhibit the presence of a comorbid disease (not the primary hospice diagnosis) that is likely to contribute to a life expectancy of 6 months or less

- Chronic obstructive pulmonary disease (COPD)
- Congestive heart failure
- Ischemic heart disease
- Diabetes mellitus
- Neurologic disease (stroke, ALS, multiple sclerosis, Parkinson's disease)
- Renal failure
- Liver disease
- Neoplasia
- Acquired immunodeficiency syndrome (AIDS/HIV)
- Dementia
- Refractory severe autoimmune disease (e.g., systemic lupus erythematosus (SLE) or rheumatoid arthritis)

To these components, CMS adds the following commentary [43]:

- A patient will be considered to have a life expectancy of 6 months and be eligible for hospice services if they meet the criteria for BOTH the above non-disease-specific baseline guidelines AND disease-specific guidelines.
- These baseline guidelines do not independently qualify a patient for hospice coverage. Refer to separate table for disease-specific guidelines to be used with these guidelines.

These statements indicate that a patient can be eligible for hospice care by meeting the criteria in Part II: Non-Disease-Specific Baseline Guidelines *plus* the disease-specific criteria for the diagnosis driving decline, but not by meeting the criteria of Part II alone, rendering the usefulness of this set of criteria somewhat limited.

In clinical practice, my hospice center has been able to qualify patients using this set of criteria by stating that the patient has *severe protein-calorie malnutrition in the setting of X (wherein X is an advanced disease with a terminal trajectory),* and by painting a picture of declining functional and metabolic status, increasing dependence for care, and worsening symptomatology. Given the reality that 80% of Americans over 65 have at least one chronic disease (with 70% having more than one), the non-disease-specific hospice criteria have the potential to catch most patients on the Frailty trajectory as they approach the end of life [136]. By providing a wide range of possible signs, symptoms, laboratory evidence, manifestations of clinical status decline, and a long list of comorbid conditions, this set of criteria provides a great deal of leeway in qualifying frail patients for hospice care.

Furthermore, highlighting the impact of cachexia (and frailty) on patient prognosis, the non-disease-specific hospice criteria potentially allow patients with organ failure, dementia, and cancer to be qualified at an earlier stage of decline than they could otherwise be qualified by using the disease-specific criteria. For example, a frail patient with heart failure who does not yet meet criteria with heart disease but who has lost 10% of their total body weight in recent months and who is exhibiting increasing dependence, fatigue, falls, and worsening appetite could be qualified by this approach, as could a patient with dementia FAST 6E with 10% of total body weight loss in the prior 12 months, as well as a patient with stage III cancer with functional, physical, and metabolic decline.

The non-disease-specific hospice criteria can also qualify patients whose comorbid conditions driving decline are not otherwise defined in the disease-specific hospice criteria. For example, a patient in my care was qualified with the autoimmune disease systemic lupus erythematosus (SLE), one of the conditions included in the comorbidity list in Part II of the non-disease-specific criteria, but for which no disease-specific criteria have been developed. This patient's SLE had caused multiple organs to fail, including the heart, liver, and kidneys. Although the patient did not meet hospice criteria by any single organ failure criteria, the patient's frequent hospitalizations and rehabilitation stays, refractory ascites and edema, worsening labs (liver function, albumin, and creatinine), and increasing need for assistance with transfers, ambulation, and other aspects of daily living easily allowed the patient to qualify.

Another patient with refractory lymphedema, whose weeping skin developed ongoing infections due to poor wound healing and whose albumin had declined below 3.0 g/dL (contributing both to poor healing and refractory edema), was qualified despite lymphedema not being included as an applicable diagnosis anywhere in the hospice criteria.

Despite the flexibility built into the non-disease-specific criteria, many of the components related to end-stage sequelae, including intractable infections, sepsis, advanced ulcers, and recurrent hospitalizations, typically occur much closer to death than six months out, putting patients at risk of being referred to hospice care far too late in their journeys.

Whole-Person Care and the Need to Un-Silo Medicine

As medicine has become increasingly specialized, conferring the benefits of a seemingly endless body of knowledge, physicians have, understandably, become myopic, and our modern practice of medicine, instead of being unified by a central dogma of whole-person care, has become increasingly siloed.

It is not at all uncommon to encounter patients with dementia who are being cared for by three or more specialists, each handling a different aspect of their diagnosis—a psychiatrist, neurologist, sleep medicine specialist, and psychologist separately treating patients' anxiety, hallucinations, insomnia, and depression, respectively. Too many cooks in the kitchen, with none acting as master chefs, often fail to recognize that the patient's various symptoms point to related aspects of their disease, for instance, the psychiatric symptoms one expects with dementia. This can leave patients and families struggling with poorly controlled symptoms, confusing polypharmacy, unappreciated disease progression, and, not uncommonly, conflicting messaging about the primary diagnosis. Despite being brain specialists, behavioral health providers, including psychiatrists, do not seem to be well-trained to recognize, assess, and support a diagnosis of dementia, which typically falls under the purview of neurologists. Patients and families, understandably, can feel helpless and stuck in this mire of medical care. Left to struggle on the sidelines of a disease wreaking havoc at center stage, they are often unprepared for the arrival of the final act, and with no lookout monitoring the forest for the trees, patients and loved ones can quickly be engulfed by flames.

To make medical choices that appropriately align their wishes with their medical care, patients and families need accurate and integrated assessments of their disease and decline. Treatment options should be discussed in a way that *accurately* reflects risk and possible outcomes, given the patient's present condition. An offer of chemotherapy, for example, to a patient who has already declined 90% of the way down the cancer trajectory cliff should be made with an honest discussion about the inherent risk of the treatment pushing the patient the rest of the way down the hill, leading to their imminent death. Patients and caregivers alike should be supported early in the course of disease with *appropriate* and *detailed education* about disease, disease progression, and the end of a journey. Rather than being surprised that the end is near, patients and families should be armed with end-of-life milestones so that they can plan, handle affairs, and make medical choices that accurately reflect their values as their quality of life and functional status change.

The palliative care approach embraced here is the course correction needed in medicine today. Based on a rich understanding of the end of life, this approach requires that providers are prepared to take a bird's eye view of a patient's circumstance; identify the disease driving patient decline; evaluate the patient's condition against hospice criteria; contextualize any metabolic, functional, and physical decline; and collaboratively discuss treatment options, priorities, and values with patients and families. Having covered the terminal trajectories and hospice criteria, we will next learn the conversational ingredients to create a safe space for collaborative and compassionate conversations.

References

1. Hamel L, Wu B, Brodie M. Views and experiences with end-of-life medical care in the U.S. 2017. https://files.kff.org/attachment/Report-Views-and-Experiences-with-End-of-Life-Medical-Care-in-the-US. Accessed 9 Jul 2022.

2. McDermott KW, Roemer M. Most frequent principal diagnoses for inpatient stays in U.S. Hospitals, 2018. 2021. https://www.hcup-us.ahrq.gov/reports/statbriefs/sb277-Top-Reasons-Hospital-Stays-2018.pdf. Accessed 12 Jun 2022.
3. Heart Disease. 2022. https://www.cdc.gov/nchs/fastats/heart-disease.htm. Accessed 15 Jun 2022.
4. Murphy SL, Kochanek KD, Xu J, Arias E. Mortality in the United States, 2020. 2021. https://www.cdc.gov/nchs/products/databriefs/db427.htm. Accessed 12 Jun 2022.
5. Emanuel EJ. Palliative and end-of-life care. In: Longo DL, Kasper DL, Jameson JL, Fauci AS, Hauser SL, Loscalzo J, editors. Harrison's principles of internal medicine. New York: McGraw-Hill, Health Professions Division; 1998. p. 67–84.
6. Lynn J. Living long in fragile health: the new demographics shape end of life care. Hastings Cent Rep. 2005:S14–8. https://doi.org/10.1353/hcr.2005.0096.
7. Rabow MW, Pantilat SZ. Palliative care & pain management. In: McPhee SJ, Papadakis MA, Rabow MW, editors. 2012 Current medical diagnosis & treatment. New York: McGraw-Hill Medical; 2012. p. 74–92.
8. Thomas K, Wilson JA, GSF Team. National Gold Standards Framework Centre in end of life care. 6th ed. GSF PIG; 2016. http://www.goldstandardsframework.org.uk.
9. Ferrell BR, Temel JS, Temin S, Alesi ER, Balboni TA, Basch EM, Firn JI, Paice JA, Peppercorn JM, Phillips T, Stovall EL, Zimmermann C, Smith TJ. Integration of palliative care into standard oncology care: American Society of Clinical Oncology clinical practice guideline update. J Clin Oncol. 2017;35(1):96–112. Epub 2016 Oct 28. https://doi.org/10.1200/JCO.2016.70.1474.
10. Carey I, Shouls S, Bristowe K, et al. Improving care for patients whose recovery is uncertain. The AMBER care bundle: design and implementation. BMJ Support Palliat Care. 2015;5:12–8.
11. Ernecoff NC, Abdel-Kader K, Cai M, Yabes J, Shah N, Schell JO, Jhamb M. Implementation of surprise question assessments using the electronic health record in older adults with advanced CKD. Kidney360. 2021;2(6):966–73. https://doi.org/10.34067/KID.0007062020.
12. Warm EJ. Fast facts and concepts #30 prognostication. 4th ed. Palliative Care Network of Wisconsin; 2015. https://www.mypcnow.org/wp-content/uploads/2019/01/FF-30-Prognostication.-3rd-Ed.pdf. Accessed 9 Jul 2022.
13. Christakis NA, Lamont EB. Extent and determinants of error in doctors' prognoses in terminally ill patients: prospective cohort study. BMJ. 2000;320(7233):469–72. PMID: 10678857; PMCID: PMC27288. https://doi.org/10.1136/bmj.320.7233.469.
14. Downar J, Goldman R, Pinto R, Englesakis M, Adhikari NK. The "surprise question" for predicting death in seriously ill patients: a systematic review and meta-analysis. CMAJ. 2017;189(13):E484–93. PMID: 28385893; PMCID: PMC5378508.
15. White N, Kupeli N, Vickerstaff V, Stone P. How accurate is the 'Surprise Question' at identifying patients at the end of life? A systematic review and meta-analysis. BMC Med. 2017;15(1):139. PMID: 28764757; PMCID: PMC5540432. https://doi.org/10.1186/s12916-017-0907-4.
16. Riley GF, Lubitz JD. Long-term trends in medicare payments in the last year of life. Health Serv Res. 2010;45(2):565–76. Epub 2010 Feb 9. PMID: 20148984; PMCID: PMC2838161. https://doi.org/10.1111/j.1475-6773.2010.01082.x.
17. Duncan I, Ahmed T, Dove H, Maxwell TL. Medicare cost at end of life. Am J Hosp Palliat Care. 2019;36(8):705–10. Epub 2019 Mar 18. PMID: 30884954; PMCID: PMC6610551.
18. Lunney JR, Lynn J, Hogan C. Profiles of older medicare decedents. J Am Geriatr Soc. 2002;50(6):1108–12. https://doi.org/10.1046/j.1532-5415.2002.50268.x.
19. Unroe KT, Greiner MA, Hernandez AF, Whellan DJ, Kaul P, Schulman KA, Peterson ED, Curtis LH. Resource use in the last 6 months of life among medicare beneficiaries with heart failure, 2000-2007. Arch Intern Med. 2011;171(3):196–203. Epub 2010 Oct 11. https://doi.org/10.1001/archinternmed.2010.371.

20. Teno JM, Gozalo PL, Bynum JP, Leland NE, Miller SC, Morden NE, Scupp T, Goodman DC, Mor V. Change in end-of-life care for Medicare beneficiaries: site of death, place of care, and health care transitions in 2000, 2005, and 2009. JAMA. 2013;309(5):470–7. PMID: 23385273; PMCID: PMC3674823. https://doi.org/10.1001/jama.2012.207624.

21. Cardona-Morrell M, Kim JCH, Turner RM, Anstey M, Mitchell IA, Hillman K. Non-beneficial treatments in hospital at the end of life: a systematic review on extent of the problem. International J Qual Health Care. 2016;28(4):456–69. https://doi.org/10.1093/intqhc/mzw060.

22. Lam MB, Zheng J, Orav EJ, Jha AK. Early accountable care organization results in end-of-life spending among cancer patients. J Natl Cancer Inst. 2019;111(12):1307–13. PMID: 30859226; PMCID: PMC6910163. https://doi.org/10.1093/jnci/djz033.

23. Kannan S, Song Z. Utilization, prices, and outcomes in intensive care units. Am J Respir Crit Care Med. 2023;207:A4213.

24. Einav L, Finkelstein A, Mullainathan S, Obermeyer Z. Predictive modeling of U.S. health care spending in late life. Science. 2018;360(6396):1462–5. PMID: 29954980; PMCID: PMC6038121. https://doi.org/10.1126/science.aar5045.

25. Siddiq Z. ChatGPT and beyond: how artificial intelligence is shaping the future of nursing home operations. 2023. https://skillednursingnews.com/2023/06/chatgpt-and-beyond-how-artificial-intelligence-is-shaping-the-future-of-nursing-home-operations/. Accessed 9 Aug 2023.

26. Jiang LY, Liu XC, Nejatian NP, et al. Health system-scale language models are all-purpose prediction engines. Nature. 2023;619:357–62. https://doi.org/10.1038/s41586-023-06160-y.

27. Rhee C, Jones TM, Hamad Y, Pande A, Varon J, O'Brien C, Anderson DJ, Warren DK, Dantes RB, Epstein L, Klompas M, Centers for Disease Control and Prevention (CDC) Prevention Epicenters Program. Prevalence, underlying causes, and preventability of sepsis-associated mortality in US Acute Care Hospitals. JAMA Netw Open. 2019;2(2):e187571. PMID: 30768188; PMCID: PMC6484603. https://doi.org/10.1001/jamanetworkopen.2018.7571.

28. NHPCO Facts and Figures Report, 2021 Edition. National Hospice and Palliative Care Organization; 2021. https://www.nhpco.org/wp-content/uploads/NHPCO-Facts-Figures-2021.pdf. Accessed 9 Jul 2022.

29. NHPCO Releases New Facts and Figures Report on Hospice Care in America. 2020. https://www.nhpco.org/hospice-facts-figures/#:~:text=The%20Median%20Length%20of%20Service,and%20dementia%20(15.6%20percent). Accessed 14 Jul 2022.

30. Walbert T. Maintaining quality of life near the end of life: hospice in neuro-oncology. Neuro Oncol. 2018;20(4):439–40. PMID: 29390139; PMCID: PMC5909631. https://doi.org/10.1093/neuonc/nox236.

31. Tatum PE, Mills SS. Hospice and palliative care: an overview. Med Clin North Am. 2020;104(3):359–73. https://doi.org/10.1016/j.mcna.2020.01.001.

32. Harrison KL, Cenzer I, Ankuda CK, Hunt LJ, Aldridge MD. Hospice improves care quality for older adults with dementia in their last month of life. Health Aff (Millwood). 2022;41(6):821–30. https://doi.org/10.1377/hlthaff.2021.01985.

33. Kavalieratos D, Corbelli J, Zhang D, Dionne-Odom JN, Ernecoff NC, Hanmer J, Hoydich ZP, Ikejiani DZ, Klein-Fedyshin M, Zimmermann C, Morton SC, Arnold RM, Heller L, Schenker Y. Association between palliative care and patient and caregiver outcomes: a systematic review and meta-analysis. JAMA. 2016;316(20):2104–14. PMID: 27893131; PMCID: PMC5226373. https://doi.org/10.1001/jama.2016.16840.

34. Patel MN, Nicolla JM, Friedman FAP, Ritz MR, Kamal AH. Hospice use among patients with cancer: trends, barriers, and future directions. JCO Oncol Pract. 2020;16(12):803–9. Epub 2020 Nov 13. https://doi.org/10.1200/OP.20.00309.

35. Meier DE, McCormick E, Lagman RL. Hospice: philosophy of care and appropriate utilization in the United States. 2022. https://www.medilib.ir/uptodate/show/2200. Accessed 7 Aug 2022.

36. Kranker K, Niedzwiecki MJ, Pohl RV, Saffer TL, Chen A, Gellar J, Forrow LV, Miescier L. Medicare care choices model improved end-of-life care, lowered Medicare expenditures, and increased hospice use. Health Aff (Millwood). 2023;42(11):1488–97. PMID: 37931188. https://doi.org/10.1377/hlthaff.2023.00465.

37. Mitchell SL, Miller SC, Teno JM, Kiely DK, Davis RB, Shaffer ML. Prediction of 6-month survival of nursing home residents with advanced dementia using ADEPT vs hospice eligibility guidelines. JAMA. 2010;304(17):1929–35. PMID: 21045099; PMCID: PMC3017367. https://doi.org/10.1001/jama.2010.1572.

38. Schonwetter RS, Han B, Small BJ, Martin B, Tope K, Haley WE. Predictors of six-month survival among patients with dementia: an evaluation of hospice Medicare guidelines. Am J Hosp Palliat Care. 2003;20(2):105–13. https://doi.org/10.1177/104990910302000208.

39. Mitchell SL, Kiely DK, Hamel MB, Park PS, Morris JN, Fries BE. Estimating prognosis for nursing home residents with advanced dementia. JAMA. 2004;291(22):2734–40. https://doi.org/10.1001/jama.291.22.2734.

40. De Vleminck A, Morrison RS, Meier DE, Aldridge MD. Hospice care for patients with dementia in the United States: a longitudinal cohort study. J Am Med Dir Assoc. 2018;19(7):633–8. Epub 2017 Nov 16. PMID: 29153752; PMCID: PMC5966338. https://doi.org/10.1016/j.jamda.2017.10.003.

41. Anderson F, Downing GM, Hill J, Casorso L, Lerch N. Palliative performance scale (PPS): a new tool. J Palliat Care. 1996;12(1):5–11.

42. Medical guidelines for determining appropriateness of hospice referral: disease-specific guidelines.   https://www.uptodate.com/contents/image?imageKey=ONC%2F61282. Accessed 12 May 2022.

43. Medical guidelines for determining appropriateness of hospice referral: non-disease-specific baseline guidelines plus comorbidities. https://www.uptodate.com/contents/image?imageKey=PALC%2F87321. Accessed 12 May 2022.

44. Longo DL. Approach to the patient with cancer. In: Longo DL, Kasper DL, Jameson JL, Fauci AS, Hauser SL, Loscalzo J, editors. Harrison's principles of internal medicine. New York: McGraw-Hill, Health Professions Division; 1998. p. 646–54.

45. Campos S, Zhang L, Sinclair E, Tsao M, Barnes EA, Danjoux C, Sahgal A, Goh P, Culleton S, Mitera G, Chow E. The palliative performance scale: examining its inter-rater reliability in an outpatient palliative radiation oncology clinic. Support Care Cancer. 2009;17(6):685–90. Epub 2008 Oct 23. https://doi.org/10.1007/s00520-008-0524-z.

46. Ho F, Lau F, Downing MG, Lesperance M. A reliability and validity study of the palliative performance scale. BMC Palliat Care. 2008;7:10. PMID: 18680590; PMCID: PMC2527603. https://doi.org/10.1186/1472-684X-7-10.

47. Ballentine JM. The five trajectories—supporting patients during serious illness. 2018. https://csupalliativecare.org/wp-content/uploads/Five-Trajectories-eBook-02.21.2018.pdf. Accessed 12 Jun 2022.

48. Lau F, Maida V, Downing M, Lesperance M, Karlson N, Kuziemsky C. Use of the palliative performance scale (PPS) for end-of-life prognostication in a palliative medicine consultation service. J Pain Symptom Manage. 2009;37(6):965–72. Epub 2009 Feb 20. https://doi.org/10.1016/j.jpainsymman.2008.08.003.

49. Prompantakorn P, Angkurawaranon C, Pinyopornpanish K, Chutarattanakul L, Aramrat C, Pateekhum C, Dejkriengkraikul N. Palliative performance scale and survival in patients with cancer and non-cancer diagnoses needing a palliative care consultation: a retrospective cohort study. BMC Palliat Care. 2021;20(1):74. PMID: 34039322; PMCID: PMC8157447. https://doi.org/10.1186/s12904-021-00773-8.

50. Weng LC, Huang HL, Wilkie DJ, Hoenig NA, Suarez ML, Marschke M, Durham J. Predicting survival with the Palliative Performance Scale in a minority-serving hospice and palliative care program. J Pain Symptom Manage. 2009;37(4):642–8. Epub 2008 Sep 26. PMID: 18823751; PMCID: PMC2699378. https://doi.org/10.1016/j.jpainsymman.2008.03.023.

51. Michaud F. Palliative pearls: how much time do I have? Part 1. [audio podcast episode]. In: Write your last chapter. No longer available online; 2020.

52. Hospice Certification/Recertification Requirements. 2021. https://www.cgsmedicare.com/hhh/coverage/coverage_guidelines/cert_recert_requirements.html. Accessed 14 Jan 2024.

53. Medicare Benefit Policy Manual. 2023. https://www.cms.gov/Regulations-and-Guidance/Guidance/Manuals/downloads/bp102c09.pdf. Accessed 14 Jan 2024.

54. Hospice Determining Terminal Status. In: Local coverage determination (LCD). 2022. https://www.cms.gov/medicare-coverage-database/view/lcd.aspx?LCDId=34538. Accessed 7 Nov 2022.

55. Blumenfeld H. Brainstem III: Internal structures and vascular supply. In: Neuroanatomy through clinical cases. 2nd ed. Sunderland, MA: Sinauer Associates; 2010. p. 613–95.

56. Jain S, Iverson LM. Glasgow Coma Scale. In: StatPearls [Internet]. Treasure Island, FL: StatPearls; 2022.

57. Hartman ME, Cheifetz IM. Pediatric emergencies and resuscitation. In: Nelson textbook of pediatrics. 1st ed. St. Louis, MO: Elsevier; 2020. p. 530–47.

58. Magee DJ, Manske RC. Orthopedic physical assessment. In: Head and face. 4th ed. St. Louis, MO: Elsevier; 2021. p. 73–163.

59. Machado C. Diagnosis of brain death. Neurol Int. 2010;2(1):e2. PMID: 21577338; PMCID: PMC3093212. https://doi.org/10.4081/ni.2010.e2.

60. Robba C, Banzato E, Rebora P, Iaquaniello C, Huang CY, Wiegers EJA, Meyfroidt G, Citerio G, Collaborative European NeuroTrauma Effectiveness Research in Traumatic Brain Injury (CENTER-TBI) ICU Participants and Investigators. Acute kidney injury in traumatic brain injury patients: results from the collaborative European NeuroTrauma effectiveness research in traumatic brain injury study. Crit Care Med. 2021;49(1):112–26. https://doi.org/10.1097/CCM.0000000000004673.

61. Moore EM, Bellomo R, Nichol A, Harley N, Macisaac C, Cooper DJ. The incidence of acute kidney injury in patients with traumatic brain injury. Ren Fail. 2010;32(9):1060–5. https://doi.org/10.3109/0886022X.2010.510234.

62. Bashore TM, Granger CB, Hranitzky P, Patel MR. Heart disease. In: McPhee SJ, Papadakis MA, Rabow MW, editors. 2012 Current medical diagnosis & treatment. New York: McGraw-Hill Medical; 2012. p. 317–419.

63. Global Initiative for Chronic Obstructive Lung Disease (GOLD) Criteria. In: Chronic obstructive pulmonary disease. https://bestpractice.bmj.com/topics/en-us/7/criteria, Accessed 3 Sept 2022.

64. Dabla PK. Renal function in diabetic nephropathy. World J Diabetes. 2010;1(2):48–56. PMID: 21537427; PMCID: PMC3083882. https://doi.org/10.4239/wjd.v1.i2.48.

65. Watnick S, Dirkx T. Kidney disease. In: McPhee SJ, Papadakis MA, Rabow MW, editors. 2012 Current medical diagnosis & treatment. New York: McGraw-Hill Medical; 2012. p. 874–911.

66. Kliger AS. Quality measures for dialysis: time for a balanced scorecard. Clin J Am Soc Nephrol. 2016;11(2):363–8. Epub 2015 Aug 27. PMID: 26316622; PMCID: PMC4741039. https://doi.org/10.2215/CJN.06010615.

67. Grubbs V, Moss AH, Cohen LM, Fischer MJ, Germain MJ, Jassal SV, Perl J, Weiner DE, Mehrotra R. Dialysis advisory Group of the American Society of nephrology. A palliative approach to dialysis care: a patient-centered transition to the end of life. Clin J Am Soc Nephrol. 2014;9(12):2203–9. Epub 2014 Aug 7. PMID: 25104274; PMCID: PMC4255391. https://doi.org/10.2215/CJN.00650114.

68. Cohen LM, Germain MJ, Poppel DM, Woods AL, Pekow PS, Kjellstrand CM. Dying well after discontinuing the life-support treatment of dialysis. Arch Intern Med. 2000;160(16):2513–8. https://doi.org/10.1001/archinte.160.16.2513.

69. Alobaidi R, Basu RK, Goldstein SL, Bagshaw SM. Sepsis-associated acute kidney injury. Semin Nephrol. 2015;35(1):2–11. PMID: 25795495; PMCID: PMC4507081. https://doi.org/10.1016/j.semnephrol.2015.01.002.

70. How to diagnose cirrhosis. https://www.hepatitis.va.gov/cirrhosis/background/how-to-diagnose.asp. Accessed 17 Oct 2022.

71. Stages of cirrhosis. https://www.hepatitis.va.gov/cirrhosis/background/stages.asp. Accessed 17 Oct 2022.

72. Liu S, Meng Q, Xu Y, Zhou J. Hepatorenal syndrome in acute-on-chronic liver failure with acute kidney injury: more questions requiring discussion. Gastroenterol Rep (Oxf). 2021;9(6):505–20. PMID: 34925848; PMCID: PMC8677535. https://doi.org/10.1093/gastro/goab040.

73. Potosek J, Curry M, Buss M, Chittenden E. Integration of palliative care in end-stage liver disease and liver transplantation. J Palliat Med. 2014;17(11):1271–7. PMID: 25390468; PMCID: PMC4229716. https://doi.org/10.1089/jpm.2013.0167.

74. McCormick PA. Improving prognosis in hepatorenal syndrome. Gut. 2000;47(2):166–7. PMID: 10896904; PMCID: PMC1727993. https://doi.org/10.1136/gut.47.2.166.

75. Engelmann C, Clària J, Szabo G, Bosch J, Bernardi M. Pathophysiology of decompensated cirrhosis: portal hypertension, circulatory dysfunction, inflammation, metabolism and mitochondrial dysfunction. J Hepatol. 2021;75(Suppl 1):S49–66. PMID: 34039492; PMCID: PMC9272511. https://doi.org/10.1016/j.jhep.2021.01.002.

76. Batra Y, Acharya SK. Acute liver failure: prognostic markers. Indian J Gastroenterol. 2003;22(Suppl 2):S66–8.

77. 9th Year of Record-Setting Liver Transplants. In: In Focus, Liver/intestine, News. 2022. https://unos.org/news/in-focus/2021-9th-record-year-liver-transplants/. Accessed 20 Oct 2022.

78. Organ Procurement & Transplantation Network Database. https://optn.transplant.hrsa.gov/data/. Accessed 20 Oct 2022.

79. Bambha K, Kamath PS. Model for end-stage liver disease (MELD). Waltham, MA: UptoDate; 2022. https://www.uptodate.com/contents/model-for-end-stage-liver-disease-meld. Accessed 22 Oct 2022.

80. Model for End-Stage Liver Disease (MELD) for ages 12 and older. https://www.hepatitisc.uw.edu/page/clinical-calculators/meld. Accessed 22 Oct 2022.

81. Dove LM, Brown RS. Liver transplantation in adults: patient selection and pretransplantation evaluation. Waltham, MA: UptoDate; 2022. https://www.uptodate.com/contents/liver-transplantation-in-adults-patient-selection-and-pretransplantation-evaluation. Accessed 22 Oct 2022.

82. Cancer Stat Facts: Common Cancer Sites. In: Reports on Cancer. 2022. https://seer.cancer.gov/statfacts/html/common.html. Accessed 24 Oct 2022.

83. Brierley J, Gospodarowicz MK, Wittekind C. Union for International Cancer Control. TNM classification of malignant tumours. 8th ed. Chichester: Wiley Blackwell; 2017.

84. National Institutes of Health. Cancer staging. In: About cancer. 2022. https://www.cancer.gov/about-cancer/diagnosis-staging/staging. Accessed 1 Feb 2024.

85. Rosen RD, Sapra A. TNM classification. In: StatPearls [internet]. Treasure Island, FL: StatPearls; 2022. https://www.ncbi.nlm.nih.gov/books/NBK553187/. Accessed 24 Oct 2022.

86. Site Specific Modules. In: SEER Training. https://training.seer.cancer.gov/modules_site_spec.html. Accessed 24 Oct 2022.

87. ECOG Performance Status Scale. https://ecog-acrin.org/resources/ecog-performance-status/. Accessed 24 Oct 2022.

88. de Kock I, Mirhosseini M, Lau F, Thai V, Downing M, Quan H, Lesperance M, Yang J. Conversion of Karnofsky performance Status (KPS) and eastern cooperative oncology group performance Status (ECOG) to palliative performance scale (PPS), and the interchangeability of PPS and KPS in prognostic tools. J Palliat Care. 2013;29(3):163–9.

89. Global HIV & AIDS statistics—Fact sheet. 2022. https://www.unaids.org/en/resources/fact-sheet. Accessed 29 Oct 2022.

90. Waymack JR, Sundareshan V. Acquired immune deficiency syndrome. In: StatPearls [internet]. Treasure Island, FL: StatPearls; 2022. https://www.ncbi.nlm.nih.gov/books/NBK537293/. Accessed 29 Oct 2022.

91. The HIV/AIDS Epidemic in the United States: The Basics. 2021. https://www.kff.org/hivaids/fact-sheet/the-hivaids-epidemic-in-the-united-states-the-basics/. Accessed 29 Oct 2022.

92. The Stages of HIV Infection. In: HIV Overview. 2021. https://hivinfo.nih.gov/understanding-hiv/fact-sheets/stages-hiv-infection. Accessed 29 Oct 2022.

93. HIV/AIDS. https://www.mayoclinic.org/diseases-conditions/hiv-aids/symptoms-causes/syc-20373524. Accessed 29 Oct 2022.

94. Fauci AS, Lane HC. Human immunodeficiency virus disease: AIDS and related disorders. In: Longo DL, Kasper DL, Jameson JL, Fauci AS, Hauser SL, Loscalzo J, editors. Harrison's principles of internal medicine. New York: McGraw-Hill, Health Professions Division; 1998. p. 1506–87.

95. T Cell Count. 2021. https://www.mountsinai.org/health-library/tests/t-cell-count. Accessed 29 Oct 2022.

96. Zolopa AR, Katz MH. HIV infection & AIDS. In: McPhee SJ, Papadakis MA, Rabow MW, editors. 2012 Current medical diagnosis & treatment. New York: McGraw-Hill Medical; 2012. p. 1285–315.

97. Wood BR. The natural history and clinical features of HIV infection in adults and adolescents. 2022. https://www.uptodate.com/contents/the-natural-history-and-clinical-features-of-hiv-infection-in-adults-and-adolescents. Accessed 1 Nov 2022.

98. Poorolajal J, Hooshmand E, Mahjub H, Esmailnasab N, Jenabi E. Survival rate of AIDS disease and mortality in HIV-infected patients: a meta-analysis. Public Health. 2016;139:3–12. Epub 2016 Jun 24. https://doi.org/10.1016/j.puhe.2016.05.004.

99. Marcus JL, Leyden WA, Alexeeff SE, Anderson AN, Hechter RC, Hu H, Lam JO, Towner WJ, Yuan Q, Horberg MA, Silverberg MJ. Comparison of overall and comorbidity-free life expectancy between insured adults with and without HIV infection, 2000-2016. JAMA Netw Open. 2020;3(6):e207954. PMID: 32539152; PMCID: PMC7296391. https://doi.org/10.1001/jamanetworkopen.2020.7954.

100. Weinberg JL, Kovarik CL. The WHO clinical staging system for HIV/AIDS. Virtual Mentor. 2010;12(3):202–6. https://journalofethics.ama-assn.org/article/who-clinical-staging-system-hivaids/2010-03. Accessed 1 Nov 2022. https://doi.org/10.1001/virtualmentor.2010.12.3.cprl1-1003.

101. Dye C, Harries AD, Maher D, et al. Tuberculosis. In: Jamison DT, Feachem RG, Makgoba MW, et al., editors. Disease and mortality in Sub-Saharan Africa. 2nd ed. Washington, DC: The International Bank for Reconstruction and Development/The World Bank; 2006. Chapter 13. https://www.ncbi.nlm.nih.gov/books/NBK2285/. Accessed 1 Nov 2022.

102. Black A, Sitas F, Chibrawara T, Gill Z, Kubanje M, Williams B. HIV-attributable causes of death in the medical ward at the Chris Hani Baragwanath Hospital, South Africa. PLoS One. 2019;14(5):e0215591. PMID: 31059528; PMCID: PMC6502348. https://doi.org/10.1371/journal.pone.0215591.

103. Chimbetete C, Shamu T, Roelens M, Bote S, Mudzviti T, Keiser O. Mortality trends and causes of death among HIV positive patients at Newlands Clinic in Harare, Zimbabwe. PLoS One. 2020;15(8):e0237904. PMID: 32853215; PMCID: PMC7451579. https://doi.org/10.1371/journal.pone.0237904.

104. Smith CJ, Ryom L, Weber R, Morlat P, Pradier C, Reiss P, Kowalska JD, de Wit S, Law M, el Sadr W, Kirk O, Friis-Moller N, Monforte AD, Phillips AN, Sabin CA, Lundgren JD, D:A:D Study Group. Trends in underlying causes of death in people with HIV from 1999 to 2011 (D:a:D): a multicohort collaboration. Lancet. 2014;384(9939):241–8. https://doi.org/10.1016/S0140-6736(14)60604-8.

105. Shen JM, Blank A, Selwyn PA. Predictors of mortality for patients with advanced disease in an HIV palliative care program. J Acquir Immune Defic Syndr. 2005;40(4):445–7. https://doi.org/10.1097/01.qai.0000185139.68848.97.

106. Gopal S, Patel MR, Yanik EL, Cole SR, Achenbach CJ, Napravnik S, Burkholder GA, Reid EG, Rodriguez B, Deeks SG, Mayer KH, Moore RD, Kitahata MM, Eron JJ, Richards KL. Temporal trends in presentation and survival for HIV-associated lymphoma in the antiretroviral therapy era. J Natl Cancer Inst. 2013;105(16):1221–9. Epub 2013 Jul 26. PMID: 23892362; PMCID: PMC3748003. https://doi.org/10.1093/jnci/djt158.

107. Li R, Duffee D, Gbadamosi-Akindele MF. CD4 count. In: StatPearls [Internet]. Treasure Island, FL: StatPearls; 2022. https://www.ncbi.nlm.nih.gov/books/NBK470231/. Accessed 5 Nov 2022.

108. Pahuga M, Merlin J, Selwyn PA. Issues in HIV/AIDS in adults in palliative care. 2022. https://www.uptodate.com/contents/issues-in-hiv-aids-in-adults-in-palliative-care. Accessed 5 Nov 2022.
109. Rhodes RL, Nazir F, Lopez S, Xuan L, Nijhawan AE, Alexander-Scott NE, Halm EA. Use and predictors of end-of-life care among HIV patients in a Safety Net Health System. J Pain Symptom Manage. 2016;51(1):120–5. Epub 2015 Sep 16. PMID: 26384554; PMCID: PMC4763921. https://doi.org/10.1016/j.jpainsymman.2015.08.010.
110. Reisberg B. Functional assessment staging (FAST). Psychopharmacol Bull. 1988;24(4):653–9.
111. Reisberg B. https://med.nyu.edu/faculty/barry-reisberg. Accessed 7 Nov 2022.
112. Reisberg B, Franssen EH, Souren LE, Auer SR, Akram I, Kenowsky S. Evidence and mechanisms of retrogenesis in Alzheimer's and other dementias: management and treatment import. Am J Alzheimers Dis Other Demen. 2002;17(4):202–12. https://doi.org/10.1177/153331750201700411.
113. Reisberg B, Franssen E, Souren LEM, Kenowsky S, Janjua KS, Veigne SW, Guillo-Benarous F, Singh S, Khizar A, Shah U, Shah RG, Bhandal A, Auer S. Alzheimer's disease. In: Moroz A, Flanagan SR, Zaretsky H, editors. Medical aspects of disability for the rehabilitation professional. New York: Springer Publishing Company, LLC; 2017. p. 31–90.
114. Wegiel J, Flory M, Kuchna I, Nowicki K, Ma SY, Wegiel J, Badmaev E, Leon M, Wisniewski T, Reisberg B. Clinicopathological staging of dynamics of neurodegeneration and neuronal loss in Alzheimer disease. J Neuropathol Exp Neurol. 2021;80(1):21–44. PMID: 33270870; PMCID: PMC7749716. https://doi.org/10.1093/jnen/nlaa140.
115. Brown MA, Sampson EL, Jones L, Barron AM. Prognostic indicators of 6-month mortality in elderly people with advanced dementia: a systematic review. Palliat Med. 2013;27(5):389–400. Epub 2012 Nov 22. PMID: 23175514; PMCID: PMC3652641. https://doi.org/10.1177/0269216312465649.
116. Dumurgier J, Sabia S. Life expectancy in dementia subtypes: exploring a leading cause of mortality. Lancet Healthy Longev. 2021;2(8):e449–50. Epub 2021 Jul 21. https://doi.org/10.1016/S2666-7568(21)00166-5.
117. Tom SE, Hubbard RA, Crane PK, Haneuse SJ, Bowen J, McCormick WC, McCurry S, Larson EB. Characterization of dementia and Alzheimer's disease in an older population: updated incidence and life expectancy with and without dementia. Am J Public Health. 2015;105(2):408–13. PMID: 25033130; PMCID: PMC4318311. https://doi.org/10.2105/AJPH.2014.301935.
118. Mitchell SL, Miller SC, Teno JM, Davis RB, Shaffer ML. The advanced dementia prognostic tool: a risk score to estimate survival in nursing home residents with advanced dementia. J Pain Symptom Manage. 2010;40(5):639–51. PMID: 20621437; PMCID: PMC2981683. https://doi.org/10.1016/j.jpainsymman.2010.02.014.
119. Fritze T, Doblhammer G, Widmann CN, Heneka MT. Time course of dementia following sepsis in German health claims data. Neurol Neuroimmunol Neuroinflamm. 2020;8(1):e911. PMID: 33293458; PMCID: PMC7803331. https://doi.org/10.1212/NXI.0000000000000911.
120. Roche JC, Rojas-Garcia R, Scott KM, Scotton W, Ellis CE, Burman R, Wijesekera L, Turner MR, Leigh PN, Shaw CE, Al-Chalabi A. A proposed staging system for amyotrophic lateral sclerosis. Brain. 2012;135(Pt 3):847–52. Epub 2012 Jan 23. PMID: 22271664; PMCID: PMC3286327. https://doi.org/10.1093/brain/awr351.
121. de Carvalho M, Matias T, Coelho F, Evangelista T, Pinto A, Luís ML. Motor neuron disease presenting with respiratory failure. J Neurol Sci. 1996;139(Suppl):117–22. https://doi.org/10.1016/0022-510x(96)00089-5.
122. Balendra R, Al Khleifat A, Fang T, Al-Chalabi A. A standard operating procedure for King's ALS clinical staging. Amyotroph Lateral Scler Frontotemporal Degener. 2019;20(3–4):159–64. Epub 2019 Feb 18. PMID: 30773950; PMCID: PMC6558284. https://doi.org/10.1080/21678421.2018.1556696.

123. Kiernan MC, Vucic S, Cheah BC, Turner MR, Eisen A, Hardiman O, Burrell JR, Zoing MC. Amyotrophic lateral sclerosis. Lancet. 2011;377(9769):942–55. Epub 2011 Feb 4. https://doi.org/10.1016/S0140-6736(10)61156-7.

124. Amytrophic lateral sclerosis. In: National amyotrophic lateral sclerosis (ALS) Registry. 2017. https://www.cdc.gov/als/WhatisALS.html. Accessed 19 Nov 2022.

125. Brown RH. Amyotrophic lateral sclerosis and other motor neuron diseases. In: Longo DL, Kasper DL, Jameson JL, Fauci AS, Hauser SL, Loscalzo J, editors. Harrison's principles of internal medicine. New York: McGraw-Hill, Health Professions Division; 1998. p. 3345–51.

126. Ferri A, Coccurello R. What is "Hyper" in the ALS hypermetabolism? Mediators Inflamm. 2017;2017:7821672. Epub 2017 Sep 7. PMID: 29081604; PMCID: PMC5610793. https://doi.org/10.1155/2017/7821672.

127. Desport JC, Preux PM, Truong TC, Vallat JM, Sautereau D, Couratier P. Nutritional status is a prognostic factor for survival in ALS patients. Neurology. 1999;53(5):1059–63. https://doi.org/10.1212/wnl.53.5.1059.

128. Procaccini NJ, Nemergut EC. Percutaneous endoscopic gastrostomy in the patient with amyotrophic lateral sclerosis: risk vs benefit? Nutrition issues in gastroenterology. 2008. https://med.virginia.edu/ginutrition/wp-content/uploads/sites/199/2015/11/ProcacciniArticle-March-08.pdf. Accessed 19 Nov 2022.

129. Chiò A, Logroscino G, Hardiman O, Swingler R, Mitchell D, Beghi E, Traynor BG, Eurals Consortium. Prognostic factors in ALS: a critical review. Amyotroph Lateral Scler. 2009;10(5-6):310–23. PMID: 19922118; PMCID: PMC3515205. https://doi.org/10.3109/17482960802566824.

130. Revised Amyotrophic Lateral Sclerosis Functional Rating Scale (ALSFRS-R). https://www.mdcalc.com/calc/10166/revised-amyotrophic-lateral-sclerosis-functional-rating-scale-alsfrs-r. Accessed 19 Nov 2022.

131. Clegg A, Young J, Iliffe S, Rikkert MO, Rockwood K. Frailty in elderly people. Lancet. 2013;381(9868):752–62. Epub 2013 Feb 8. Erratum in: Lancet. 2013 Oct 19;382(9901):1328. PMID: 23395245; PMCID: PMC4098658. https://doi.org/10.1016/S0140-6736(12)62167-9.

132. Morley JE, Vellas B, van Kan GA, Anker SD, Bauer JM, Bernabei R, Cesari M, Chumlea WC, Doehner W, Evans J, Fried LP, Guralnik JM, Katz PR, Malmstrom TK, McCarter RJ, Gutierrez Robledo LM, Rockwood K, von Haehling S, Vandewoude MF, Walston J. Frailty consensus: a call to action. J Am Med Dir Assoc. 2013;14(6):392–7. PMID: 23764209; PMCID: PMC4084863. https://doi.org/10.1016/j.jamda.2013.03.022.

133. Ali S, Garcia JM. Sarcopenia, cachexia and aging: diagnosis, mechanisms and therapeutic options—a mini-review. Gerontology. 2014;60(4):294–305. Epub 2014 Apr 8. PMID: 24731978; PMCID: PMC4112511. https://doi.org/10.1159/000356760.

134. Morley JE. Treatment of sarcopenia: the road to the future. J Cachexia Sarcopenia Muscle. 2018;9(7):1196–9. PMID: 30697982; PMCID: PMC6351669. https://doi.org/10.1002/jcsm.12386.

135. Adhiyaman V, Chattopadhyay I. Is it appropriate to link 'old age' to certain causes of death on the medical certificate of cause of death? Future Healthc J. 2021;8(3):e686–8. PMID: 34888466; PMCID: PMC8651340. https://doi.org/10.7861/fhj.2021-0050.

136. Get the Facts on Healthy Aging. 2021. https://www.ncoa.org/article/get-the-facts-on-healthy-aging. Accessed 3 Dec 2022.

Part II

Ground Rules for Compassionate Conversations

Illness, Disease, and Sickness: Three Dimensions of a Diagnosis

When we consider what matters most and how best to help people as they traverse the landscape of a diagnosis, we must keep in mind that patients and their families are an intertwined set of individuals with rich, varied, complicated, and interesting lives and relationships.

One of my patients, when I asked, "What would a good death be like for you?" shared a surprising desire to be shot by a jealous husband. In contrast, most people tell me they want to pass away in their sleep, a comforting expectation in its simplicity. But here was a man, nearing the end of his life and dying of old age, who appeared to be hiding a veritable treasure trove of dreams, passions, experience, and conviction. If only I had time for a much longer interview with him, certainly an engaging memoir would have been forthcoming.

This patient demonstrated an essential truth in medicine: that every patient's unique and special story lies below the surface if we only inquire more deeply. Out of sight, unless we ask, resides the purpose, meaning, pains, and pleasures of a human life.

Think of the proverbial iceberg. On the surface, visible above the water, a patient's clinical story exists, which tends to be where the medical community focuses its energy and time, being most comfortable and efficient in a space dedicated to diagnosis and treatment.

However, patients are much greater than the sum of their lab values and imaging results. In our exuberance to identify and manage the various medical mysteries of the human body, it can be easy to miss the immense and complex human story entirely, submerged but frequently on the verge of crisis, just beneath the confusion and chaos of a new or developing diagnosis.

A neurology colleague shared an often-reported concern of her patients admitted with stroke or seizure or some other worrisome disorder, "Who will feed my dog while I'm in the hospital?" Less concerned are many patients with their health and well-being than they are with the practical impact of their diagnoses on the lives of their loved ones, spouses, children, and pets. This is an excellent reminder that patients are complex beings with rich, complete, and meaningful lives.

© The Author(s), under exclusive license to Springer Nature Switzerland AG 2024   161
A. Shaw, PA, *The Arc of Conversation*,
https://doi.org/10.1007/978-3-031-70495-6_6

In 1975, Marshall Marinker, writing in the *Journal of Medical Ethics*, defined "three modes of unhealth"—disease, illness, and sickness—to illuminate the critical dimensions of a diagnosis that patients experience [1]. Using the metaphor of an iceberg, Fig. 6.1 illustrates the relationship between these three dimensions, highlighting the divergence in focus that often occurs between the medical system and that of the patient and family.

Marinker defines **disease** as "a deviation from a biological norm" or "a pathological process." [1] Because physicians are almost exclusively trained in the identification, staging, and treatment of disease and because economic pressures insist that physicians see patients as quickly as possible, nearly all of physician time and energy is spent addressing disease.

On the end of this continuum exist physicians with little to no bedside manner who barely acknowledge the patient in the room. Such interactions showcase Marinker's commentary that "the patient has often been described as the 'accident of the disease.'" [1]. Fortunately, business practices focusing on the customer service aspect of medicine along with the move toward patient-centered care in the last half-century have had an impact in correcting this un-patient-friendly approach. And yet, that healthcare systems still need to provide training to teach physicians how to listen to patients and respond with empathy speaks to the reality that nearly 50 years after Marinker's commentary, disease continues to be "valued as the central fact in the medical view." [1].

The reality, however, is that for patients and families, disease is *not* the central fact in their medical view and is *not* what matters most. Away from our clinic, hospital, and procedure rooms, people experience the impact of disease in every area of their lives all day—at home, at work, and in the world. The specific way that disease manifests and impacts the ability of patients to navigate their lives *is* what matters most to patients and families.

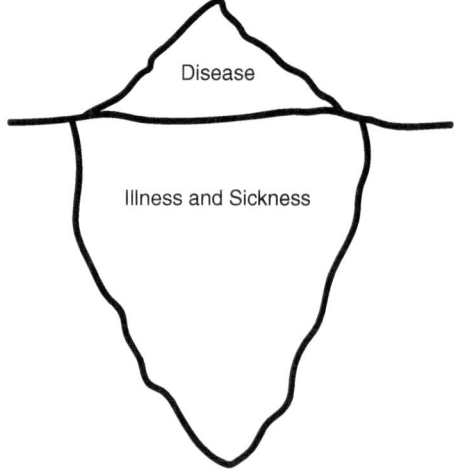

Three Dimensions of a Diagnosis

Disease

Illness and Sickness

Fig. 6.1 Three dimensions of a diagnosis. Marinker describes three diagnosis dimensions: disease, illness, and sickness [1]. If we think of a diagnosis as an iceberg, disease is most salient and the central focus for the medical community, but for patients and families, personal experience of disease (illness) and the societal role patients and families assume (sickness) matter most

This "personal experience of disease," what Marinker calls **illness** [1], is the particular way that disease shows up in a patient's life and can affect every domain and activity of daily living. As a diagnosis progresses, disease will impact patient relationships, marriages, and family dynamics, as well as self-esteem and self-image. In the case of a disease like dementia, it will affect a patient's ability to handle their finances and medications, to participate in activities they previously enjoyed, and to work, hobby, and love. Illness is the nitty-gritty, individual, and granular impact of disease on the business of living, and this is the dimension that matters most to patients and families.

Marinker points out that an illness without a diagnosis can be particularly uncomfortable for patients and providers, creating particular problems for each [1]. Illness in the absence of any identifiable mechanical or structural dysfunction is often given a psychiatric label or called "functional," [1] which can leave patients and families feeling unsupported or invalidated, and can leave physicians feeling incompetent or frustrated. Once illness is diagnosed, both patients and physicians can feel relief. Still, while patients will continue to experience their illness, physicians often ensconce themselves once again in the realm of patient disease, more comfortable with objective measurements and treatment algorithms than with tending to patient and family emotional, social, and practical needs. Physicians must continually work against this natural inclination to focus on disease and continuously work to remain focused on the human dimension of a diagnosis.

For it is in the personal experience of disease that patient and family lives either flourish or degrade, as every aspect of a diagnosis, from symptom management to the demands for caregiver support, will reverberate down and through a family like the stressors that calve a glacier, often turning people's lives on end. As Ira Byock, MD, leading palliative care physician, author, and advocate, points out in his book, *The Best Care Possible*, "When one person gets a diagnosis, their family gets an illness." [2]. The impact of disease is felt not only by the patient but by the entire family system.

How illness unfolds for a patient and family will depend on their unique psychosocial, economic, and physical realities, further informed by their hopes, fears, priorities, and values.

For instance, a treatment as seemingly simple as starting a new blood pressure medication can ripple through a family system like a boulder dropped onto a calm lake. I care for an elderly patient with dementia who lives at home with his wife. He is deep into the personal care stage of his journey, so his wife has had to take over managing their finances, medications, appointments, home, housework, transportation, and shopping. She must remind her husband to take a shower and help him pick out and change his clothes. She still works, in part, so that she can get a mental and physical break from the care of her husband, whose needs have exhausted her, elevating her blood pressure.

The wife's primary care physician, eager to address her hypertension, started her on a diuretic, hydrochlorothiazide (HCTZ), which causes her to frequently need to use the restroom, which in turn disturbs her sleep. The medication also disrupts her potassium level, requiring that she take a large potassium supplement three times a day, one more thing she must remember to do. Her poor sleep had further exhausted her so that when we met, she was in crisis, tearful, and expressing a wish for it to all be over. We discussed many forms of support, including a medication change from HCTZ to amlodipine, which would control her blood pressure without affecting her bladder, and eliminate the need for the potassium supplement. We also discussed counseling, starting an antidepressant, hiring a home care agency for some immediate help in the home, and, in the long term, considering a move into an independent living facility, where she would have additional help in managing their basic living needs, including cooking, driving, and housework.

Although the primary care physician technically did nothing wrong in choosing HCTZ to manage the wife's high blood pressure, by focusing solely on her diagnosis (HTN) while not considering her need to help navigate her husband's disease (dementia), the physician inadvertently worsened the patient's experience of her disease and risked that of her husband's. I cannot think of a better example to illustrate the importance of elevating illness—the personal experience of a patient or family member's diagnosis—to the level of consideration warranted by disease.

Closely connected to the illness dimension of a diagnosis and also hidden unless we ask, is the dimension of **sickness**, what Marinker defines as "a social role, a status, a negotiated position in the world, a bargain struck between the person henceforward called 'sick,' and a society which is prepared to recognize and sustain him." [1].

The social role of disease is either self-adopted or imposed on patients by society. Think of the "disabled person," "cancer survivor," "drug-seeker," "drug addict," and "alcoholic" labels applied to patients (with or without their consent) by society that inform the way patients are treated by society. Sickness roles are superimposed on top of disease and illness, often go unacknowledged, interact with a patient or family's sense of self-worth and identity, and can augment suffering.

Cancer and mental illness diagnoses carry two very different sickness roles that profoundly impact the way patients and families experience these diseases. Consider the following two vignettes: true stories of actual patient and family lives.

Imagine a family with a 16-year-old child who receives a devastating diagnosis of cancer. Within hours of the diagnosis, the parents share their child's story on Facebook, asking for prayers, and receive more than 250 messages of love and support. Updates across the child's journey are shared publicly, with pictures of the family surrounding the child during and after chemotherapy appointments posted for everyone to see. Extended family members shave their heads in solidarity with the child when the child begins to lose their hair. Other messages of love and support pour in from the community, from far and wide, including care packages from professional sports teams in neighboring cities that include signed jerseys, pennants, and photographs. The family is supported during cancer treatment visits by a nonprofit organization that pays for their hotel room stays, and the parents attend every single visit with the child, advocating for their child by interacting with the doctors to better help their child navigate this difficult journey. During the first few weeks of care, the child's mother never leaves the child's side. When, thankfully, months later, the child is declared cancer-free, the family hosts a community celebration, the child is honored at school, and the family is sent on an all-expense-paid trip to a fun resort by a national foundation.

Now imagine a very different family, with a 19-year-old experiencing their first year of college, with anxiety severe enough to prevent completion of the school year. Suicidal thoughts lead the child to the emergency room, but because the child is 19 and the condition is psychiatric, the parents are not allowed into the child's room. Instead, they must wait in the waiting room to see and support their child only during visiting hours, just two hours each day. The child experiences the overnight emergency room stay alone, isolated in the psychiatric ward, and away from their familial support during a terrifying first interaction with the medical system.

In subsequent months, the child is seen by a psychiatrist, a counselor, and a neuropsychologist and eventually diagnosed with a significant mental health disorder, which prevents the child from holding a job, returning to college, or living on their own. Because the child is legally an adult, and because of the way treatment works within the mental health domain, but mainly because the child's particular disorder causes the psychiatric symptoms of paranoia, the parents are not allowed to attend appointments with their child. The parents have a difficult time learning about the child's diagnosis and treatment options, which continue to evolve, further complicating the child's recovery. Experiencing incredible strain on their marriage, the parents do not publicly share their child's diagnosis, and no care packages, community or foundation support, nursing navigation, or family therapy are part of their child's journey. Before receiving a formal diagnosis labeling their child's condition, the parents file for divorce.

I can think of no stronger contrast than between the sickness roles of cancer and mental health. In the United States, a warrior ethic in the "fight against cancer" encourages patients to experience public journeys that are often well-supported and cheered on from the sidelines. By contrast, patients and families with mental disease struggle in silence, frequently having a very difficult, frustrating, and unsupported time navigating the behavioral health system. The experience of mental disease can also intersect with the civil and criminal justice systems, further adding to the internal sense of shame and societal abandonment patients and families can experience. As these vignettes illustrate, the sickness roles accompanying these two diagnoses impact how patients and families navigate the healthcare system, their identities, relationships, and sense of community.

Every illness carries with it a particular sickness role, with a hierarchy of disease that prioritizes youth, curability, structural dysfunction, and the retention of independence above advanced age, terminality, functional or psychiatric dysfunction, and the loss of independence [1]. Sickness frequently intersects with illness, as in the vignettes above, or in the example of patients with significant functional loss who need but are too ashamed to ask for ADA-friendly parking tags.

While it is always necessary to be aware of a patient's sickness role, addressing the sickness role for patients and families with diagnoses that carry a negative emotional valence like shame, fear, distrust, or embarrassment is particularly important. For those with issues of mental illness, substance abuse, disability, loss of independence, and especially for those nearing the end of their lives with any of these conditions, it is essential to offer compassionate words that validate, normalize, and humanize patient and family experiences and emotions.

Getting to the heart of this matter, writing in 1974, psychoanalyst Michael Balint, in his book, *The Physician, His Patient, and the Illness*, points out that "every illness is also the vehicle for a plea for love and attention." [3]. I could not agree more.

Patients and families seeking medical care bring their disease, illness, and sickness, needing and deserving tenderness and care in each dimension. Medical professionals must bring sensitivity and awareness of these facets of patient experience to care for the whole patient, which also means caring for caregivers and loved ones.

In its simplest definition, patient-centered care means putting the needs of the patient before the needs of the physician. Recalling our metaphor of the iceberg, patient-centered care requires that we turn our approach on end, prioritizing the human dimensions of a diagnosis (illness and sickness) and ensuring that medical recommendations for treating disease remain grounded in patient and family values and goals. More than merely arriving at an accurate diagnosis, we must always keep in mind what matters most to patients and families.

References

1. Marinker M. Why make people patients? J Med Ethics. 1975;1(2):81–4. https://doi.org/10.1136/jme.1.2.81. PMID: 1177270; PMCID: PMC1154460
2. Byock I. The best care possible: a physician's guide to transform care through the end of life. Penguin Group; 2012.
3. Balint M. The doctor, his patient, and the illness. London: Pitman; 1974.

Holding Space: Creating a Compassionate and Collaborative Environment

In the weeks and months following my divorce, as my life unraveled and reknit anew, my friends taught me the essential lessons of this chapter, for they were my physicians, and I their patient, seeking the balms of friendship—love, affection, attention, and affirmation. As my heart broke, time and again, as I experienced each solitary first during that initial year on my own, learning to navigate my new reality, my friends held space and treated me with boundless compassion that helped me survive what can only be described as the most painful experience of my life.

Yoga teacher and author, Adam Brady, describes the act of holding space as the "conscious act of being present, open, allowing, and protective of what another needs in each moment" or the "principle of *surrounding the environment with your awareness in a way that provides comfort and compassion for all.*" [1]. Author, Amy Wright Glenn, in her wonderfully insightful and tender book, *Holding Space: On Loving, Dying, and Letting Go*, speaks of holding space as the act of companioning, explaining that, "When we companion, we walk alongside the bereaved. We offer our open-hearted and gentle presence. We listen." [2]. In common parlance, holding space means "being there" for people [1], just as my friends were for me.

Despite this painful reference point, I can hardly begin to imagine what it feels like to be facing one's mortality. Yet, that is precisely what is asked of us when we sit with patients and families in their anxieties, fear, and grief over a new or developing illness. That we can open our hearts to our patients' anguish and let our experience of their pain motivate us in our provision of care is the fundamental calling of medicine.

Empathy—the ability to experience the suffering of others—is the necessary ingredient for **compassion**—the motivation to help that arises from the shared experience of another's pain. So central is compassion to the practice of medicine that it appears in the American Medical Association's (AMA) first principle of medical ethics immediately after the call to administer care:

> A physician shall be dedicated to providing competent medical care, with compassion and respect for human dignity and rights [3].

A. Shaw, PA, *The Arc of Conversation*,
https://doi.org/10.1007/978-3-031-70495-6_7

As discussed earlier in this book, patient-centered care requires that patient choice springs from an accurate understanding of the patient's medical reality in the context of the patient's values and goals. Creating a space for this to happen naturally for people requires a commitment to both compassion and **collaboration**—the integration of patient and family values and priorities with treatment recommendations that are discussed and decided on through a process of shared decision making that involves the patient, caregivers, and other members of the medical team [4]. Collaboration, thus, is the highest expression of patient-centered care, reflecting a complete shift from the "traditional hierarchical model based on physician power and control toward a more equal partnership- and relationship-based model." [5].

The way my friends "treated" me in the wake of my divorce was a beautiful example of the relationship-based model of care, wherein I received loving support, helpful advice, and gentle empowerment, all while being met where I was in my grief and healing process by my friends' abundant empathy and compassion.

Compassionate Collaborative Care (The Triple C) Model and Framework

The relationship-based model of care was codified in 2014 into a standard of patient-centered medical care called the Compassionate Collaborative Care (The Triple C) Model and Framework [6]. Developed by an expert panel convened by the Schwartz Center for Compassionate Healthcare and the Arnold P. Gold Foundation, "The Triple C" model marries the twin engines of compassion and collaboration to support the "quadruple aim" of healthcare—improving patient health, improving patient experience, reducing cost, and supporting provider well-being [7]. "The Triple C" Model and Framework is available for inclusion in healthcare curricula and business model development at www.theschwartzcenter.org [4].

Being grounded in the understanding that "communication is the medium by which compassion and collaboration are expressed," [7] "The Triple C" Model and Framework

> is based on (1) the ability to experience and act on one's compassion, (2) the ability to collaborate, communicate and partner with patients and family members to the extent they need and desire, (3) the commitment of all who provide and support healthcare to communicate and collaborate with each other, and (4) the resilience and wellbeing of professional and family caregivers [4].

"The Triple C" Model and Framework articulates the following 14 attributes of compassionate and collaborative care, which form the foundation of this chapter [4]. To this list, I have added Holding space; Acceptance; Normalizing, validating, and reassuring; Acknowledging, respecting, and accepting patient beliefs; the "Wish, Worry, Wonder" technique for responding to patient beliefs and wishes; Not making assumptions; and Checking in.

- Direction and focus of one's attention
- Recognition of nonverbal cues

- Asking about emotions, concerns, and distress
- Responding to emotions, concerns, and distress
- Nonjudgmentally valuing each person
- Fostering well-being and resilience
- Showing interest in the "whole person"
- Demonstrating trustworthiness
- Active listening
- Sharing information and decision making
- Communicating with colleagues and adjusting actions
- Practicing self-reflection
- Attending to relationships
- Attending to one's own well-being

Holding Space

Together, these attributes enable medical professionals at every level of the health-care system, including clinical and non-clinical staff, as well as leadership [4], to **hold space** for patients and families, creating the patient-centered milieu through which we can guide patients and families in an exploration of their personal experience and understanding of disease; empowering them to articulate their wishes, fears, and concerns; and working with them to arrive at medical decisions that continually align with their values.

Attention

The first ingredient of holding space is our "intention, attention, and energy." [1] To fully hold space, we must clear our hearts and minds and the physical environment of distractions to focus entirely on the patient and family. We must leave our worries at the door and be aware of and manage our internal emotional state to remain patient, kind, and generous in our communications.

Attention requires both non-verbal and verbal mastery. Non-verbally, we must make and maintain eye contact, as culturally appropriate. We should remain seated throughout our consultations, sitting with an open posture, leaning in, and mirroring our patients' body language and speech patterns to convey our complete presence and acceptance of who and how they are. We should continually monitor and interpret patients' and families' body language and facial expressions, which can communicate a wide range of emotions, as well as concern, confusion, or acceptance. At the same time, we must also manage our body language and facial expressions to communicate a concentrated, compassionate focus on those in our care.

Verbally, we must allow patients and family members to speak without interruption, controlling the impulse to rush in with our questions, comments, or responses [1], which can make people feel hurried, unheard, or unvalued. Instead, we must manage our verbal and nonverbal responses to show that we are keeping pace with the conversation, are eager to hear more, and accept, rather than judge, what is being said. A head nod or phrase like "Uh huh," "Sure," "Yes," "Makes sense," "Go on," "Tell me more," "Okay," or "What do you mean by that?" are excellent ways of conveying our ongoing interest and engagement. By modulating our tone of voice and choice of words, we can continually communicate our humility, gentle inquiry, nonjudgment, empathy, acceptance, and authentic interest.

We must develop a deep comfort with silence, resisting the compulsion to fill the quiet moments with our words [1], which can inadvertently communicate our discomfort with patients' emotions and stifle their trust and openness. It must be understood that silence is the pause in which patients and families experience or process their feelings or the information being discussed. The time needed for people to process medical revelations must be respected and honored, for ultimately, patient choice needs to arise from the internal sensibilities of the patient and family, not from external force. The time required for patients and families to arrive at decisions that make sense to them must be granted, even when it takes days, weeks, or months.

Interest in and Tending to Emotions, Concerns, and Distress

Silence is often heavily laden with emotion, as when a patient's eyes well up with tears and their voice catches in their throat. Emotion, like silence, must always be honored, embraced, and tenderly acknowledged, never ignored or rushed, which communicates a lack of comfort with or even disrespect for a patient's interior world. Offering words like, "I'm sorry," "This must be so difficult," or a soothing touch (as culturally appropriate) or empathetic facial expression is often all that is needed to ensure that patients continue to feel comfortable experiencing and expressing emotion in our presence.

Inquiries such as, "How are you feeling?", "How are you doing with this information?" and "I know that was a lot to cover. How are you doing?" are helpful ways of acknowledging the potential heaviness of a situation and providing time for patients and family members to experience, process, and share their emotions.

Sometimes, patients or family members say one thing, but their intonation, body language, or facial expressions indicate a different meaning. Always pause to ask for clarification with a gentle inquiry such as, "Tell me what you're thinking," providing plenty of time for an answer, which may reveal difficult or conflicting emotions, thoughts, or concerns.

Asking directly about concerns is especially important because fears that patients and families are embarrassed by or afraid to express can become insurmountable obstacles to a successful and collaborative conversation. While writing this book, I received worrisome results of a mammogram requiring I return for further testing on account of microcalcifications concerning for breast cancer. Suddenly faced with a cancer scare, I became consumed with worry about not being able to complete my manuscript on account of "chemo brain," the sluggish cognitive side-effect common to chemotherapy. Beside myself with worry, I called a dear friend, who is a women's diagnostic radiologist, for advice. Upon hearing my situation, she immediately provided the much-needed reassurance that in the worst-case scenario, I would need only surgery and radiation but no chemotherapy. I was relieved that I would be able to complete my manuscript, and the possibility of having breast cancer was much less scary. Fortunately, my imaging and biopsy results were benign, and I finished writing my book without impediment.

This experience was a good reminder that when discussing anything potentially worrisome, it is best to ask patients and families upfront about any concerns they might have so that they can be addressed immediately. "Before we begin, I'd like to address any specific concerns or worries you might have" is an encouraging invitation, and for those who demur, "Please feel free to interrupt me with questions or concerns" shows interest in what is important to them.

Emotions, concerns, or distress that patients and family members express must always be immediately acknowledged, validated, and responded to with empathy. Responses such as, "I'm so sorry," "That must be so hard," "Thank you for sharing that," and "I'm glad you told me that was so important to you" go a long way toward helping patients and loved ones feel heard, seen, and validated. For those times when it is not best to address a patient's concern right away, offer your intention to address it later by saying, "I heard your concern and will help make sense of (or navigate) that in a bit."

A note about identifying with people's emotions: while it is important to acknowledge patient and family emotions and even to mirror their emotions by shedding a tear or laughing with them, it is risky business to express a sentiment of *understanding exactly what a patient or family member is going through*. Statements like, "I can understand how hard this is," risk offending patients because the reality is that no one, except the patient themself, can truly understand what they are experiencing. Each patient's approach to the end of life is unique—they are the *only* person who will ever have experienced their particular journey. Instead, empathize by saying, "I can imagine this must be very difficult."

Nonjudgment and Acceptance

Holding space means creating a fully accepting and nonjudgmental environment in which patients and family members can feel safe to explore medical decisions in the context of their personal values, wishes, and concerns. To create such an environment, we must put aside our egos, biases, and personal values so that we can be present to the emotional, spiritual, and physical needs of patients and family members, never passing judgment or inserting our own needs, but rather, extending comfort and solace while remaining humble, loving, and kind. Because patient-centered care is never about us, we must leave our personal opinions, beliefs, and preferences out of their equation. The only exception is when providing validation, which is an important means of empowering patients and families on their challenging journeys.

To communicate our acceptance and nonjudgment, we must continuously manage our facial expressions and body language so we don't inadvertently communicate criticism, frustration, impatience, or discomfort. The goal is to remain a compassionate and impartial sounding board for patients and families to express, explore, and evaluate their wishes, needs, and priorities with respect to medical options.

Particularly when patients and families make brave decisions to forego or stop treatments, which are almost always fraught, we must honor their decisions and humanity by keeping dissenting personal beliefs or opinions out of our responses. Several patients of mine have communicated a sense of feeling abandoned, disrespected, discarded, and disdained by their physicians when they chose to focus on quality of life over the *potential* for additional quantity of life by deciding to stop chemotherapy, avoid a leg amputation, enroll in hospice care, etc. Patients and family members should *never* walk away from medical interactions feeling diminished in this way, and such responses by physicians fly in the face of the call to provide "competent medical care, with compassion and respect for human dignity and rights." [3]. Patient choice, especially when made from a place of earnest consideration of personal values and priorities, must always be deeply respected, honored, and validated by the medical community.

For those who have made brave decisions to stop or forego treatment, offer words that honor their bravery in the face of cultural messaging that frequently encourages them to "never give up," validating their choices and acknowledging what could only have been very difficult decisions to make.

Normalizing, Validating, and Reassuring

Offering words that generously acknowledge, normalize, validate, and reassure the patients' and families' emotional, physical, and spiritual struggles is one of the most powerful ways of expressing acceptance and nonjudgment. Such words, offered encouragingly and authentically, are a means of tending to patients' and family members' emotional and spiritual well-being and resilience. This loving-kindness should be extended at every opportunity. Learning that they are not alone in their challenges and hearing that their concerns are valid provides patients and loved ones much-needed relief and a source of empowerment.

To spouses and other caregivers, make a point of telling them, when appropriate, that their loved one is doing so well because of their incredible care. Explain that disease often takes its greatest toll on caregivers, especially spouses and intimate partners, validating the caregiver's need for self-care, respite, and grieving. Offer to write a prescription for self-care and join in as caregivers laugh appreciatively.

Reassure patients and families that they are not alone in their worries and experiences, offering support groups or counseling referrals when possible. When sharing a concern about caregiver strain or burnout, explain that it is normal to feel overwhelmed by caregiving and that it is both important and necessary that caregivers find a way to prioritize their own health, as the health and well-being of their loved ones depend on *their* health and well-being. Alleviating caregivers from the burdens of shame and guilt that can accompany the need and desire for self-care or respite by acknowledging and validating their exhaustion is often the first permission caregivers receive to rest, make time for themselves, and ask for help.

Patient care is the perfect setting to provide the kind of normalization, validation, and reassurance we would give to friends reaching out to us for support.

Interest in the "Whole Person"

Holding space in a way that empowers patients and families to make decisions that align with their values requires an authentic interest in the **whole person** by extending our concern beyond patient symptoms and disease to explore the socioeconomic, cultural, spiritual, religious, and ethnic realities of patient and family life. This is done by asking open-ended questions and encouraging patients and families to "Tell us more," inquiring about caregiver health and well-being, day-to-day experiences at home and in the world, family dynamics, financial and nutritional resources, transportation stressors, etc. so that we can better understand, assess, and make recommendations that fit the needs of the patient and family.

For example, learning that a patient is caring for a loved one at home and needs high-quality, regular sleep to maintain resilience to the threat of caregiver strain should guide recommendations for blood pressure management. Diuretics, which can interrupt a good night of sleep, might not be the best option for this patient-who-is-also-a-primary-caregiver.

Extending our interest beyond the patient is necessary when providing patient-centered care because patients do not experience a diagnosis alone. Family members, particularly spouses or intimate partners, are always profoundly impacted by a patient's disease. The patient-centered care model requires that we consider the **family**, not merely the patient, the primary unit of care.[1] This is particularly true for families experiencing the dementia journey, which so heavily taxes caregivers, who may be friends, neighbors, or relatives. Most of the care I provide to patients with dementia is directed toward their caregivers.

Acknowledging, Respecting, and Accepting Patient Beliefs

Open-ended questions investigating the "whole person" will frequently reveal beliefs (and belief systems) held by patients and families. Beliefs are ideas, opinions, or tenets that people accept as truth and help organize their understanding of the world and personal experience. Uncovering patient and family beliefs, particularly about theological and medical matters, is critically important. As we will learn in later chapters about the *Arc of Conversation* technique, before we can share information with patients and families, we must first understand what they believe to be true about their health, healing, and mortality.

---

[1] Note that families can be made up of friends rather than relations by blood or marriage.

Part of caring for patients is to inquire about their spiritual well-being, which can be done by asking, "Do you have any spiritual or religious beliefs or practices that bring you comfort?" This is a gentle way of investigating people's theological beliefs, which often dictate or influence their medical beliefs.

When asked this question, patients often respond by telling me they are comfortable with where they are going, reflecting an optimistic expectation about the afterlife. To clarify and avoid making inaccurate assumptions, I will ask whether they are "afraid of the dying process" or "of being dead." These two very distinct questions must be addressed and can reveal a patient's spiritual beliefs or acceptance or fears about their mortality.

As with emotion, beliefs must be honored, accepted, and respected. It is never appropriate to directly dispute, confront, oppose, or unravel a patient or family member's beliefs. This includes beliefs about medical matters, such as where they are in their journey, their life expectancy or prognosis, and how a higher power may determine medical matters. Even beliefs about small medical realities, like why weight loss occurs toward the end of life, should be handled gently and lovingly so as not to force a confrontation with or unkindly undo patient or family beliefs.

Beliefs likely to be more robust and long-standing, such as about who or what is in charge of the timing of the end of life, must be handled with expert care. Statements offered by patients, such as, "Only God knows when my time will be up," reveal important information about how willing they may be to trust the medical community's knowledge about prognostication and timing of end-of-life care.

Some patients and family members will express belief or hopes for medical miracles, which are, by definition, events that oppose what humans expect to be possible according to natural laws of physics or biology and are thought to be accomplished by divine or supernatural intervention. Although belief in miracles may seem to directly oppose a belief in medicine, science, and biology, these beliefs must also be respected, accepted, and gently honored.

The "Wish, Worry, Wonder" Technique to Respond to Patient Beliefs or Wishes

A valuable technique for responding to patient beliefs or wishes that do not match up with what might be expected given the medical reality is one I learned from a palliative and hospice care physician, Dr. Faryal Michaud, on her podcast, "Write Your Last Chapter." [8]. The "Wish, Worry, Wonder" technique that Dr. Michaud describes supports holding space, companioning our patients, and providing compassionate and collaborative care as a friend might do. This technique is similar to the "wish…worry," "hope…worry" method in the *Serious Illness Conversation Guide* published by Ariadne Labs [9].

The first step of the "Wish, Worry, Wonder" technique is to be aware of and sensitive to any contradiction between the patient's beliefs or wishes and the medical reality. Let's imagine a previously very fit 89-year-old patient who has lost 25% of their body weight in the previous six months (despite appropriate mealtime support), is suffering from frequent falls and an increasing need for assistance across the day, currently meets hospice criteria, and responds to the question, "What are you expecting going forward?", by saying, "I want to get strong enough that I can hike the Pacific Coast Trail with my grandson next year."

This patient's answer reveals a medical belief about the body's ability to heal that is inconsistent with what we know about aging, metabolic decline, and mortality risk once a patient meets hospice criteria. Holding space for patients means we must respect, acknowledge, and respond to such beliefs gently and kindly. The "Wish, Worry, Wonder" technique provides an excellent scaffolding for doing so.

Starting with a **wish**, offer a statement that aligns your hopes for the patient with their wishes, such as, "Oh, I **wish** that could be possible for you too. That sounds amazing." Placing you next to the patient in a companionate role rather than in a position of medical authority, this type of response supports, affirms and validates the patient's hopes, dreams, and aspirations.

Next, share a **worry**, which gently relates the patient's medical reality to the unlikelihood of their wish coming to fruition. "I **worry**, though, given your age and how much weight you have lost, and how frail you have become, that getting back to a point where you could do such a strenuous hike might be difficult." This type of statement gently acknowledges the discordance between the patient's wish and their medical situation but in a kind and respectful way that allows them to arrive at their own conclusion and to relinquish their wish in their own time.

Remember, patient wishes that wildly misalign with their medical reality indicate an internal struggle with their mortality that has not yet been resolved, a Herculean, once-in-a-lifetime task for which no one can adequately prepare. Watching patients bravely face their mortality is something to cherish, respect, and learn from. Acknowledging their grace by saying, "You are so brave. I can't imagine how difficult this must be," provides much-needed encouragement and reassurance for an unimaginably challenging effort.

Sometimes, I will follow up a **worry** statement with the question, "Do you **worry** about that too?" providing an opportunity for patients to investigate their doubts about their original wish. Affirmative responses to this question provide a stepping stone that can be relied on later in the conversation when it is time to deliver delicate information about where a patient is in their journey, such as the fact that they meet hospice criteria.

Before doing that, it is important to offer a **wonder** statement, which includes an alternative proposition that aligns with some aspect of the patient's original wish. For the patient in our example, who was hoping to regain the strength he enjoyed when he was younger in order to experience a life-affirming adventure with a beloved grandchild, you might offer, "I wonder if instead of going on the Pacific Coast Trail, you and your grandson could get together and share stories and pictures of your last trip, or maybe you could help him plan his next hike." A suggestion like this acknowledges and tends to the patient's humanity while helping to reimagine their original intent in a way that more effectively works given their current health status.

The "Wish, Worry, Wonder" technique is an important tool in our toolkit of rapport-, trust-, and safety-building with patients, allowing us to continually validate and reassure our patients' interior lives.

Rapport, Trust, and Safety

Rapport, trust, and safety, all critical components of the patient-provider relationship, develop early when we set the stage and expectations for how we will interact with patients and caregivers. Rapport reflects a relationship characterized by friendliness and harmony, a beautiful foundation for a patient-centered relationship in which trust and safety can flourish. Once patients and family members feel a sense of rapport, they can feel safe enough to let down their guards and trust us with their wishes, cares, values, and concerns.

One of the easiest ways to establish rapport with other people is by offering our humanity. This can be done by appropriately sharing the burden of patient emotion through the expression of empathy or mirrored emotion (it is okay to tear up or laugh when patients and family members do, so long as our emotions don't take center stage); by sharing an anecdote of our own experience, an act of humility that can both validate and empower patients and their loved ones; or by interjecting a well-timed joke, which can lighten the mood and alleviate the heaviness of a situation. Rapport with patients, like with friends, develops from the generosity of authenticity, vulnerability, and a sense of shared humanity.

Trustworthiness

An important contributor to the development of trust and safety is our trustworthiness, which requires more than just competent medical care [4]. In addition to honesty and integrity, trustworthiness requires that we consistently work to improve patient and family physical and mental well-being and quality of life, willingly advocate for patients and families, go the extra mile to help them navigate the complexity of disease and the healthcare system, follow through on what we say we will do, and apologize for our mistakes or those of the medical community [4]. Trustworthiness becomes a safety net for patients and families, helping to ensure that their experience of the healthcare system and their disease journey adds to their quality of life instead of diminishing it. An essential part of the customer service aspect of health care, trustworthiness is felt by patients and families when they consistently receive both competent and compassionate medical care [4].

Active Listening and Not Making Assumptions

Another vital aspect of holding space involves a conversational skill called **active listening**, an important means of building rapport, safety, and trust. A communication mode that centers patient and family experiences and concerns, active listening is grounded in full and impartial attention, comfort with patient silence, and the provision of encouraging or comforting verbal and nonverbal responses to whatever has been said [4]. Active listening is an *active* form of communication that requires our continuous engagement with the emotions and narratives that patients and families feel comfortable sharing and also requires that we remain fully present and focused.

Tending to others actively in conversations requires that we respond to what was just said [4] (either verbally or nonverbally) with empathy or in a way that allows for a smooth transition in the conversation. When patients are expressing or experiencing emotion or delivering a narrative, we should respond with **continuers** [4]. Continuers are verbal and nonverbal conversational tidbits that encourage patients and families to "Go on," "Tell us more," or communicate that we are keeping pace with what they are saying, for example, "Uh huh," "Wow," "Amazing," "Oh my gosh," or a head nod, a lifted eyebrow, or a smile. When asking patients or family members to elaborate on something they've said, encouraging inquiries can be made, such as, "Can you explain that to me?", "What was that experience like for you?" or "How did that make you feel?"

When we need to move patients from one point in a conversation to another, such as from a discussion of their personal experience of their illness at home to a discussion about their stage of disease and treatment options, we can summarize where we've been and where we're heading, by saying something like, "Thank you for sharing how things have been going at home. I want to move us into a discussion about your wishes, but first, I'd like us to talk about where you are in your journey with your heart disease." Summarizing what you've already accomplished and what you would yet like to accomplish is a wonderful way of keeping families aligned with the goals and trajectory of the conversation. It also sets the stage for them to share any conversational wishes that they might have.

Reflective listening skills, in which we summarize, rephrase, or paraphrase what patients and families have said, fall under the active listening skillset, and at times, these skills can be beneficial, as in the example immediately above illustrating how to summarize a discussion to move it forward. However, because conversations about disease, disease progression, and end-of-life wishes are emotionally fraught, it can be very easy to offend people by incorrectly paraphrasing what they've said.

Paraphrasing means to put what someone else has said into different words. Paraphrasing assumes understanding, and at times, our understanding will be wrong. What we think a person *meant* to say often differs from what they *intended*. Paraphrasing, by definition, is the act of leaping from something heard to a separate conclusion about meaning. Rather than assuming you understand what someone means by what they've said, it is best to ask for clarification.

For example, you might be tempted to assume from the comment, "I'm going down," that a patient means that they are declining, maybe even approaching the end of their life. Yet the patient may have no insight into any possible decline and might be offended to hear you paraphrase their words in that manner. I learned this lesson the hard way.

When I paraphrased the comment, "I'm going down," by saying to a patient, "I heard you say that you are declining," the patient became noticeably offended and physically and emotionally withdrew from our conversation. Rather than assuming I knew what the patient meant, I learned to ask for clarification, quoting the patient's words directly, "What did you mean when you said, 'I'm going down.'?" Other ways of asking for clarification include, "Can you tell me what you meant by what you just said?" or "Can you tell me more?"

A patient may answer a request for clarification about the comment, "I'm going down," in two very different ways. My patient meant, "I've lost 25 pounds in the last two months. I can no longer lift my laundry basket, and I need help preparing meals." which is a description of their personal *experience* of disease. I mistakenly assumed they were commenting about their *understanding* of where they were in their journey, as in, "I'm getting to the end of my life." Had I asked for clarification rather than assuming, I would have avoided offending this patient's internal beliefs.

For this reason, I recommend taking notes of exact patient phrasing so that you can refer to their words when delving more deeply into their understanding of their health journey. Any summaries, rephrasing, or paraphrasing should be done gently and sensitively to the possibility of unintended offense. Often, a disclaimer such as, "I can't remember exactly how you phrased this, but what I think you said was X. Please correct me if I'm wrong. Did I get that right?" can head off an unfortunate interaction. When we speak to patients and families, we must always be mindful to maintain a respectful and sensitive demeanor.

Sharing Information and Decision Making

At no point in conversation is this more important than when we share information and decision making with our patients and their families. Remember that the purpose of holding space is to empower patients and family members to act in their own best interests as equal members of the medical decision making team and that medical decisions that align with their values must arise from an accurate understanding of their disease, its trajectory, and where they are in their journey.

As we will learn in the later chapters of this book that describe the *Arc of Conversation* approach to having goals of care conversations with patients and families, the first step in sharing information is ascertaining what patients and families already understand about their disease and treatment options. There is no sense, for example, in telling a patient about the need for a heart catheterization to investigate the cause of their heart failure if they have no idea how heart disease can result in shortness of breath and edema, the symptoms that initially caused their admission to the hospital. Were we to begin talking to this patient about heart procedures before first understanding what they think is causing their symptoms and what they know about heart failure, we might offend their beliefs, speak beyond their medical literacy level, or they may be left wondering why they are being told about their heart instead of their lungs and feet. Confused about why we are discussing their heart, the patient might miss important details they need to understand.

Thus, it is crucial, as we will learn, to start in an *investigative* mode to ascertain what patients and families understand about their personal experience, how they are making sense of it, where they think they are in their journey, what they understand about their specific diagnosis, and what they are expecting ahead. Once we understand the ballpark of a patient's understanding, we can offer to "fill in the gaps of their understanding to help make sense of what they've been experiencing," providing *education* about disease and treatment options in a way that promotes a collaborative discussion. This respectful and gentle approach to guiding patients and their loved ones through challenging conversations ensures that we provide information that can truly be heard so that decisions can come from a place of accurate understanding.

Sharing information with patients and family members requires that we are effective at translating complicated medical and physiologic information into language that they can understand when we discuss their diagnoses, treatment options, the pros and cons of their options, alternative choices, and our recommendations, our own experiences, and the scientific evidence available [4].

Sharing decision making with patients and families requires that we encourage them to participate fully in the conversations and decisions by eliciting and responding to their input (including their priorities, values, concerns, expectations, and preferences), discuss the patient and family's ability or willingness to follow through on decisions, and help them navigate considerations about how decisions will impact their goals, priorities, and quality of life [4].

As providers, we must be willing to encourage deferral of decisions when appropriate [4], such as when more information is required, and be able to facilitate decisions to forego tests and procedures when the outcomes would suggest treatments that would not align with patient wishes and priorities. Questions like "What will you do with that information?" or "How will that information help you?" gently guide patients and families to consider the usefulness of testing, whether the patient could tolerate treatment or procedure recommendations made with that information, or the requirements during the recovery or rehabilitation period. Leading patients and families through such conversations is critical to helping them make decisions that align with their values and goals.

One very effective way of empowering patients and families to participate fully in their decisions is to lessen the emotional weight of the responsibility for making decisions that can be life-changing, by providing the reassurance that "There is no right answer, only the answer that is right for you." and encouraging them to "Take all the time you need. There is no urgency."[2] I offer these words early and often in

---

[2] There are situations in which healthcare decisions must be made urgently, in which case the statement "There is no urgency" would be inappropriate.

discussions about medical wishes and have noticed the visible relief these words provide in reducing the expectation that decisions are either easy to make or must be made quickly.

Decision-Making Capacity

To share decision making with patients, we must first determine whether they have decision-making capacity. Developing the ability to assess a patient's decision-making capacity is an important skill all providers must hone, especially those working with older adults. In addition to honing our ability to assess a patient's decision-making capacity, providers should value and investigate the concerns of any family or medical team member about a patient's memory or cognitive function, including certified nursing assistants (CNAs) and registered nurses (RNs), who often have insight about patient capacity for handling the mechanics of toileting, bathing, dressing, and feeding themselves.

Cognition is the underlying skill for decision-making capacity; thus, because psychiatric illnesses (e.g., depression or schizophrenia), stroke, traumatic brain injury (TBI), or any of the neurodegenerative diseases (e.g., Alzheimer's disease, Parkinson's disease, or vascular dementia) can affect cognition, decision-making capacity should be evaluated continually in patients with these conditions [10]. Likewise, decision-making capacity should be evaluated for patients experiencing illness or infection causing delirium.

Because dementia is so prominent in the aging population and increases in prevalence with increasing age, a decision-making capacity assessment should be considered for all older adults, especially those hospitalized or being seen in the ER. Older adults being seen should have a family member present to confirm pertinent details about their history, especially when a diagnosis of dementia or medications like donepezil or memantine appear in the patient's chart.

A diagnosis of dementia should prompt an evaluation by a team with robust expertise in the dementia journey to assess where the patient is in their journey and to provide valuable insight into the patient's cognitive function and medical decision-making capacity. Of course, capacity decisions should be reassessed daily in circumstances where mental status is fluctuating, such as those with delirium.

Understanding, Appreciating, Reasoning, and Communicating a Choice

To have **decisional capacity**—the ability to make medical decisions—patients must have four competencies, including understanding, appreciating, reasoning, and communicating a choice.

Understanding is the ability of the patient to summarize the meaning inherent to the important details of the situation or choice [10]. By asking patients to "Explain to me what I just explained to you," you can assess whether the patient is capturing the important information upon which a decision must be made [10].

Appreciating means the ability of the patient to relate the information at hand to themselves [10]. A patient must appreciate how the information they are considering relates to their situation. Again, this relies on an accurate appreciation of their situation. "Can you tell me what you understand about your condition or diagnosis?" [10] becomes the starting point to assess patient competency, which is an essential aspect of the technique taught in this book.

If patients are being asked to weigh a treatment decision, then we must also inquire about their understanding of the risks and benefits by questioning, "Can you tell me how this treatment option might benefit you?" or "Can you tell me how this treatment option might harm you?" [10].

Reasoning means understanding the consequences of their decisions through a comparative analysis of the choices offered [10]. Asking, "How would X be better for you than Y?" or "How is this choice going to affect your daily life?" are important questions for assessing the patient's understanding of the consequences of their decisions [10].

Finally, patients must be able to **communicate a choice**: to speak their decision out loud or convey it by appropriate assistive means. For patients who don't speak English, using a skilled medical interpreter—not family members who might inadvertently or purposefully alter a patient's words—is essential. Ask plainly, "Given what we've just discussed, what would you want for yourself?" [10].

An important principle to remember is that decisional capacity is "decision specific," meaning the degree of capacity required to make a given decision varies with the decision itself. A patient might have plenty of capacity to decide what to have for dinner or whether they want to see a particular visitor but not to consent to major surgery or accept or refuse an invasive treatment. Capacity assessment is not a simple one-and-done exercise; it may have to be repeated according to the need and the nature of the decision to ensure full respect for patient autonomy.

It is incredible to watch a patient with dementia who has lost the ability to work through this process of understanding, appreciating, reasoning, and communicating a choice. Their **foundational motivation** and **foundational humanity** (see Chap. 4) come into play in these instances, either resulting in their deferral of opinions and choice to their appointed surrogates or, if their underlying sense of competence, capability, and control has been offended, in reacting defensively. Alternatively, they may answer definitively to one question, for instance, an inquiry about a resuscitation attempt by saying, "If I'm dead, I'm dead," but to follow-up questions like, "Do you know what effort I'm talking about when I mention a resuscitation attempt?" or "Can you tell me how you would feel if following a resuscitation attempt you were to end up on a breathing machine?", they are often unable to respond at all, indicating an inability to do the cognitive labor involved in such complicated and abstract decisions.

Remember, complicated medical decisions involve the ability to store and recall new pieces of information (recent memory) and the ability to manipulate that information using the skills contained in the prefrontal cortex (logic, reason, abstract thinking, planning, judgment, anticipation, and computation). These skills are lost early in the dementia journey. Patients who are losing their ability to perform instrumental activities of daily living (IADLs), which include cooking, cleaning, driving, shopping, and managing appointments, medications, mealtime, finances, the home, and pets, all of which rely on these cognitive capacities, are often unable to make complex medical decisions for themselves or others.

Because cognition degrades across a dementia journey but can be preserved very early on, patient capacity must be continually reevaluated for patients with dementia, particularly because dementia can mask itself so well, even into the end stage. Also, patients in the hospital are not allowed, for the most part, to do any of their own personal care (i.e., to protect them from falling, patients must be assisted by CNAs with dressing, bathing, and toileting), and there is no need in the hospital to perform IADLs. Therefore, assessments based purely on hospital staff reports or observations garnered from superficial conversations with patients are not always accurate. We must involve families at home or staff at care facilities to report on patient baseline for tasks such as bathing, toileting, continence, mealtime management, etc., to assess patient baseline and recent disease progression.

Finally, although cognitive assessment scores cannot be used as a substitute for a conversation-based assessment of a disease trajectory and cognitive capacity, lower scores on tests such as the Montreal Cognitive Assessment (MoCA) and the Mini-Mental Status Examination (MMSE) generally correlate with a reduced capacity for decision making. A 32-study review of patients with Alzheimer's disease revealed that MMSE scores < 16 were consistent with a loss of decision-making capacity [10]. Likewise, a study evaluating MoCA scores in Parkinson's disease patients showed that a score < 22 was highly sensitive (90%) for patient loss of ability to provide consent [10].

Concerning decision-making capacity, I find it helpful to ask spouses and caregivers of patients showing cognitive decline whether they think their loved ones can make complicated medical decisions. In my experience, their answers are almost always congruous with my assessment of the patient's capacity. Asking families to weigh in this way involves them as equal participants in a shared decision-making model and reinforces or validates their experience of their loved one's journey. Ultimately, a shared evaluation of the patient's loss of medical decision-making capacity empowers those legally authorized to take on the role of surrogate decision-maker for their loved ones.

Communicating with Colleagues and Adjusting Actions

Ideally, treatment options identified by primary care providers, oncologists, orthopedists, surgeons, ICU physicians, hospitalists, etc., would be discussed in a team-like, collaborative space that involves the important participants (medical providers, patients, and caregivers), wherein all of the patient-related considerations are known *before* treatments are offered. These considerations would include medical details about any acute issue, but also, and more importantly, medical details about the patient's long-term trajectory, functional status, and any recent decline, the patient's proximity to meeting hospice criteria, and patient and family values, preferences, and wishes, particularly for end-of-life care.

We know that many patients want to pass away at home at the end of their lives and that families do not want their loved ones to suffer from unnecessary, nonbeneficial, or distressing treatments. The further a patient is into a terminal trajectory, the more critical it is to ensure an evaluation by a provider empowered to have the in-depth conversations required to accurately assess the patient's overall health journey and to uncover the patient's and family's values and wishes. Such conversations should be a standard part of medical care for all adults, particularly for those who are hospitalized, admitted for rehabilitation or nursing home care, and those with a chronic or terminal disease.

As mentioned earlier in this book, discharge recommendations made by physical and occupational therapists are often made without consideration of the patient's disease trajectory or where they are in their journey. A snapshot recommendation by occupational or physical therapy that a patient is appropriate for discharge home with family support might be valid for a patient expected to recover fully. However, for patients approaching or already meeting hospice criteria who are expected to decline in the coming days and weeks, such recommendations ignore the caregiver's capacity to address the patient's expected physical and functional decline and risk patient and caregiver safety and well-being.

Too often, my palliative care team observes discharge plans being made by hospitalists relying primarily on physical and occupational therapy recommendations while ignoring the progressive and terminal nature of the patient's disease trajectory and the increasing need for patient support at home or at a care facility. This frequently occurs because a provider has yet to acknowledge where the patient is in their overall journey or because treatment and discharge recommendations have been made before such an assessment. While both situations can lead to a misalignment of patient wishes and medical care, the latter situation can leave families feeling frustrated and can undermine their sense of confidence in the medical community.

Recently, I had a patient living alone who, at a baseline, required help with all aspects of daily living due to significant deficits in cognition but whose verbal fluency and short-term memory were preserved. This patient was recommended for discharge home based on a speech and language therapy (SLT) cognitive assessment using a cognitive screening instrument (e.g., MoCA or MMSE) that determined they only had moderate cognitive impairment.

Although a cognitive assessment using a cognitive screening instrument is an important aspect of evaluating a patient with cognitive decline, it should not be relied on as the *only* component of their cognitive evaluation. Because dementia is a progressive loss of one's ability to make it through the day without help, an accurate assessment of a dementia journey requires that the story of the patient's ongoing day-to-day functional loss be revealed, which often requires a lengthy discussion with caregivers. In this case, our team spoke at length with the family and friends who had known the patient for years and provided much-needed assistance in the home to ensure the patient's survival. During this conversation, our team learned that the family and friends were experiencing significant caregiver strain and were worried that the care they were providing, though necessary, was not enough, as the patient was home alone most of the time. Their concerns were spot on.

Based on the SLT recommendation, which was made without the story of the patient's dementia journey and caregiver concerns, the hospitalist planned to discharge this patient back to their home with home health care (HHC) support. Although HHC can provide intermittent visits by physical, occupational, and speech and language therapists, certified nursing assistants (CNAs), and registered nurses (RNs), the patient would still experience most hours of each day at home alone, at risk of being unable to navigate the day-to-day tasks required to remain safe. Had our team not gotten involved in assessing the patient's status in their dementia journey (near end stage), the discharge plans would have wildly missed the mark of recommending the appropriate level of care (skilled nursing or memory care) for this patient. Because not all cognitive screening instruments evaluate patient capacity to handle IADLs and ADLs, results can be misleading or inconsistent with the story of the patient's need for assistance throughout the day—the most important assessment for patients on the dementia journey.

This is but one example of how medical recommendations that fail to involve the important participants and to consider the critical information about a patient's health status *as well as* family values, preferences, and concerns, can lead to inappropriate or undesired recommendations for the patient and caregivers. The medical community must better integrate acute and long-term medical knowledge and patient and family wishes by assessing the patient's health status and discussing patient and family values *before* making treatment recommendations.

Collaborating with colleagues also means providing courtesy communications before ascertaining patients' and families' wishes and discussing treatment options. One day, I learned this important lesson when I pursued a conversation with a family member without informing the hospitalist that I would be doing so. By the end of my discussion, the family member was hospice minded for their loved one. However, the discharge plans were already set to send the patient to a rehabilitation facility. Understandably, the hospitalist was upset by the unexpected change in course, and the family member's confidence in the medical community's competence was diminished.

Whereas "collaboration without compassion may result in technically correct but depersonalized care that fails to meet the unique emotional and psychosocial needs of all involved," [7] it is equally true that "compassion without collaboration may result in uncoordinated care." [7]. Frustrating both my hospitalist colleague and the patient's caregiver by failing to collaborate with *every* member of the patient care team resulted in less-than-ideal compassionate care.

Rather than pursuing my conversation with this family member to its logical end, I learned to pause my discussion after arriving at my assessment of the patient's health status and reaching out to the hospitalist with this information before offering to pursue further conversations. Ideally, in turn, my colleague, recognizing that my assessment was missing from their evaluation, would welcome my input and my offer to pursue patient and family medical wishes, as well as remain open to adjusting patient treatment plans based on what I learned about their values, hopes, priorities, and concerns.

This is to say that genuinely collaborative and compassionate patient-centered care requires bidirectional communication with colleagues, patients, and families that is timely, considerate, and accompanied by a willingness to adjust actions (i.e., treatment options, discharge plans, etc.) accordingly.

Practicing Self-Reflection

As I mentioned in this book's introduction (Chap. 1), I learned to speak with patients and families about disease and end-of-life wishes through much trial and error and a heaping dose of self-reflection. Whenever I felt that I had pushed patients or family members too quickly, far, or fast through a conversation, I reflected on my actions and adjusted my approach in future interactions.

The reality of practicing medicine is that we must constantly self-reflect to improve our approach. Practice makes perfect, as they say, and we should endorse an attitude of self-compassion to appreciate the reality that we will make mistakes but can get better over time. It might be surprising to learn that the lesson in collaborating compassionately that I mentioned above was one that I learned just a couple of months before writing this chapter. Perfect timing and an excellent reminder that I still have much to learn!

Just as crucial as self-reflection, we must also be open to eliciting and implementing feedback from colleagues [4], which at times can be difficult but is a necessary ingredient of self-improvement. It was my hospitalist colleague's respectful and kind feedback that allowed me to learn the important lesson about coordinating compassionate care.

Attending to Relationships

It is true that to best support patients and families across their complex medical journeys, we must work continuously to hold space for *everyone*—patients, family, other caregivers, and medical professionals across the healthcare system—so that everyone can feel safe and empowered to share their knowledge, experience, opinions, recommendations, and emotions [4]. Such an environment, based on compassionate respect for each care team member's unique contributions and limitations (patients and families included), will naturally result in partnership, relationship, and teamwork [4].

A partnership-, relationship-, and teamwork-based milieu is based on a deep respect for differing cultures, contributions, ideas, beliefs, and expertise, [4] and on communication grounded in respect, compassion, and collaboration, even in disagreement [4]. This requires mindfulness of how hierarchy and power differentials affect relationships [4], willingness to share, and confidence. It also requires intentionality in encouraging team members across the healthcare hierarchy to feel empowered to speak up.

Not long ago, a nurse at an assisted living care facility expressed reluctance to share with her patients' families her recommendations for their care. This situation came to light when I sought the nurse's help with a mutual patient's daughter, who was considering an involved surgery for her father's facial skin cancer. Sharing my concern that the patient's advanced dementia would prevent him from remembering to leave his bandages alone and follow the post-procedure instructions, I asked the nurse for her thoughts. While she agreed with my concerns, she felt reluctant to share them with the patient's daughter, explaining that she worried her opinions and experience might inappropriately sway the daughter's decision. Rather than being inappropriate, I reassured her that her advice was *exactly* the information the daughter needed as she struggled to make the best decision for her dad.

The reality is that everyone in healthcare, including CNAs, RNs, physical therapists, the billing department, the valet service, etc., has vital information to contribute concerning patient and family perceptions, beliefs, preferences, and wishes. Everyone's input should be acknowledged, respected, and respectfully included in patient-centered care.

The ability for everyone in the patient's sphere to be and do their best requires not only that we care for each other in our interactions, for example, by delivering feedback to colleagues that is compassionate, gentle, and preserves their dignity, but we must also continue to learn independently and collaboratively (for example, by mentoring). We must also encourage each participant to take good care of themselves [4]. Self-care is one of the most essential aspects of well-being. Again, *everyone*—patients, caregivers, family members, and clinical and non-clinical medical staff—should be encouraged to acknowledge compassion fatigue, take respite in the form of personal time off (PTO) or breaks from caregiving, to care for their physical bodies with enough nutrition, hydration, exercise, and rest, and to care for their spiritual bodies in whatever ways fill their cup.

Attending to One's Own Well-being

Self-care is singled out as a specific attribute of the compassionate, collaborative care model, highlighting the importance of this critical ingredient of patient-centered care [4]. To remain compassionate and caring in our interactions with patients and family members, we must ensure that our cup of well-being is full. If we don't, compassion fatigue, which reduces our ability to experience and act on empathy, can occur. In essence, self-care is the act of holding space for ourselves.

First appearing in the literature to describe the negative emotional toll on hospital nurses of repeated exposure to their patients' emergencies [11], *compassion fatigue* results from the effort of caring for others over time [12] and is common to those working in the helping professions, such as firefighters, police officers, social workers, palliative and hospice care workers, and paramedics [13]. Research suggests that compassion fatigue is comprised of two "negative aspects of caring,": *burnout* and *secondary traumatic stress* [14].

Burnout, which can occur in any profession, is physical, emotional, or mental exhaustion that limits one's capacity to respond to the environment [15] and can reduce one's sense of accomplishment [16]. Secondary traumatic stress is trauma-related stress that occurs because of ongoing exposure to other people's "stressful events and suffering." [14] Compassion fatigue, burnout, and secondary traumatic stress can lead to depression, self-neglect, and an increased risk of suicide [14].

Warning signs of compassion fatigue include but are not limited to feelings of hopelessness, helplessness, anger, sadness, anxiety, irritability, numbness, nausea, hypersensitivity, insensitivity, insomnia, nightmares, anhedonia (reduced pleasure from enjoyable activities), poor decision making, poor concentration, relationship conflict, problems at work, issues managing tasks at home, self-medicating with drugs or alcohol, and social isolation and withdrawal [17].

The Professional Quality of Life (ProQOL) Scale, developed by traumatic stress researcher Dr. Beth Hudnall Stamm, measures the work-related impact of helping others [18]. Assessing the two negative aspects of compassion fatigue (burnout and secondary traumatic stress) and the positive aspect of *compassion satisfaction* (the pleasure derived from the work of helping others) [14], the ProQOL is currently free and available online at https://proqol.org.

To prevent compassion fatigue, we must acknowledge our limitations, keep healthy boundaries for demands and expectations (both of ourselves and from others), continually revisit our plan for self-care, realize how our losses and grief can impact our ability to care for others, maintain healthy and supportive relationships, and give ourselves time to experience joy, rest, and reward, all of which deliver a "sense of renewal." [4].

In the wake of my divorce, I readily shared with my patients and their families what I was experiencing, allowing them to pour their coffee and compassion for me in equal measure. Many of my patients became my caregivers during those months, and I do not doubt that their loving tenderness toward me gave them a sense of reward and purpose that touched their sense of renewal. We are all in this together, as the saying goes, and there is no shame in being vulnerable with our patients as long as our issues don't take center stage.[3]

Also, in the wake of my divorce, I had to acknowledge my limitations of time, compassion, and attention as I deeply experienced and shared with colleagues, friends, and family members my depths of sorrow, despair, and disconnection. Over the months, in therapy and in friendship, as I acknowledged my failings in my marriage, I learned to love myself compassionately and gently, and by sharing my

---

[3] In her book *Dare to Lead*, Brené Brown clarifies that being vulnerable does not mean "oversharing, indiscriminate disclosure…or vulnerability for vulnerability's sake." While sharing details of one's life with patients to communicate one's humanity is okay, it is important to be mindful of appropriate boundaries. Brown writes, "Vulnerability minus boundaries is not vulnerability. It's confession, manipulation, desperation, or shock and awe, but it's not vulnerability." (Brown B. Dare to lead. Vermilion; 2018.)

stories with others, I felt a deeper connection to many friends and family members who had shared similar experiences in life. Self-compassion requires that we do all this, including embracing our suffering, nonjudgmentally acknowledging our faults, and seeing ourselves as part of the greater human family [4].

We must also engage in a healthy and ongoing practice of self-regulation and self-monitoring [4]. We must remain constantly aware of how our personal beliefs (cultural, religious, political, etc.) or biases can impact our attitudes and behaviors when interacting with others, ask for help or step away whenever these beliefs or biases interfere with our ability to remain compassionate and caring, create healthy boundaries when we begin to over-identify with a patient or situation, and equally important, monitor ourselves when we begin to detach from a patient or situation [4]. Monitoring and regulating ourselves also requires that we understand when we are approaching our breaking point, when compassion fatigue is beginning to set in, and when we are experiencing signs or symptoms of mental health issues or personal grief or strain [4]. As I often remind caregivers, we cannot care for others unless we first care for ourselves.

Compassion fatigue happens to me fairly often, especially when I encounter patients and family members whom I experience as overbearing and demanding or who exhibit traits of narcissistic or borderline personality, which can leave me feeling drained. Recently, when a scheduling mix-up occurred wherein a patient's family member showed up for an appointment when I was across town seeing another patient, I felt myself reach the bottom of my generosity barrel as I heard her say, "I'm having a tough time. I am a very important part of my mother's care, and you should be ministering to me." At that point in my week, I was fresh out of ministrations, and although she was not wrong, the demand in her voice triggered irritation instead of empathy. It was all I could do to kindly apologize for the error and share my willingness to reschedule with her. How ironic to hear the message of my book echoed back to me by a family member as I felt the dregs of compassion evaporating from my spirit at the exact moment that I was completing this chapter. The reality is that compassion fatigue can happen to any of us at any time. Noticing myself feeling annoyed, frustrated, or short in my replies serves as a reminder to schedule a day off, time in nature, or an evening out with my friends.

Checking In

There is no doubt about it; conversations about disease and end-of-life are often emotionally draining and time-consuming. We ask a lot of patients and families when we ask them to face their mortality or changing family dynamics and to sit with us in a discussion about a diagnosis or medical wishes. To avoid pushing people too quickly, too far, or too fast into challenging terrain, we must periodically check in with them and take their emotional temperature by asking, "How are you doing so far?"

This question gently communicates to patients and families our concern for their interior lives and our wish for them to feel comfortable in our conversation, and their answers provide meaningful feedback about whether it is safe for us to continue. I suspect the asking helps bolster people's confidence in pushing onward through difficult terrain. This question can safely be repeated several times during a challenging conversation.

Likewise, when wrapping up a difficult conversation, offer a final check-in with the question, "How are you feeling about our conversation?" This will give patients and families a moment to reflect on the emotional labor they've just performed. Their answers will let you know if you are leaving them in a better condition than when you started. I find that if I've done an excellent job in remaining compassionate and collaborative, properly respecting people's willingness to move forward with me in our conversation, and providing information gently and kindly that respects their beliefs, medical literacy, and values, patients and families will thank me for the information I've shared and voice their gratitude for a challenging, but necessary, discussion. Most people want to discuss these topics and are grateful for the opportunity.

Bedside Manner and "The Triple C" Model of Care

One of the highest medical accolades is for a patient or family member to claim that a practitioner has an excellent bedside manner. Capturing the compassionate aspect of the AMA's first principle of medical ethics, bedside manner refers to a physician's humanity, ability to listen, and responsive engagement with the patient and family. Providers who can readily bridge the gap between scientific endeavor and the human patient, make accessible what is so often clinical, and individual what is so often impersonal, can be said to have excellent bedside manner.

The attributes of "The Triple C" Model and Framework, fleshed out in this chapter, serve as a blueprint for developing bedside manner, allowing providers to properly companion patients and families as they journey through some of the most challenging terrain imaginable. As we will see in the coming chapters, the *Arc of Conversation* technique is grounded in the ability to successfully hold space for patients and their families as we guide them through the rugged landscape of disease, its progression, and decisions about the end of life.

References

1. Brady A. Holding space: the art of being present with others. 2018. https://chopra.com/articles/holding-space-the-art-of-being-present-with-others. Accessed 8 Feb 2023.
2. Glenn AW. Holding space: on loving, dying, and letting go. Berkeley, CA: Parallax Press; 2017.
3. AMA principles of medical ethics. 2001. https://code-medical-ethics.ama-assn.org/principles. Accessed 31 Jan 2023.
4. Lown B, McIntosh S, McGuinn K, Aschenbrener C, Chou C, King A, Irons M, Baldwin D, Schwartzberg J, D H. Advancing compassionate, patient-and family-centered-care through interprofessional education for collaborative practice: compassion, collaborative care

model and framework. https://www.theschwartzcenter.org/media/FINAL-CCC-Model-and-Framework.pdf. Accessed 4 Feb 2023.

5. Pfaff K, Markaki A. Compassionate collaborative care: an integrative review of quality indicators in end-of-life care. BMC Palliat Care. 2017;16(1):65. https://doi.org/10.1186/s12904-017-0246-4. PMID: 29191185; PMCID: PMC5709969

6. Recommendations from a conference on: advancing compassionate, person- and family-centered care through interprofessional education for collaborative practice. 2014. https://www.theschwartzcenter.org/media/FINAL-Triple-C-Conference-Recommendations-Report.pdf. Accessed 4 Feb 2023.

7. Lown BA, McIntosh S, Gaines ME, McGuinn K, Hatem DS. Integrating compassionate, collaborative care (the "triple C") into health professional education to advance the triple aim of health care. Acad Med. 2016;91(3):310–6. https://doi.org/10.1097/ACM.0000000000001077.

8. Michaud F (Host). (2020, Aug 28). Wish worry wonder. [Audio podcast episode]. In Write your last chapter. Accessed 4 Mar 2023.

9. Serious Illness Conversation Guide. April 2017. https://www.ariadnelabs.org/wp-content/uploads/2017/05/SI-CG-2017-04-21_FINAL.pdf. Accessed 4 Mar 2023.

10. Karlawish J. Assessment of decision-making capacity in adults. 2023. https://www.uptodate.com/contents/assessment-of-decision-making-capacity-in-adults. Assessed 19 Feb 2023.

11. Joinson C. Coping with compassion fatigue. Nursing. 1992;22(4):116. 118-9, 120

12. McHolm F. Rx for compassion fatigue. J Christ Nurs. 2006;23:12–9.

13. Figley CR. Catastrophes: an overview of family reactions. In: Figley CR, McCubbin HL, editors. Stress and the family: coping with catastrophe, vol. 2. New York, NY: Brunner/Mazel; 1983. p. 3–21.

14. Huggard P, Stamm BH, Pearlman LA. Physician stress: compassion satisfaction, compassion fatigue and vicarious traumatization. In: First do no self harm: understanding and promoting physician stress resilience. Oxford Academic; 23 Jan. 2014 [cited 26 Jan. 2024]. [online]; 2013. https://doi.org/10.1093/acprof:oso/9780195383263.003.0007.

15. Maslach C, Leiter M. The truth about burnout: how organizations cause personal stress and what to do about it. San Francisco, CA: Jossey-Bass; 1998.

16. Canadian Medical Association. Compassion fatigue: signs, symptoms, and how to cope. In: Physician Wellness Hub. 2020. [cited 2024 Jan 26]. Available from: https://www.cma.ca/physician-wellness-hub/content/compassion-fatigue-signs-symptoms-and-how-cope .

17. Centre for Addiction and Mental Health (CAMH). Is there a cost to protecting, caring for and saving others? Beware of Compassion Fatigue. In: CAMH News and Stories [Internet]. [accessed 26 Jan 2024]. Available from: https://www.camh.ca/en/camh-news-and-stories/is-there-a-cost-to-protecting-caring-for-and-saving-others-beware-of-compassion-fatigue .

18. Stamm BH. The ProQOL manual. 2005. [cited 2024 Jan 26]. Available from: https://compassionfatigue.org/pages/ProQOLManualOct05.pdf.

Part III

The Arc of Conversation

The Arc of Conversation: Foundations of the Technique

8

As the owner of a wedding photography studio in Southern California, where the clientele was sophisticated and fashion-forward, I quickly realized that I needed an approach to my initial consultation that would allow me to showcase my work without the sense that I was trying to sell anything. At the higher price point where my studio was positioned, my clients were the kind of people who wanted their life experiences to be, well, *experiences*. They wanted their wedding photographer to be an affable and hip addition to their wedding day, someone with whom their friends and family would feel comfortable being themselves. As important as their photos would be, my clients placed equal importance on the experience I would help to create as I captured their special day. Although mindful of value, they were more dedicated to making a decision that would provide the reliability, comfort, and quality they desired.

So, I developed an approach to my initial client visit that would gently traverse a conversational landscape centered on the couple, their envisioned wedding experience, family traditions, values, priorities, and important relationships. Positioning myself as an investigator of their vision, I started our visit by asking them to share their story—how they met, how they became engaged, and how their wedding planning had been going so far. As they spoke, I listened for personal tidbits that conveyed their sense of style, personality, and the overall tenor of the wedding day they wanted to create for themselves, their friends, and their families.

After learning as much as I could about the couple, I moved the conversation into an exploration of their photography wishes, including their desired photographic style and any ideas they might have for their engagement photos and portraits on their big day. As I listened, determining whether the couple's vision matched my artistic approach, I also addressed their fears and concerns, collaboratively brainstorming ideas for achieving their goals on film. Only at the end of our conversation did I introduce my packages and pricing, avoiding any pressure on them to decide.

While it was always a cause for celebration when the couple decided to book me on the spot, I learned to let go of such expectations, recognizing that a considered decision to hire me more often represented a compatible alignment of the couple's

A. Shaw, PA, *The Arc of Conversation*,
https://doi.org/10.1007/978-3-031-70495-6_8

wishes and budget with what I had to offer. I learned that each "No" was as critical to my business success and client satisfaction as every "Yes."

Learning to be a savvy business owner in a nonmedical milieu prepared me to work with patients and families in palliative care. Not only did weddings provide basic training for compassionately navigating people through one of life's most challenging milestones, but the initial client appointment provided a valuable framework for developing the collaborative conversational approach that I call the Arc of Conversation.

The Arc of Conversation

The Arc of Conversation is based on a very simple premise—that an **investigation** of patient and family **experience** of illness and **understanding** of a diagnosis must occur before providing **education** about disease, because medical decisions that best reflect patient and family values come from an accurate understanding of patient health status (Fig. 8.1).

The flow directed by the Arc of Conversation diagram follows that of an English-language book, moving from left to right and from top to bottom. Four distinct, colorful arcs of focus are approached in the following order: **Illness Arc, Disease Arc, End-of-Life Wishes Arc,** and **Hospice Care Arc.** In each arc, **investigation** of patient and family **experience** and **understanding** occurs before providing **education**. As we move from one arc to the next, we get closer and closer to the heart of the matter—patient and family wishes for medical care.

Like a rainbow, the Arc of Conversation relies on certain atmospheric conditions—empathy, patience, and expertise about the end of life. Just as a rainbow can quickly disappear when the atmosphere shifts, the Arc of Conversation can disintegrate before our eyes if we don't manage ourselves and others in the room appropriately. The skills discussed in prior chapters enable us to create the

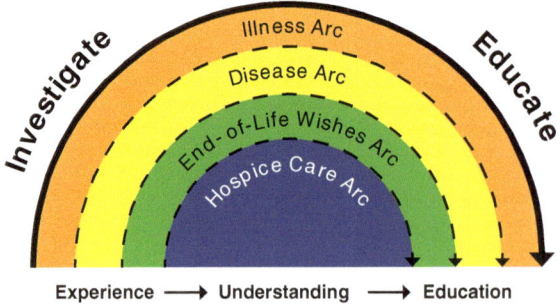

Fig. 8.1 The Arc of Conversation. The Arc of Conversation technique is based on the premise that an investigation of patient and family experience of illness and understanding of a diagnosis must occur before providing education about disease because medical decisions that best reflect patient and family values come from an accurate understanding of patient health status

compassionate and collaborative milieu required to guide patients and families through the Arc of Conversation.

The Role of the Clinician as Guide

If we think of the patient and family as travelers on a medical journey, then I can think of no better metaphor for the job of a physician than a guide, ushering those in our care through the landscape of a diagnosis by helping to make sense of where they've been so that they can better plan for the journey ahead.

According to Dictionary.com, a **guide** is "a person who guides, especially one hired to guide travelers," and **to guide** means "to assist (a person) to travel through, or reach a destination in, an unfamiliar area, as by accompanying or giving directions to the person," or "to accompany (a sightseer) to show points of interest and to explain their meaning or significance." [1].

For most people, the landscape of illness and disease represents unfamiliar and uncomfortable territory. Many lack a rich understanding of why a disease causes its symptoms, how a diagnosis will impact their lives, and what they can expect as their disease progresses. Death—that elusive surprise ending—though ever on the horizon, is experienced out of sight, something that happens to *other people* but never to *them*. As the sun sets on people's lives and the horizon nears, patients and families often flounder in this foreign and frightful terrain. With no one to help make sense of their experiences, people can feel lost, abandoned by the world, physically and psychologically diminished, and confused by medical options that don't seem to be "working." A sense of helplessness can lead to anxiety, depression, frustration, and disconnection, transforming a potentially spiritually rich time of life into a jungle of chaos and fear.

As guides, our role is to lead people through a personal exploration of this landscape, attending to their spiritual selves by holding space as they process and express their feelings during this sacred stage of life. We are not peddlers or pushers, nor are we dealers selling hospice—or any other treatment option—to those in desperate need. Although a colleague once barked at me, "If you ask someone 99 times, the 100th time they're going to say 'Yes' to hospice," browbeating patients is not at all our role.

Instead, our role is to metaphorically take our patients' and families' hands and lead them through an examination of personal wishes, values, cares, and concerns as we guide them through a rich conversational odyssey of illness, disease, and end-of-life choices. We revisit the conversation when disease progresses or when we recognize that the level of care a patient requires exceeds the physical or emotional capacity of their caregivers.

As we guide people through conversation, guiding them from one arc to the next, we continually assess their willingness to move further with us in our exploration. When we find they are reluctant, resistant, or unable to move forward, we pause, back up, or start again, patiently exploring their experiences, understanding, and wishes more deeply, and tending to their emotional and spiritual needs. Like a tour guide leading hungry or weary travelers, we must adjust our plan for the day when our patients and their loved ones cannot venture further. At no point do we ever compel, coerce, or persuade.

If we feel frustrated, we must take a deep breath and reflect. Our expectations of the patient or family are likely out of sync with their understanding or emotional processing; they may need more time. Or it might be that we are centering ourselves instead of those in our care. Lack of understanding or insight by the patient or family can also mean we must fully orient ourselves to their perspective. We must slow down, listen more deeply, and kindly and patiently continue our gentle investigation. Only when the patient and family have expressed their willingness to proceed should we lead them forward in the conversation.

For those ready to move on, we gently lead the way. As we travel deeper into the conversation, we reference patient and family experiences to gently open doors to allow insight to arise naturally from the linkage of their personal experience of illness with the medical reality we are describing. We can also foster mental connection by gently posing questions about patient and family understanding or related experiences, softly planting seeds of insight with our words.

Education about disease is only provided after assessing patient and family understanding of a diagnosis, where they think they are in their journey, and what is ahead. This ensures that our education can be tailored to the patients' and families' medical literacy level and existing points of reference and, thus, can serve as an architectural framework on which they can arrange or organize their bits of knowledge and experience. Listening for indications of confusion, ignorance, or misunderstanding, we offer to "help make sense" of inquiries as we "fill in the gaps" of their understanding by "painting a picture" of the patient's specific disease trajectory and what is ahead.

Guiding patients and families through difficult conversations in this manner facilitates natural understanding and empowers people to make decisions from the authenticity of their innermost sanctums. A decision to transition to hospice care, for instance, is best made when patients and families genuinely believe that the patient is getting to the end of their journey. This reflects an internal compass reading that best derives from a personal sense of confidence and comfort with the patient's and family's knowledgebase and experience—from what *they* know to be true—not from a directive articulated by a provider, or, worse, from the resigned acceptance that comes from knowing that no other treatment options are available.

Understandably, this type of insight takes time to develop. It is not reasonable to expect that patients and families can arrive at a decision for hospice care after just one conversation. Often, the shift in emotional and spiritual orientation toward medical interventions required to make such a decision takes days, weeks, or even months. This is because authentic insight and acceptance of a new understanding rely on a foundation of personal experience, which takes time for patients and families to accrue. More importantly, insight about the end of life, especially the realization that a person is arriving at the end of their journey, is a spiritual undertaking that cannot be measured. If we are lucky, this effort will be required just once for each of us, yet the task is Herculean. Grace, time and space, and infinite compassion are needed to empower and enable patients and their loved ones to complete this quest successfully.

Illness Arc

A goals of care conversation begins in the Illness Arc, focusing on the patient and family's personal experience of a diagnosis (see Chap. 6). The **investigation** of patient and family **experience** is begun with the inquiry,

- "Can you paint a picture of how things have been going?"

Most people find it easy to provide plenty of detail in response to this request, and as soon the floodgates are opened, most are eager to share. Willingness on the part of the patient and family to describe specific details about their personal experience provides an excellent opportunity to build rapport and trust through active listening and holding space. It also provides the opportunity to assess patient medical literacy and to take their emotional temperature.

In addition to building rapport, the priority during the Illness Arc is to identify the disease that is driving patient decline and to assess where the patient is in their disease trajectory, including whether they meet hospice criteria. A robust understanding of the primary disease trajectories that patients follow as they approach the end of life and a working knowledge of hospice criteria are required to accurately make this assessment (see Chap. 4 and Chap. 5).

After completing this assessment, the clinician begins the **investigation** of how patients and families are **understanding** their experiences by asking,

- "How are you making sense of the changes you just described?"

Answers to this question will shed light on patient and family medical literacy and their conceptualization of the situation. Hearing the patient or caregiver name the diagnosis believed to be responsible for their decline is the cue to transition the conversation into the Disease Arc. Because patients and families are the experts on their own experience of a diagnosis, the Illness Arc is the only space where no education is provided.

Disease Arc

In the Disease Arc, the focus is on the diagnosis driving patient decline. The **investigation** of patient and family **experience** is begun by asking,

- "Have you ever seen someone go through the (*diagnosis*) journey?"
- "Can you tell me what you saw?"

It is amazing how people will accurately describe the terminal decline patterns depicted by the disease trajectory diagrams in Chaps. 4 and 5. For instance, people describing a loved one who died of cancer often describe a journey that "went very quickly at the end."

The **investigation** of patient and family **understanding** of the patient's diagnosis begins by asking questions that shed light on their conceptualization of the disease as a terminal trajectory with an expected endpoint of death. At a minimum, this includes asking,

- "Can you tell me what you understand about the (diagnosis) journey?"
- "Where do you think you are in your overall journey with your health?"
- "What are you expecting going forward?"

Collectively, these questions provide a better understanding of how the patient and family are making sense of their diagnosis as it relates to the patient's life expectancy and anticipated future experiences.

Once we understand what the patient and family believe to be true about where the patient is in their journey, we can begin to "fill in the gaps of their understanding" and to "help make sense of what they've been experiencing" by providing **education** about the patient's disease trajectory, where the patient is in their journey, and what can be expected ahead. By connecting a discussion of the diagnosis and its trajectory to the patient's experience, we gently open the doors to allow insight to arise naturally *on its own* for patients and families so that our acknowledgment of the patient's health status, including whether they meet hospice criteria, should not come as a surprise. Template language that can be used to teach patients and families about the various disease trajectories can be found in Chap. 15.

During this part of the conversation, we will gently deliver the news that the patient meets hospice criteria, if that is the case. This is much easier to do if the patient and family have verbalized earlier in the conversation that they believe the patient's time is limited. Immediately after delivering your assessment that a patient meets hospice criteria, it is important to check in with the patient and family by asking,

- "Does that surprise you to hear?"

It is important to monitor facial expressions and body language and tend to any emotional discomfort before moving on.

End-of-Life Wishes Arc

By this point in the conversation, the patient and family should accurately understand where the patient is in their overall journey with their health, including whether they meet hospice criteria. This understanding is the foundation for patients and loved ones to make medical care decisions that reflect their values.

The End-of-Life Wishes Arc comprises two significant tasks related to eliciting personal wishes for medical care. The first is to discuss end-of-life care wishes grounded in patient and family hopes for the future; the second is to investigate advance care directive wishes.

The **investigation** of what the patient and family hope for in the end-of-life **experience** is done by asking questions that include,

- "Knowing what we just talked about and what you can expect with your disease going forward, what are you hoping for in whatever time you have left?"
- "Where do you want to be at the end of your life?"
- "What would a good death be like for you?"

Space must be carefully held during this discussion, as many people have yet to be previously asked to contemplate these matters, and the emotional and spiritual labor involved can be significant.

To better enable patients and families to specify their wishes for the end of life, it can be helpful to **investigate** their **understanding** of this time of life by asking questions that can include,

- "Can you tell me what you expect the end of life to be like?"
- "Have you ever seen someone die of (*diagnosis*)?"
- "Do you know how much help you will need when you reach the end of your journey?"
- "Who will be able to help care for you when you reach the end of your journey?"

Many people do not know what to expect at the end of a human life. For those who do not know what to expect, it is helpful to provide **education** by "painting a picture" of the final weeks of life. It can also be beneficial to explain what can happen if patients or families do not make a choice early enough in the patient's journey to transition to hospice care. Many patients with heart or lung failure, for instance, do not understand that as their disease progresses toward the end of life, interventions in the hospital become increasingly invasive, to the point that patients without hospice support can be expected to pass away in the hospital during a final exacerbation.

The second task of the End-of-Life Wishes Arc is to investigate advance directive wishes, including who patients would want to be their surrogate medical decision maker if they cannot make medical decisions for themselves, as well as living will considerations, code status wishes, and their preferences for medical interventions. Waiting until this point in the conversation to discuss these crucial considerations allows patient and family decisions to arise from an accurate understanding of the patient's health status. Template language that can be used to discuss these topics can be found in Chap. 16.

Patients not supported by palliative care who are close to meeting hospice criteria, who meet hospice criteria but are not hospice minded, or who are hospice minded but do not yet meet hospice criteria should be offered a referral to palliative care. Template language that can be used to discuss palliative care can be found in Chap. 11.

Hospice Care Arc

For patients who meet hospice criteria, the primary goal of the Arc of Conversation is to arrive at the Hospice Care Arc to discuss hospice care in a way that enables patients and families to more readily consider this treatment option as one that may meet their values and needs. Many people want to be at home at the end of their lives. Hospice agencies care for patients in private homes, assisted living or nursing facilities, and sometimes dedicated inpatient hospice residencies. If we can guide patients and families to this point in the conversation kindly and compassionately, most will be able to carefully consider whether hospice care represents an alignment of their wishes with the kind of medical care they want and where they wish to receive it.

The **investigation** of patient and family **experience** of hospice care begins by asking,

- "Do you have any personal experience with hospice?"
- "Do you know anyone who received hospice care at the end of their lives?"

The **investigation** of patient and family **understanding** of hospice care begins by asking,

- "What does the word *hospice* mean to you?"

The answer to this question will reveal perceptions of hospice care, including fears, prejudices, and sometimes negative experiences of hospice care, all of which should be addressed before providing education about hospice care.

Once particular concerns about hospice care have been addressed for patients and families, **education** can be provided by offering to "paint a picture of what hospice care looks like." Although specifics should be confirmed with local hospice teams, general template language that can be used to teach patients and families about hospice care can be found in Chap. 17.

For most patients and families, the subject of hospice care is laden with uncertainty and discomfort. Holding space so people can process their experiences and emotions is never as important as during a discussion about hospice care. Plenty of time should be provided for patients and family members to work through their feelings, ask questions, and consider their options, along with offering the reassurance that there is no urgency to decide and that "There is no right answer, only the answer that is right for you." For patients ready for hospice care, helping to ensure a smooth and easy transition is also essential to our compassionate care.

Investigation Before Education with Any New Topic

The foundational technique of the Arc of Conversation—**investigation before education**—should be engaged with any new topic in conversation with patients and families. Suppose a patient asks questions about a new subject or expresses a misunderstanding. Before providing an informative explanation, we must take a moment to ask what they already know or have experienced about that topic. Then, we must determine the appropriate time to provide an explanation, recognizing that explanations provided without ascertaining what a patient and family already understand about a topic can be unhelpful and even counterproductive. If it is not best to explain (or correct a misconception) immediately, we must validate the person's beliefs and experience and offer to explain later. A recent conversation with a wife about her husband's dementia illustrates.

While listening to this patient's wife describe the history of her husband's memory loss, when we were yet in the Illness Arc, she mentioned an episode in which the patient had what she called a "stroke," describing his difficulty talking and right arm weakness that began abruptly one morning when they were eating breakfast. Recognizing that something was wrong, the wife contacted a friend who used some "biofeedback therapy" over the phone to "manage the patient's artery." According to the wife, this treatment resolved the patient's medical issue within the hour. The medical community did not see the patient, and no formal diagnosis was made.

Rather than a stroke, I surmised that this patient had probably had a transient ischemic attack (TIA), what we generally call a "mini-stroke," as these events tend to resolve within a few hours without formal intervention. Although it was clear that the patient's wife lacked a medical appreciation for the significance of a stroke and how a stroke might relate to her husband's memory loss, I investigated her understanding further by explicitly asking, "Do you know what causes a stroke?" and "Do you know how strokes might relate to memory loss?" Not yet knowing if the wife understood that the patient had *dementia*, I avoided the use of that term right then in our conversation.

When the patient's wife answered negatively to both questions, wanting to preserve her dignity, I provided reassurance by responding, "Okay, very good. Many people don't understand how these things relate. I will help make sense of this in a bit, okay?" Offering my questions and responses in a kind and friendly manner, I watched her facial expressions and body language for signs of offense. Noting none, I felt satisfied that I could proceed with the investigation of her husband's illness.

Later, when we got to the Disease Arc, while providing education about her husband's diagnosis, I first described general brain anatomy and function, vascular dementia, and the pathophysiology of strokes and TIAs. I then linked the event that her husband had experienced and the evidence of "widespread ischemia" noted on his recent brain scan (indicating extensive damage due to poor blood flow) to his cognitive decline. Knowing the limits of the wife's medical understanding better prepared me to relate my education about dementia to the reference points of her experience and understanding.

The basic technique of the Arc of Conversation—investigation before education—provides a valuable framework for engaging patients and families in a collaborative conversation about medical wishes and end-of-life care. Over the following four chapters, we will explore each of the four primary arcs of the Arc of Conversation in greater detail.

Reference

1. Guide. Collins English Dictionary—complete & unabridged 2012 Digital Edition. 2012. http://www.dictionary.com/browse/guide. Accessed 23 Mar 2023.

The Illness Arc: Exploring Personal Experience and Understanding of Illness with Patients and Families

9

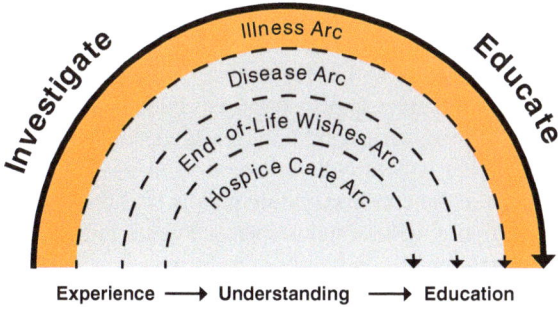

Fig. 9.1 The Illness Arc

> **Objectives During the Illness Arc (Fig. 9.1)**
> - Establish a compassionate and collaborative conversational space
> - Investigate patient and family experience of illness
> - Identify the disease driving patient decline
> - Evaluate disease progression with respect to hospice criteria
> - Investigate patient and family understanding of illness

Investigate Patient and Family Experience of Illness

Question:
- Can you paint a picture of how things have been going?

A goals of care conversation is begun in a way similar to any other patient encounter, with a friendly "hello" and introduction, followed by the inquiry,

- "Can you paint a picture of how things have been going?"

The initial priority is establishing a compassionate and collaborative conversational milieu—to *hold space*—for patients and families to share their personal values, wishes, and goals (see Chap. 7). The best place to start a conversation is where patients and families are the experts, in their own personal **experience** of the patient's **illness** (see Chap. 6). By responding empathetically to the story that the patient and family share, and by respectfully acknowledging and validating their experiences, we position ourselves as trusted allies and companions in this collaborative, conversational venture.

Starting a conversation with an open-ended inquiry, such as,

- "How have things been going at home?"

keeps the emotional stakes low for patients and families, as it can be scary to learn that the purpose of a visit with a provider is to discuss end-of-life wishes.[1] Even (or perhaps especially) when it is clear that a patient meets hospice criteria and that the purpose of the visit is to discuss hospice care, it is necessary to start a conversation in a low-key manner and to prioritize building rapport and trust. Time spent nourishing the atmospheric conditions required to successfully usher a patient and family through an emotionally charged conversation is always fruitful. Shortcutting this part of the conversation frequently backfires, as patients and families can be leery of divulging personal wishes or worries or accepting difficult news before the proper relational groundwork is established.

Another low-key way of asking patients to share their experience is to cue them to,

- "Catch me up on how things have been going at home."

Open-ended inquiries invite patients and families to begin where they believe the patient's recent history became compelling, which provides important information about their appreciation and understanding of the patient's journey. It is a good sign when, for instance, the family of a patient suspected of having end-stage dementia begins by describing the problems the patient had while still working 10 years earlier, indicating that they have some awareness that the patient's current condition is the result of a decade-long process of decline. On the other hand, if the same family

---

[1] Because patients and families can be offended by the involvement of palliative care, assuming incorrectly that palliative means hospice care, our palliative care department followed the lead of the MD Anderson Cancer Center in changing our name to Supportive Care. Most people, particularly those experiencing or supporting a loved one with a chronic or terminal disease, intuitively understand how they might benefit from "an extra layer of support," which is our informal tagline. (Dalal S, Palla S, Hui D, Nguyen L, Chacko R, Li Z, Fadul N, Scott C, Thornton V, Coldman B, Amin Y, Bruera E. Association between a name change from palliative to supportive care and the timing of patient referrals at a comprehensive cancer center. Oncologist. 2011;16(1):105-11. doi: 10.1634/theoncologist.2010-0161. Epub 2011 Jan 6. PMID: 21212438; PMCID: PMC3228056.)

starts by detailing an incident just one week earlier, this is a sign that we will need to be more directive with our questions to uncover the patient's complete and pertinent history.

When listening to the patient's story, begin to target the disease suspected to be driving the patient's decline, asking questions that reveal further details about the story of disease progression that would be expected with that trajectory. For instance, when talking to a family of a loved one with dementia, ask questions that follow the FAST Scale progression (see Chap. 5), inquiring about recent memory issues (e.g., repeating questions and stories, forgetting for new pieces of information), cognitive function loss (e.g., needing assistance with cooking, cleaning, driving, shopping and with managing appointments, medications, finances, mealtime, the home, and pets), personal care task loss (e.g., needing reminders to bathe and change clothes, and needing assistance with dressing, bathing, and toileting), and evidence of physical function loss (e.g., bladder and bowel incontinence, weight loss, declining appetite, weakness, mobility issues and falls, trouble chewing, swallowing or taking pills, needing assistance with transferring or walking, sleeping more across the day, and a reduced vocabulary). Also, ask about psychiatric symptoms (e.g., anxiety, depression, agitation, apathy, delusions, hallucinations, insomnia, and sun-downing), and screen the patient for safety issues, the family for financial strain, and the primary caregiver for caregiver strain. Together, this information should allow you to determine where a patient with dementia is in their overall journey, whether they meet hospice criteria, and whether the family is in crisis.

This part of the conversation can and should take significant time, particularly when the patient and family are new to us. Building rapport and trust requires a down payment of our time upfront. It also takes good old-fashioned time to learn the level of detail needed to accurately assess where a patient is in their journey with their health and to understand their symptom progression and physical and functional decline at a granular enough level to determine whether the patient meets hospice criteria. This is not something that can be accomplished in a 15-minute office visit. In my practice, this conversation arc routinely takes between 30 and 60 minutes. Only when I have known the patient for months or years, and the detail required to catch up on their experiences since the last time we met is limited, does this part of the conversation not require that much time. During our initial visit, however, I would have spent whatever time was needed to learn the complete patient and family history.

This shared knowledge of the patient and family experience becomes the foundation of our collaborative relationship, and there is no way to short this investment. During this arc, we must allow patients and families to share whatever level of detail they believe to be pertinent without interrupting them, but rather, expressing our eager interest and attention. The details that appear unimportant or redundant will often become the specifics we will reference later when connecting education about the patient's disease trajectory to the patient's experience.

Furthermore, targeting our questions to the disease trajectory the patient is following and providing the opportunity for patients and families to recall and explain the details of their experience allows them to illustrate the story of disease progression and decline for us, an exercise that provides the groundwork for patients and families to recognize and determine what matters most. Later in the conversation, we will connect the patient's story, including specific details of their experiences, to our education of patients and families about the disease trajectory the patient is following, providing the opportunity for insight to arise as they recognize and acknowledge *on their own* where the patient is in their overall journey with their health. Ultimately, this is what we hope to enable—insight to arise naturally within patient and family hearts, minds, and souls that touches their values and personal preferences and empowers them to make decisions about their lives from a place of authenticity.

We must not shortcut this part of the conversation because the visceral experience of tying their personally felt history to the expected story of disease progression makes the patient's medical status real to patients and families. No amount of explaining can replace the personal understanding that comes from the experience of insight arising on its own. Providing the time and compassionate space for the details of the patient and family experience of disease progression to be laid out before us *is* the work of this arc.

Identify the Disease Driving Patient Decline and Evaluate its Progression

While allowing patients and families to share their experiences, we must identify the disease driving patient decline and assess where the patient is in their disease trajectory, including whether they meet hospice criteria. A robust understanding of the primary disease trajectories that patients follow as they approach the end of life and a working knowledge of hospice criteria are required to accurately make this assessment (see Chap. 4 and Chap. 5)

Because patients need an accurate assessment of their overall health to make decisions about their medical care that appropriately reflect their values, and because death is not a surprise ending of a human life, all providers should be concerned with disease progression and whether patients meet hospice criteria. Primary care providers, intensive care unit (ICU) physicians, and hospitalists should have a robust working knowledge of all hospice criteria, and specialty providers should be well-versed in the hospice criteria related to their specialties. Surgeons and ER providers should be familiar with the approach to qualifying patients for hospice exhibiting age-related decline or frailty, at a minimum. Geriatricians (including providers who work in care facilities) and palliative and hospice care providers should be experts in using all of the hospice criteria, as should hospice and palliative-certified clinicians.

Identifying the disease that is driving patient decline can often be accomplished before the patient visit by reviewing the patient's chart and recent medical history. Patients following the Organ Failure trajectory are easy to recognize by their repeated hospital admissions for exacerbations, as are patients following the Cancer trajectory, who are frequently hospitalized for sepsis, dehydration, or treatment-induced anemia or thrombocytopenia. Following a significant trauma or stroke, patients following the Catastrophic Event trajectory will often experience an ICU or hospital admission, and when able to recover from the acute event, will experience a stay in a rehabilitation facility or a move to a skilled nursing home. Although identifying the Frailty/Dementia trajectory sometimes requires a more detailed conversation with caregivers and spouses, this trajectory can also be evident from a chart review by looking for weight loss, a declining albumin level, time spent in rehabilitation facilities (i.e., the hospital-to-rehab cycle), and hospitalizations for urinary tract infections (UTIs), aspiration pneumonia, sepsis, hip fractures, and failure to thrive.

A chart review can also often determine whether a patient meets hospice criteria. Heart failure patients qualify for hospice with New York Heart Association (NYHA) Class IV symptoms, which cardiologists often document. A review of lab values can determine liver and kidney failure qualification. Kidney failure patients receiving dialysis qualify at the time that they decide to stop dialysis treatments, as do cancer patients when they choose to forego further cancer treatment. A simple scan of weight loss in the preceding 6 to 12 months and a glance at the serum albumin level on the comprehensive metabolic panel provide a rapid screen of all patients for hospice criteria with cachexia related to the Cancer, Organ Failure, and Frailty/Dementia trajectories. Infections of any type should prompt a review of the primary disease trajectory to contextualize any infection as a potential indicator of end-stage disease.

Maintaining an open mind when speaking with patients and families about their experience of the patient's illness is essential. Sometimes, what looked on chart review to be age-related decline will be COPD progression, or vice versa. As patients and families describe their experiences, listen for descriptors that match the disease trajectory diagrams detailed in Chap. 4. Patients with organ failure will often report that "Every time I go to the hospital, I am a little worse when I get back home, and I don't seem to bounce back to where I was before," detailing the downward trend of the Organ Failure trajectory, punctuated by exacerbations. Patients following the Cancer trajectory will often identify the moment in their journey when they began to transition down the very steep cliff, identifying a treatment, illness, or hospitalization that marked that shift. Mentally note these details to reference later when connecting education about the patient's disease trajectory to their experiences.

With the disease trajectory diagrams and hospice criteria in mind, assess where the patient is in their journey by targeting questions to further understand the extent of patient symptoms, metabolic decline (e.g., weight loss, appetite loss, increasing fatigue, falls, and decreasing strength, stamina, and speed), functional decline (i.e., increasing need for assistance across the day), healthcare system utilization (e.g., ER visits, hospital admissions, ICU stays, procedures, surgeries, and stays in rehabilitation), and loss of independence requiring a move to a care facility (i.e., from home to independent living, assisted living, skilled nursing, or memory care). Converting this information into the patient's Palliative Performance Scale (PPS) score, remember that patients following a terminal trajectory with a PPS score of 50% or less have reached the point in their journey where they *may* meet hospice criteria, and those with a score of 40% or less *likely* meet criteria.

Sometimes, patients will have multiple contributing diagnoses, any one of which could qualify them for hospice criteria, but none of which stand out as the primary driver of overall decline. These patients may meet hospice criteria by a *decline in clinical status* or *non-disease-specific indication* (see Chap. 5), in which the overall picture of progressive physical and functional decline is a result of multiple, difficult-to-control diagnoses at play. Patients with multiple organ failure caused by autoimmune diseases, such as sarcoidosis or rheumatoid arthritis, may also qualify in this manner, often earlier than they would otherwise be eligible for any single organ failure diagnosis.

Continue to inquire about the patient and family's experience, symptoms, and functional and physical status until confident about the disease driving patient decline, where the patient is in their journey, and whether the patient meets hospice criteria.

Investigate Patient and Family Understanding of Illness

Questions:
- How are you making sense of the changes you just described?
- Do you know what diagnosis[2] is responsible for these changes?

After completing this assessment, begin to **investigate** how patients and families are **understanding** their experiences by asking,

- "How are you making sense of the changes you just described?"

Answers to this question will shed light on patient and family medical literacy and their conceptualization of the situation. During this part of the conversation, the objective is to learn whether the patient understands that their decline is related to the disease we believe to be responsible.

Often, patients and families will have no idea how to answer the question of how they are making sense of the changes they've been experiencing. Realizing that this may be the first time patients and families have been asked to make sense of their

---

[2] The words *illness, disease,* and *diagnosis* refer to different aspects of a medical concern. *Illness* refers to the personal experience of disease, *disease* refers to the pathological process at play, and *diagnosis* is the label for that pathology. Any one of these words can be used in place of the word *diagnosis* in this question. Often, more important than the literal meaning of a word when communicating with patients and families is its connotation—the feeling it conveys. Whereas *disease* conveys heavy permanence and terminality, and *illness* conveys a softer, less permanence, *diagnosis* conveys technical specificity with detached neutrality. Use the word appropriate to the emotional tenor of the conversation.

experiences, it is important to provide plenty of time for their consideration. If the question doesn't make sense to them, we can ask it differently, such as,

- "Do you know what diagnosis[2] is responsible for these changes?"

Many times, patients and families will answer in the negative by saying, "I have no idea." The reality is that many patients and families do not know how to make sense of their experiences.

When this happens, we can gently probe to learn whether patients and families know that the illness they are struggling with has a formal name and has been identified or diagnosed. For patients with any organ failure, dementia, or other specific terminal illness (e.g., AIDS, sarcoidosis, rheumatoid arthritis, multiple sclerosis, Parkinson's disease, etc.), we can gently probe to learn whether they are aware that the patient has been diagnosed with x, y, or z. The following examples provide template language for posing this question gently and respectfully to patients and families.

For a patient with dementia, we might ask any of the following questions:

- Has anyone ever mentioned a diagnosis of dementia?
- Are you aware that your loved one has dementia?
- Has anyone mentioned Alzheimer's disease?

For a patient with COPD, we might ask:

- Have you been diagnosed with any lung disease?
- Has anyone ever mentioned a diagnosis called COPD?

And getting more basic than this, we might ask a patient with COPD:

- Do you know why you wear oxygen?
- Do you know why you have such a hard time breathing?
- Do you know what diagnosis[2] is making it hard for you to breathe?

At this point in the conversation, the purpose is to define the patient and family's ballpark of understanding about what is happening with the patient's health. The priority is to learn whether they know that the patient carries the diagnosis we believe to be responsible and whether they are tying that diagnosis to the changes the patient has been experiencing. Later, in the Disease Arc, we will more thoroughly investigate what they understand about the disease journey the patient is following, where the patient is in that journey, and what they are expecting ahead. For now, we simply need to tease out whether the patient and family know that the diagnosis we believe to be responsible for the patient's decline is playing a role in the patient's health.

Patients following the Frailty trajectory often speculate about the cause of their decline by saying, "I'm old!" Families may say, "This is what we expect when someone gets as old as they are, isn't it?" These answers, which label the patient's age as the culprit, satisfy our objective during this part of the conversation.

Patients following the Cancer trajectory often have a tough time making sense of what may appear to be unrelated symptoms of physical and functional decline, including weight loss, declining appetite, mobility issues and falls, and infections. Despite cancer-related cachexia being a well-documented experience and part of the cancer journey for most patients with advanced cancer [1], many cancer patients do not have a robust understanding of how this physical and metabolic decline relates to their cancer diagnosis.

Sometimes, patients with cancer experience this constellation of symptoms despite their imaging and lab work indicating what appears to be well-controlled disease. In other circumstances, patients will surmise that their cancer is cured or at least well-controlled despite imaging studies revealing that the disease, in the form of tumors, is still present in their bodies. Patients with cancer seem to hold separate their diagnosis of cancer from their overall health, not understanding the Cancer trajectory or what to expect at the end and lacking an appreciation for the significance of their functional and physical decline. Because they have not been educated about what to expect as their disease progresses, patients with advancing cancer often have a challenging time reconciling what they hear in clinic visits with their experience at home. With this in mind, we must tread lightly anytime we recognize that the patient and family's appreciation of the patient's cancer status misaligns with the medical reality so as not to forcibly confront their beliefs.

Plant a Seed of Connection to Allow Insight to Arise on its Own

If, when asked, "What diagnosis do you think is responsible for the changes you just described?" patients with cancer do not name their cancer as the possible cause, we can gently plant the seed of connection between their cancer and their decline by asking any of the following questions:

- Do you know how your cancer might be responsible for these changes?
- What about your cancer? How do you think that might be playing a role?
- Do you know how weight loss and fatigue are related to cancer?

This is a valuable strategy that can be used when introducing an idea, especially when we need to make a connection between seemingly disparate pieces of clinical information. Gently posed questions, in which we ask whether the patient and family understand how disease and symptoms relate, become a kind and loving way to introduce the possibility of a connection without talking at people, explaining, or educating. Asking people to look to their knowledge or experience to tell us how two things might be connected positions them as equal partners in this conversational endeavor, keeping us aligned beside them instead of above them. Remember that we want to *companion* patients and families, not position ourselves as authorities.

The goal of the **investigation** phase of each conversational arc is to *plant a seed for insight to arise on its own*. By asking what the patient and family already know, from experience or knowledge, we can custom tailor our education to their worldview and reference points. Ideally, when learning about disease and its expected progression, patients and families will realize *on their own* where a patient is in their overall journey with their health so medical decisions can arise naturally in alignment with their values and goals.

Gently asking questions also allows us as practitioners to remain humble. Maintaining empathy, sympathy, and compassion for others is much easier when we understand the reference points and beliefs guiding patient and family decisions. Offering medicine to patients and families in a way that truly adds to their quality of life requires that we shift our approach to one that centers *their* experience, knowledge, and personal reference points and which positions our treatment options and general approach with respect to *their* world.

Often, patients with cancer and frailty, when asked how they are making sense of the changes they've experienced, will answer by saying, "I'm just not hungry," or families may conjecture, "They aren't eating or exercising enough." This answer provides important insight into patient and family understanding (or lack thereof) of the relationship between metabolic decline and strength building in advanced age or disease settings.

Later, when we fill in the gaps in their understanding, we will explain that while it seems that patients should eat and exercise more to get stronger, the relationship is reversed. The body becomes unable to utilize the nutrition the patient is taking in and then loses its interest in eating while losing muscle mass. As we explain the metabolic shift as a critical part of end-stage disease, regardless of diagnosis, we can help families accommodate to the idea that at some point in the patient's journey, no amount of nutritional intake is going to reverse this trend; at that point, even forcing nutrition on the body cannot make the body utilize the nutrition it receives.

This education, which maintains a respectful awareness of patient and family beliefs and medical knowledge, can help them accommodate this new medical reality and alleviate them from the often very compelling cultural drive to show love by providing nourishment. Permitting family members to let go of trying to control a patient's intake at mealtime and to accept where a loved one is in their journey, especially concerning their desire to eat, can improve the patient's and family's quality of life. Permitting spouses and caregivers to let go of this form of advocacy who have otherwise spent their lives ensuring that their partners eat supports the well-being of the entire patient and family unit because it targets the *illness* area of disease, meaning real-life experiences at home, where living and loving happens for people.

Imagine if, instead of asking this question and learning this answer, we skipped right over this part of the conversation, never appreciating that patients and families often believe that eating less is the cause of patient decline. It is easy to imagine that people with this belief might have a difficult time accepting the reality that their loved one is getting to the end of life naturally. It is also easy to imagine that they might also believe that the medical community should be doing more, including offering a feeding tube to support their loved one's nutrition.

It is important to recognize that family members often feel driven by a strong responsibility to *do everything possible* to ensure quality and quantity of life for their loved ones. Without a complete and accurate picture of a patient's medical status, including the reality that metabolic decline is an expected part of the end of life and that a medical treatment such as a feeding tube at that time may introduce adverse side effects (e.g., aspiration pneumonia, edema, pleural effusions, weeping skin, etc.), families may make decisions in direct opposition to what we know most people work toward on behalf of loved ones reaching the end of their lives.

Not uncovering patients' and families' underlying beliefs about the relationship between eating and weight loss can lead to real problems. Families can be frustrated and confused when we refuse to offer treatments they believe might help and when we provide treatments that turn out not to help. At the same time, healthcare providers can feel obligated to offer treatments believed to be nonbeneficial out of an authentic desire to help, even knowing that the risks will outweigh the benefits. The solution to these problems is to increase our interest in patients' and families' understanding of medical knowledge. Then, our discussion of treatment options, including risks and benefits, can better align with the patient's medical reality, but in a way that kindly and lovingly addresses important misconceptions frequently held by patients and families.

Rather than Making Assumptions, Ask for Clarification

Sometimes, when asked how they are making sense of things, patients will comment, "I'm going downhill." Before assuming that the patient means that they are declining, ask for clarification, quoting the patient's words directly,

- "What do you mean when you say, 'I'm going downhill'?"

A patient may answer this request for clarification in two very different ways. They may provide further information about their **experience** of disease by adding, "I've lost 25 pounds in the last two months, I can no longer lift my laundry basket, and I need help preparing meals," or they may share insight into their **understanding** of where they are in their journey, as in, "I'm getting to the end of my life."

When patients answer by sharing information about *where they think they are in their overall journey with their health*—meaningful information about their understanding of their life expectancy—we still need to understand if patients and families know what disease or diagnosis is responsible for the patient's decline. We must not leave the Illness Arc until we have accomplished that task.

Once the diagnosis that we believe to be driving the patient's decline has been named in the conversation as having some relationship to the story of decline shared by the patient and family, either named by the patient and family or by being gently introduced by us, we can proceed into the next part of the conversation, where we will focus on the patient's disease. Because patients and families are the experts in their personal experience and understanding of illness, the Illness Arc is the only space where no education is provided.

Reference

1. von Haehling S, Anker SD. Prevalence, incidence and clinical impact of cachexia: facts and numbers-update 2014. J Cachexia Sarcopenia Muscle. 2014;5(4):261–3. https://doi.org/10.1007/s13539-014-0164-8. PMID: 25384990; PMCID: PMC4248411

The Disease Arc: Exploring Disease, Disease Progression, and the End of a Journey with Patients and Families

10

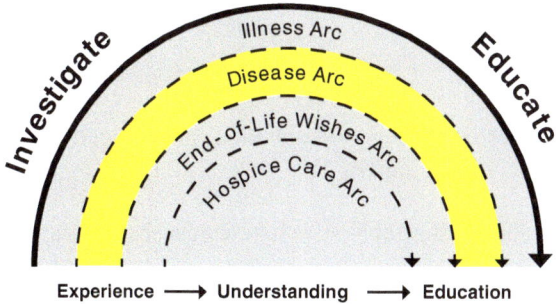

Fig. 10.1 The Disease Arc

Objectives During the Disease Arc (Fig. 10.1)
- Investigate patient and family experience of disease
- Investigate patient and family understanding of disease, including:
    - Their understanding of the disease process
    - Where they think the patient is in their journey
    - What they are expecting ahead
- Educate patient and family about disease, including
    - The disease trajectory the patient is following*
    - Where the patient is in their journey
    - What is ahead*
    - Whether the patient meets hospice criteria

*Chapter 15 provides template language for this part of the conversation.

© The Author(s), under exclusive license to Springer Nature Switzerland AG 2024
A. Shaw, PA, *The Arc of Conversation*,
https://doi.org/10.1007/978-3-031-70495-6_10

Having established that the patient and family understand a connection between the patient's overall decline and the diagnosis believed to be responsible, we can safely transition the conversation into the Disease Arc. The overarching objective of this part of the conversation is to explore and discuss the patient's disease as a terminal trajectory with an expected endpoint of death.

Investigate Patient and Family Experience of Disease

Start to **investigate** the patient and family's prior **experience** of the disease by asking if they know anyone who experienced a similar journey. When asking about Dementia, Organ Failure, or Cancer, inquire,

Question:
- Have you seen anyone go through the [diagnosis] journey?

- "Have you seen anyone go through the dementia journey?" or "heart failure journey?" or "cancer journey?"

When asking about Catastrophic Event, reference the specific event, for example,

- "Have you seen what can happen to someone following a stroke?"

When asking about Frailty, use plain language that most people can appreciate and readily understand,

- "Have you seen anyone 'die of old age'?"

To this question, patients and families will often reveal the experiences of a spouse, parent, sibling, or close friend. Ask them to describe what they saw and listen for a picture of a loved one's experience that closely resembles one of the disease trajectories described in Chap. 4.

Pay close attention to indicators of frustration along the loved one's journey, which provide an opportunity to express sympathy and to address worries for the patient's journey ahead. Often, families will describe end-of-life healthcare utilization, including emergency room (ER) visits, hospital admissions, escalations of care in the intensive care unit (ICU), and stays in rehabilitation facilities that were frustrating, nonbeneficial, and ultimately not in line with what they know the patient would have wanted. Families often share experiences about hospice care, which we will investigate further in the Hospice Care Arc. Because witnessing and experiencing other people's journeys often informs future choices, we must create the opportunity for patients and families to describe their experiences.

Using the word "journey" when referencing the patient's diagnosis during the Disease Arc serves to gently introduce the idea that the patient has a progressive illness with an expected endpoint. The purposeful use of language in this way opens a doorway for insight to arise on its own about what is happening, creating an opportunity for patients and families to connect the dots between what they witnessed in someone else's journey and what they see on the patient's journey. Using the word "journey" also maintains respect for patient and family beliefs about a medical diagnosis that may differ from the medical community's understanding and expectations.

When patients and families share their lack of prior experience with the disease journey being discussed, provide reassurance, saying something like,

- "Okay, very good. Many people have not seen someone go through this journey. I will help make sense of things in a bit."

Understand that people without reference points to a disease journey are likely to harbor fears or worries about what is ahead; not knowing is often as scary, if not scarier, than knowing.

Investigate Patient and Family Understanding of Disease

Questions:
- Can you tell me what you understand about your [diagnosis] journey?
- Where do you think you are in your overall journey with your health?
- What are you expecting ahead?

Our next objective is to **investigate** patients' and families' **understanding** of disease as a progressive and terminal medical journey, including where the patient is in their journey and what they are expecting ahead.

The questions in this part of the conversation can be asked quickly, one immediately following the other, to learn the general ballpark of patient and family understanding of disease. Doing so will often reveal a disconnect between what people understand about a disease journey and how they are making sense of the patient's particular medical experiences. Because we will target our education about disease to the patient and family experience and understanding, spending time investigating exactly what they believe to be true is crucial.

Begin with the first question, referencing the terminal diagnosis or disease trajectory that the patient is following, by asking,

- "Can you tell me what you understand about the heart failure journey?" or "Can you tell me what you understand about the journey of 'dying of old age'?"

We hope to hear an answer that reveals some level of understanding by the patient and family that the disease in question is progressive and terminal. This is often the response for those with dementia, heart failure, COPD, frailty, and cancer, with people offering descriptions like, "Dementia is a progressive loss of memory and cognitive function that results in an increasing need for care," "Eventually my lungs (or heart) are going to give out, and I'm going to die," "I think she's going to continue to get weaker and weaker until her body just gives out and she eventually just goes to sleep," or "Eventually, my cancer is going to kill me."

Sometimes, patients and families will express a lack of understanding, saying, "I don't know." Provide reassurance, offering to "help make sense of things in a bit," noting the gap in their understanding. This will be addressed in the next part of the conversation when providing education about the patient's disease.

Once we have learned the high-level conceptual understanding the patient and family have about the disease journey the patient is experiencing, we next need to understand where they believe the patient is in that journey by asking,

- "Where do you think you are in your overall journey with your health?"

Some patients will need clarification on this question. In that case, the question can be asked differently,

- "On a range from someone healthy to someone close to dying, where do you think you are in your journey with your health?"

To help illustrate the idea of a continuum, I will spread my arms apart, motioning to the healthy end of the spectrum with one hand and the terminal end with the other.

Patients without insight into their decline often share their belief that they are in the middle of their journey. Inquire further into their understanding by asking,

- "Can you tell me more?" or "Can you tell me how much time you think you might have left?"

This line of inquiry is essential for patients who meet hospice criteria and have limited time remaining. Because we want to manage our communications to avoid directly confronting or dismantling patient beliefs about longevity and mortality, we must ascertain their beliefs about these matters before providing any education or our assessment of where we think the patient is in their journey. For more information about respecting patient beliefs, see Chap. 7.

Patients with insight into their decline will usually answer the question of where they believe they are in their overall journey with their health in a way that continues the metaphor, saying, "I'm getting to the end," or "I'm more than halfway there." Before assuming that the patient means that they are getting to the end of their life, remember to ask for clarification, quoting the patient's words directly,

- "What do you mean when you say, 'I'm getting to the end'?"

Most patients will then clarify, offering a more direct indication that they believe they are close to death.

When patients look saddened or frightened by this reality, take the time to comfort and validate them, offering, "I'm so sorry," or "You're so brave." Observing concern on a patient's face in response to the question of what is ahead is also a suitable and appropriate moment to ask two important and distinct questions,

- "Are you afraid of being dead?"
- "Are you afraid of the dying process?"

These questions target potential spiritual distress regarding personal salvation and the afterlife and fearful anticipation of physical suffering, respectively.

When patients confirm fears about the spiritual realm, ask,

- "Do you have a spiritual or religious faith or belief system that gives you comfort?" and "Would you like to talk to a chaplain or spiritual advisor?"

Be prepared to follow up with a referral or connection, knowing that hospice services are required to provide chaplain services to patients and families enrolled in hospice care and will often make other forms of support, such as grief groups, bereavement support, counseling, etc., available to the community regardless of hospice enrollment status.

Those with cancer and COPD understandably frequently have significant fears about worsening symptoms, including pain or the panic of not being able to breathe. When patients confirm fears about the physical nature of dying, ask them to explain precisely what symptoms they are worried about. Then, provide the reassurance that medications are available to help ensure that when their time comes, they will pass peacefully and with dignity, without pain or other symptoms. Template language for addressing specific concerns patients frequently voice about dying, including responses to various misconceptions of hospice care, are included in Chap. 17. Note that most concerns about end-of-life care are best addressed later in the conversation, during the Hospice Care Arc, after providing education about disease and investigating patient wishes for end-of-life care, which will be done in the End-of-Life Wishes Arc.

The final inquiry to be made about patient and family understanding of the disease process is to ask,

- "What are you expecting ahead?"

This question seeks to uncover patient and family expectations, fears, and concerns about the future.

To this question, patients with organ failure and frailty and families of those with dementia will often express an understanding that the disease will continue to worsen until the patient passes. However, patients and families will not infrequently express a lack of understanding, saying, "I have no idea what to expect." Provide reassurance, offering to "help make sense of things in a bit," noting the gap in their understanding. This will be addressed in the next part of the conversation when providing education about the patient's disease.

Again, patients may reveal fears about dying or concerns about their place in the afterlife with their facial expressions or tone of voice. Offer comfort by saying, "I'm so sorry," or "This must be so hard." If it hasn't already been done, inquire about their fears of dying and of being dead using the questions and responses discussed above.

Sometimes, patients will respond to the question of what they are expecting ahead by indicating that they are hoping or even expecting to get better. When patients share unlikely hopes for physical and functional improvement, it is important to inquire further about their wishes by asking them to "Tell me more." Often, patients will reveal wishes that convey a fundamental misunderstanding of where they are in their medical journey, expressing desires that do not align with what they seem to understand about the disease process or that contradict what they shared about where they believe the patient to be in their overall journey with their health.

When patients express hopes and wishes for possibilities misaligned with what appears to be medically possible, engage the "Wish, Worry, Wonder" technique discussed in Chap. 7. An example illustrating the use of this technique will be provided shortly.

To reiterate, the purpose of the questions in this part of the conversation is to discover what the patient and family understand about the biological process of the disease driving the patient's decline. When patients and families lack an understanding of a disease process, or when their answers convey a disconnect between their understanding of the disease process and where they understand the patient to be in their journey, we must pause and investigate further by determining the exact ballpark of their understanding, including the limits of their medical knowledge about disease, symptom evolution, and disease progression. Because this gap in understanding is responsible for much of the discord between what patients and families want and what the medical community believes to be reasonable regarding treatment options, we must take the time to investigate this space thoroughly.

Patients with alcoholic liver failure provide an excellent example to illustrate this important point. I have found that this population tends to have very limited understanding of their disease, including why their failing liver creates the symptoms it does, what their symptoms signify about how advanced their disease is, the likelihood of their recovery given their current state, and how little time they have left. This makes sense because the liver does so many jobs, yet most people would be hard-pressed to explain exactly how the liver functions. More importantly, even if someone does understand that liver failure can turn a person's skin yellow, for instance, most people likely cannot explain why, or what yellow skin in the setting of liver failure signifies in terms of prognosis. Even less seemingly related to liver disease are the symptoms of abdominal edema, esophageal varices, and bleeding and clotting events.

Yet, without ensuring that patients with liver failure are working from a rational understanding of the medical facts of their disease, we are essentially asking them to trust us *on faith* that our assertion that they are dying is correct. Instead, when we take the time to understand the patient's medical understanding, including the limits of their knowledge, we can tailor our education to their needs. I have found that bridging this medical literacy gap is the most effective strategy for supporting patients in making choices that align with their values.

For a patient with liver failure, we might begin an investigation of their understanding of a diagnosis by starting with a very general question,

- "Can you tell me what you understand about liver failure?"

Often, this question is so broad and high level as to be relatively meaningless, but it serves as a transition to a deeper line of inquiry. Following are various questions that might be asked to investigate a patient's understanding of liver disease, examining the relationship between liver function and symptomatology, as well as symptom development and disease progression:

- Can you tell me what the liver does?
- Can you tell me what "liver failure" means?
- Can you tell me what "cirrhosis" means?
- Do you know why your abdomen keeps filling up with fluid?
- Do you know how the fluid that is building up in your abdomen is related to your liver failure?
- Do you have an expectation about whether the fluid building up in your abdomen is going to continue to happen?
- Do you know what needing to have fluid removed from your abdomen on a routine basis means about how advanced your liver disease is?
- Do you know why your skin is yellow and how that relates to your liver?
- Do you know what esophageal varices are?
- Do you know what procedure the physician is doing when treating your esophagus?
- Do you know how the problem in your esophagus is related to your liver disease?
- Do you know why you are bruising and bleeding so easily?
- Do you know why problems with bleeding or clotting are related to your liver?

Taking the time to investigate the limits of patient and family understanding of a disease can be very illuminating. The reality is that frequently, people do not understand why disease causes symptoms or what symptom evolution means about disease progression and prognosis. This can lead patients with near-terminal diseases to errantly expect to make a full recovery, making it nearly impossible for them to choose care that aligns with what they would want if they authentically believed they were close to the end.

A poignant example is a patient with stage IV colon cancer with a large, complex, and inoperable tumor that had invaded his kidneys, prostate, bladder, and rectum. To provide comfort in his final weeks, an ostomy had been placed, from which blood had begun exuding several days before my visit, an ominous sign. With a Palliative Performance Scale (PPS) score of 40%, the patient had experienced significant recent physical and functional decline and was spending most of his days asleep in his bed. No longer a candidate for cancer therapy, the patient was imminently terminal; I expected he would pass within days to weeks. Yet, not appreciating his medical reality, he remained hopeful about recovering his strength and returning to the mile-long walks he once enjoyed with his wife.

Listening to the couple describe their recent experiences and share their wishes, I recognized the immense disconnect between their medical understanding and the patient's medical reality, which, in truth, initially showed up for me as frustration at what I erroneously labeled as their "denial." Aware of my internal state and heeding my own advice, I paused the conversation, dropped any expectations about how long I might be there, backed up, and started again.

As I began to inquire about basic cancer-related medical facts that I had initially mistakenly assumed were understood by the patient and his wife, something magical happened. Uncovering the extent of their lack of understanding recalibrated my frustration, an alchemy that converted my internal annoyance into heartfelt compassion. My conversation was the first time anyone had taken the time to uncover and bridge the gap in their medical understanding. It took more than two hours but resulted in their willingness to enroll in hospice care by the end of our visit.

Despite their sorrow at recognizing that the patient had arrived at the final leg of his journey, the patient and his wife were incredibly grateful for my compassionate approach, thanking me for my patience in kindly explaining things to them in a way they could easily understand. Moreover, they were relieved to finally know where the patient was in his journey and to have arrived at a place where their wishes for his comfortable and dignified passing could be appropriately supported at home.

The following are the questions I asked during this part of our conversation:

- Do you know where your cancer started? In what organ?
- Do you know if your cancer has spread, and if so, to where?
- Do you know what stage your cancer is?
- Can you tell me what "stage IV" means?
- Can you tell me what "stage IV" means in terms of your cancer's curability?
- Do you know what the word "metastasis" means?
- Can you tell me what "metastatic" means in terms of your cancer's curability?
- Do you know how large your tumor is?
- Can you tell me what you know about how cancer grows or progresses?
- Can you tell me what it means when a tumor is small versus large?
- Can you tell me what having a large tumor says about how advanced a cancer is?
- Can you tell me what having a large tumor that cannot be removed from your body means about your cancer?
- Do you know why you have blood in your ostomy bag?

- Do you know how the bleeding in your ostomy might be related to your cancer?
- Do you know how bleeding or clotting can be related to cancer?
- Do you know why you are tired, weak, and less interested in eating?
- Do you know how your fatigue, weakness, loss of strength, and loss of weight and appetite might be related to your cancer?
- Do you know what happens to a person with untreated cancer inside their body?

As I tailored my questions to the level of their understanding, I came to realize that this patient and his wife knew very little about cancer. It made perfect sense that they hadn't chosen hospice care prior to our conversation. Without even a basic understanding of how cancer progresses, they were unable to recognize the importance of the size of his tumor or its inoperability, and they were unable to reconcile those facts with his physical and functional decline. Although they knew that his cancer would eventually result in his death, it made sense that from their vantage point, he might yet survive for many months or even years. Only by discovering the ballpark of understanding from which they were operating was I able to effectively educate them about his disease in a way that compassionately corrected their misconceptions.

When this patient and his wife answered my question about what they expected ahead by articulating their wish for a recovery of his strength, I responded by utilizing the "Wish, Worry, Wonder" technique to gently open the door to the possibility that their wish might not be possible.

Knowing by this point in our conversation that the patient's hope for recovery derived from his inability to make sense of his medical experiences, I replied by compassionately aligning myself with the patient's wish, saying,

- "I wish that could happen for you too."

This response validated the patient's desire while gently suggesting that it might not be possible without directly articulating that certainty.

I continued slowly by sharing my concern as a speculative worry, saying,

- "But I worry about the amount of decline you have experienced lately, with the amount of weight you have lost, how poor your appetite is, how much you're sleeping every day, and how exhausted you become after even what sounds like just a little bit of exertion. Given the fact that you have a large tumor in your abdomen that is not being presently treated and that has begun to bleed into your gut, it might be too tall of an order for your body to be able to become strong enough for you to take long walks again."

These words, offered in a kind, humble, and tentative manner, as opposed to being offered from a position of direct and confrontational authority, reiterated the exact details of physical and functional decline shared by the patient and wife during the Illness Arc, as well as the pertinent medical facts about his cancer that I knew the couple had been unable to reconcile. Doing this purposefully but gently suggested that these facts were related and carried more significance than had been presumed, opening the door for awareness by the patient and wife that the situation was more dire than they realized, but without directly confronting their innocence with a statement of fact.

Immediately next, I followed up by checking in, asking,

- "Have you been worried about this?"

I provided plenty of time for a response and, more importantly, the opportunity to process what I had just shared.

I have found that if I have done an excellent job of remaining patient and compassionate to this point in the conversation, not pushing patients and families further than they are willing to travel with me, almost everyone will answer in the affirmative to this question, which revealed to me long ago a crucial clinical pearl that the medical community should appreciate.

Patients and families are almost always correct in their assessment of where a patient is in their overall journey with their health. Often, they are waiting for a provider to be brave and skilled enough to compassionately ask about and articulate what they already believe to be true.

In the case of the patient with advanced colon cancer, the answer to my final inquiry using the "Wish, Worry, Wonder" technique was the first time the patient and his wife had collectively voiced a concern that the patient might not survive or recover in the way they had hoped. They were both terrified that this worry might be true, but they were shielding themselves from this possibility with hopeful optimism. Capitalizing on this agreement between their understanding and my assessment of the patient's medical status, I articulated for the first time in our conversation my concern that the patient may not continue to survive for much longer, offering in a very loving, kind, and compassionate voice,

- "Me too. I worry you're much further into your journey than you might have realized."

To this, they both nodded their heads in agreement.

Learning that a patient who meets hospice criteria also believes they are getting to the end of their journey is the permission we need to move forward in the conversation. Mark this transition by gently saying the following,

- "Okay, I'm going to try to make sense of what you've been experiencing and share where I think you are in your journey so that we can talk about your wishes."

Monitor the facial expressions and body language of the patient and family for acceptance of these words and check in with their emotional status by asking,

- "How are you doing?"

Give pause for their internal assessment. For patients who articulate a desire to stop the conversation, offer to do just that, providing reassurance that,

- "I know this is a tough conversation. You're doing a great job. I'm so sorry this is such hard work. We can revisit this conversation when you're ready."

Understand that this type of conversation represents a magnificent emotional undertaking for patients and families that can alter their entire perception of reality. Sometimes, these conversations take days, weeks, and even months. Being compassionate, understanding, and patient as people face their greatest fears is an absolute necessity and requirement of the job.

Educate Patient and Family About Disease

Our next objective is to **educate** the patient and family about the disease trajectory the patient is following, including sharing our assessment of where the patient is in their journey and, when appropriate, delivering the news that the patient meets hospice criteria. Template language to use when discussing these topics is included in Chap. 15.

It is important to understand that many patients and families have limited experience with the end of life. Whereas 100 years ago, most people died at home in the care of relatives, that pattern began to change with the rise of hospitals and nursing facilities. Today, many people do not know what to expect or how to interpret patterns of decline at the end of life.

Because predictability is comforting, our task at this stage of the conversation is to present the end-of-life decline many people have witnessed as relatives and friends have passed as easy-to-understand categories of experience and then to tie the patient's personal experience to the trajectory driving their decline. Although doing so may feel like extensive or unnecessary explaining, this effort will pay off in spades. Providing a framework for the terminal phase of life allows patients and families to understand their own experiences, enables them to accept the end of a patient's journey as a natural development of a common experience and part of the human condition, and empowers people to make choices about medical wishes that reflect their values.

Introduce the Disease Trajectories

The general approach to this part of the conversation is first to introduce the idea of a disease trajectory and then describe the five terminal trajectories, starting with the four patterns the patient is not following and finishing with the trajectory driving patient decline.

Begin by introducing the idea that there are a limited number of recognizable patterns of end-of-life decline by saying,

- "We know what it looks like as patients approach the end of their lives. It might be surprising to learn that we don't die from every diagnosis possible. Rather, there are a limited number of diagnoses that most people die from. End of life can be described by just five patterns of decline, with most of us following just one of three patterns at the end of life."

Next, provide brief descriptions of the five trajectories, starting with the Sudden Death pattern, which most patients will not follow, explaining that,

- "About 1 in 10 of us will die suddenly, following a major medical event or accident, such as a massive heart attack or car accident."

Then, work through the remaining trajectories, ending with the pattern the patient is following. When describing the trajectories, it can be helpful to point to a diagram or draw each pattern presented in Chap. 4.

As most patients will not follow the Catastrophic Event trajectory, it can be helpful to describe this trajectory next, sharing that,

- "Uncommonly, patients will pass away following some type of catastrophic event in which the medical community saves our life, but often at a greatly diminished capacity to live on our own, with our family faced with the decision to withdraw treatment, after which we typically pass away in the ICU."

If the patient is following this trajectory, this trajectory should be discussed last.

Assuming that the patient is not following the Catastrophic Event trajectory, continue by introducing the Organ Failure, Cancer, and Frailty/Dementia trajectories, explaining that,

- "The rest of us will follow just one of three patterns of decline."

Then, work through these trajectories, leaving the one the patient is following for last. Template language for introducing each trajectory is provided in Chap. 15.

When describing each trajectory, provide a patient example, making the stories of decline real. I typically describe examples of family members' deaths from my family tree, illustrating the point that most of us have experience with most of the terminal trajectories, recognizable if we know what we're seeing.

When describing the Organ Failure, Cancer, and Frailty/Dementia trajectories, it is critically important to introduce the idea that,

- "At some point, the patient will progress beyond the medical community's capacity to control disease or symptoms, at which point the patient can be said to *meet hospice criteria*, meaning we would worry that the patient's time is limited."

Tying the disease trajectory to the expected endpoint of death by gently introducing the phrase "hospice criteria" is the goal during this introductory phase of education. Because this step provides the foundation for connecting the patient's physical and functional decline to their expected mortality, skipping this important part of the message can be detrimental.

The following is an example of a description of the Organ Failure trajectory that could be provided to a patient with chronic obstructive pulmonary disease (COPD).

- "Approximately 1 in 5 of us will die of some type of organ failure. Heart failure is the most common cause of death for humans, with lung failure close behind. Patients following this type of journey will experience progressive decline over several years that is punctuated by periods of worsening symptoms when the organ that is failing struggles to get itself back into harmony. Often, during these episodes, called "exacerbations," symptoms become severe enough that patients need to go to the hospital to be helped to feel better. Many times, patients are initially diagnosed with heart failure or COPD during one of these exacerbations. Eventually, as the organ continues to fail, patients need an increasing level of support at the hospital to feel better, until eventually, they get to the point in their journey where the organ fails beyond the medical community's ability to manage their symptoms, at which point any next hospitalization may be the last time they'll leave their home."

The critical information that should be conveyed when describing the disease trajectory driving patient decline includes the following:

- How common the trajectory is,
- The general pattern of decline that can be expected, and
- The idea that disease will progress until the patient meets hospice criteria, at which point we worry that the patient's time is limited.

See Chap. 15 for template language to describe the five disease trajectories.

Connect the Patient's Illness Experience to the Disease Trajectory Driving the Patient's Decline

After introducing the general pattern of decline that the patient is following, the next task is to connect the patient's experiences, detailed by the patient and family during the Illness Arc, to the trajectory just described. For the patient with COPD, this part of the conversation might go as follows:

- "It sounds like your COPD was diagnosed during an exacerbation in which you developed pneumonia and needed steroids, intravenous (IV) antibiotics, and oxygen support. You described multiple trips back to the hospital for episodes of bronchitis, pneumonia, and even COVID-19 over the last several years. Each of these episodes and hospitalizations represents an exacerbation, which is an expected, normal experience with COPD. You mentioned earlier that you noticed your difficulty in bouncing back to the way you felt before each hospitalization, which is also very common and expected for patients on this type of journey and represents your ongoing loss of physical and functional stamina. It sounds like as your oxygen needs at home have increased, your ability to walk short distances has decreased, and your need for assistance at home has increased."

Watching for signs that the patient and family are keeping pace with your narrative, note and address any emotional content conveyed by their facial expressions, verbalizations, or body language. If they are keeping pace and don't appear skeptical, it is okay to continue. It is never a bad idea, even for those who do not appear skeptical, to check in by asking,

- "Does that make sense?" or "Does it surprise you to hear this?"

If a patient or family member expresses a disagreement, such as, "I don't think that is what is happening," it is senseless to continue. Instead, pause the conversation and back up, investigating their understanding of disease and their beliefs about what is happening before attempting again to discuss the disease trajectory, and certainly before sharing the news that the patient meets hospice criteria. People who do not believe they are getting to the end of their lives will not hear this message, or if they do, it can so offend their beliefs that it results in a damaged or dismantled sense of rapport and trust, undermining the compassionate and collaborative milieu that has been established.

Inform the Patient and Family that the Patient Meets Hospice Criteria

For patients and families who are keeping pace with and appear to be agreeing with the discussion, the next step is to deliver the assessment that the patient meets hospice criteria. This messaging should be accomplished in three steps:

- Introduce the idea of hospice criteria,
- Share the assessment that the patient meets hospice criteria, and
- Check in with the patient and family to learn whether they are surprised by this information.

Because most people are unaware that hospice criteria exist, it is important to introduce the idea of hospice criteria as a legitimate mechanism for determining when patients have arrived at a point in their journey where their time is limited. This can be done by providing a simple introduction that people can understand,

- "Just as we have criteria to diagnose and stage disease, we also have criteria that enable us to recognize when a patient has reached the point in their journey where the medical community can no longer alter the course of their disease."

By this point in the conversation, the patient and family will have heard the phrase "hospice criteria" or some gentle description of "getting to the point in the journey where the medical community can no longer alter the course of disease" twice, which is a benign way of introducing difficult information without directly sharing an assertion like, "You have two weeks left to live," a jarring, unkind, and inappropriate approach to sharing such life-altering news.

After reintroducing the idea of hospice criteria, it is time to deliver the most delicate news of the conversation—the assessment that the patient meets hospice criteria. This message should be delivered with compassion, kindness, and caring and by referencing the components of the hospice criteria for the disease driving the patient's decline. Continuing with the example of a patient with end-stage COPD, we might say,

- "With the number of exacerbations you have had recently, how difficult it is for you to breathe even at rest, how limited your capacity to walk has become, and the fact that you are spending most of your day either in your chair or in your bed, you have reached the point in your journey where you now meet hospice criteria."

It is important to directly state that the patient "has now reached the point in their journey where they meet hospice criteria." Avoid inexplicit or ambiguous messaging, as that only further confuses the matter. Patients and families deserve and need compassionate and kind but direct communication about the patient's health status to make medical decisions that reflect their values.

Continue, explaining that,

- "This means that you have arrived at a point in your lung failure journey where we worry that your time is limited and where we, the medical community, will be unable to fix or alter the course of your disease beyond controlling your symptoms."

Pause here, providing the patient and family time to process what they have just heard. Monitor their facial expressions and tend to their emotional needs, for instance, providing a tissue when people tear up or offering encouraging kindness, such as,

- "I'm sorry. This is so hard. You are so brave."

Finally, check in with the patient and family by asking,

- "Does it surprise you to hear me say this?"

If you have had to tend to their emotions,

- "Does it surprise you to hear me share my assessment that you've reached the point in your journey where I am worried that your time is limited?"

Do Not Skip Over This Question Collaborative communication requires that we keep pace with the patient and family, never pushing beyond their spiritual or emotional capacity or willingness to process what we're saying.

Again, I have found that if I have done an excellent job of remaining patient and compassionate to this point in the conversation, not pushing patients and families further than they are willing to travel with me, almost everyone will answer "No" to this question. The reality is that patients and families often know before the medical community is willing to bring it up in conversation that the patient has reached the end of their journey.

Hearing from the patient and family that they are not surprised to learn that the patient has arrived at the end of their journey is the permission we need to move forward in the conversation. During the next part of the conversation, the End-of-Life Wishes Arc, we will explore more fully the patient and family wishes for the end of life.

When Patients Do Not Meet Hospice Criteria

For patients who do not yet meet hospice criteria, the goal of this part of the conversation is a little different. Rather than informing the patient that they meet hospice criteria, the objective is to provide an assessment of where the patient is in their disease trajectory, to educate them about how disease can progress, and to help anticipate expected concerns. Goals for this part of the conversation further depend on the specific trajectory the patient is following and how advanced the disease is. Guidance for the Organ Failure, Cancer, Dementia, and Frailty trajectories, including what should be accomplished for patients with early- and late-stage disease, follows.

See Chap. 15 for template language to provide general descriptions of the five disease trajectories.

Organ Failure

For patients with well-controlled or early-stage Organ Failure, the goal is to provide:

- A general overview of the disease journey
- Reassurance that the patient is early in their journey

– Education about what to expect as disease progresses
– Instructions for monitoring symptoms to prevent hospitalizations for expected exacerbations

For example, a patient newly diagnosed with COPD who does not require oxygen, who can walk up to five miles a day without shortness of breath, and who has no functional or physical limitations would be positioned at the earliest point of the disease trajectory diagram. Following the general description of the Organ Failure trajectory (see Chap. 15), it would be appropriate to say,

- "Given your high level of function, your ability to walk far, and the fact that you aren't experiencing any symptoms and don't require oxygen, I think you are very early in your journey. Because exacerbations are an expected part of organ failure that can lead to hospitalizations, I would like to teach you about how to monitor your symptoms and what to do if symptoms develop so that we can try to keep you out of the hospital."

Further discussion would teach patients about the various symptoms that can occur with an exacerbation, the importance of monitoring symptoms so that treatment for an exacerbation with steroids and antibiotics can be started as quickly as possible, plus encouragement to quit smoking, if applicable, and education about how consistency with taking maintenance medications can support lung function and prevent exacerbations. It can also be helpful to gently paint a picture of the expected decline and to suggest that a change in health status or a decline in functional status would be an appropriate opportunity to revisit a conversation about medical wishes. Most patients will be grateful for this type of education, particularly advice that can help prevent hospitalizations.

For patients with more advanced Organ Failure, a discussion should include the following:

– A general overview of the disease journey,
– An assessment of where the patient is in their disease course,
– Education about what to expect as disease progresses,
– Instructions for monitoring symptoms to prevent hospitalizations for expected exacerbations,
– The expectation that, at some point, the patient will meet hospice criteria, as well as a description of the criteria so that the patient and family know what to watch for, and
– A discussion of medical care that the patient and family should consider as that point approaches.

For example, a patient with advanced COPD, whose PPS score is 50%, who can still walk around the block, but who has begun to use the store-provided electric scooters while shopping, and who needs assistance at home with some instrumental activities of daily living (IADLs), would be positioned on the disease trajectory diagram about half-way down the y-axis, at the point that corresponds to a PPS score of 50%. Because patients with a PPS score of 50% *can* be appropriate for hospice care, talking about hospice criteria with such patients is not only appropriate but is critically important to supporting patient and family autonomy and aligning patient end-of-life wishes with their care.

For a patient with advanced COPD, following the general description of the Organ Failure trajectory (see Chap. 15), it would be appropriate to say,

- "Your need to use the scooter when shopping and your inability to walk more than a few steps before becoming short of breath tells me that your lung disease is advanced. As your disease progresses, I would expect you to be able to walk shorter and shorter distances before needing to rest or before becoming short of breath."
- "Because exacerbations are an expected part of organ failure that can lead to hospitalizations, I would like to teach you about how to monitor your symptoms and what to do if symptoms develop so that we can try to keep you out of the hospital. Additionally, it is important to know that having any advanced disease can make it more difficult to bounce back from an insult or injury, such as pneumonia, a urinary tract infection, or COVID-19."
- "I will keep a close eye on you to watch for disease progression so that I can try to identify the point where you meet hospice criteria, that is, the point when we would worry that your time is limited. For patients with lung failure, that point occurs when you start having symptoms at rest, when you are spending most of your day in your bed or chair because even minimal exertion wears you out or causes shortness of breath, or when you lose a significant amount of weight unintentionally in a short amount of time."
- "Whenever you have advanced disease, it is important to think about the kinds of medical interventions you would or would not want because treatments that might have been helpful when you were younger and healthier may not be as effective with advanced disease. Some treatments can be what we call "nonbeneficial" and could even shorten your life. An example would be major surgery with general anesthesia in a patient with end-stage lung disease. Patients with very advanced lung disease might not even be a candidate for surgery because the anesthesia could compromise their breathing to the point of respiratory failure and death in the operating room."
- "Also, as lung disease progresses, patients tend to need increasingly invasive oxygen support during exacerbations. Although right now, your exacerbations are controlled by increasing the oxygen setting through your nasal cannula, as lung failure worsens, patients can require BiPAP support (which is an oxygen mask that is strapped to your head and which forces air into your lungs) or intubation (which is the tube that goes down your windpipe and keeps your airway open) and mechanical ventilation support (which is the machine that breathes for you)."

- "Eventually, patients with lung disease will get to a point where any next exacerbation may be the last time they'll leave their house. Because most people want to be at home at the end of their lives, it is important to know what to expect so that you can make decisions about care that align with your wishes and values before it becomes too late."
- "Does all of that make sense?"

Cancer

For patients following the Cancer trajectory, whose disease is well controlled, who have early-stage disease, or whose disease is expected to be cured, the goal is to provide,

- A general overview of the cancer journey,
- Reassurance that the patient is early in their journey,
- Education about what to expect if disease progresses, and
- Discussion of the fact that end-of-life decline can occur rapidly.

Many people have little to no idea of what to expect on a cancer journey, and painting a picture of what can happen can be a powerful way of preparing them to articulate their threshold for stopping treatment and transitioning to hospice care.

Note that these recommendations are designed for use with adult cancer patients. It would not be appropriate to discuss end-of-life disease trajectory with parents of pediatric patients expected to be cured of disease. Any attempt to adopt this method with parents of pediatric patients whose disease progresses beyond the medical community's ability to control disease should be done with extraordinary compassion, care, kindness, patience, and consideration and by providers who have built considerable trust and rapport with the patient's family.

Consider a patient with prostate cancer whose disease is well-controlled, whose appetite and energy level are robust, who is not losing weight or who has not lost a clinically significant amount of weight, and who can fully participate in their life. This patient would have a PPS score that places them on the plateau at the top of the Cancer trajectory.

Following the general description of the Cancer trajectory (see Chap. 15), it would be appropriate to say,

- "Given your high energy level, ability to fully participate in your life, and the fact that your disease is well-controlled, I think you are up on top of the plateau, and as long as your treatment continues to control your cancer, I would expect you to stay there. We'll continue to monitor your energy, appetite, weight, and need for assistance across the day. If those things start to change, we'll reevaluate and have further discussions about your wishes."

This is a gentle and kind way of acknowledging the possibility of disease progression and the need to revisit wishes should that happen without robbing the patient and family of all hope for continued longevity or a cure.

When a patient's cancer is expected to be cured, it is not necessary to go into lengthy discussions about cancer's progression. However, for patients who are frail, who are elderly, or who have other contributing comorbidities, it is important to prepare them for the possibility that their disease can change quickly and that significant decline in the setting of a cancer journey can be challenging to recover from.

For patients whose cancer is more advanced or is progressing despite continued treatment, or for those who have already made the transition down the Cancer trajectory cliff, and for any patient with advanced cancer who would meet hospice criteria should they choose to forego treatment, a discussion should include the following:

- A general overview of the disease journey,
- An assessment of where the patient is in their disease course,
- Education about what to expect as disease progresses,
- Discussion of the fact that end-of-life decline can occur rapidly, and
- Discussion of medical care that the patient and family should consider as that point approaches.

For example, consider a patient with metastatic cancer and these other features:

- PPS score of 50%,
- Needs assistance with many household chores,
- Reduced appetite and oral intake,
- Body weight declined by 20% in the prior 12 months,
- Able to participate at a reduced level in their daily life, and
- Not yet ready to stop treatment.

This patient would be positioned somewhere down the Cancer trajectory cliff. Such a patient meets hospice criteria due to their weight loss, but because they are still receiving treatment for their cancer, they would not be eligible to receive hospice care.

Following the general description of the Cancer trajectory (see Chap. 15), it would be appropriate to say,

- "Given your weight loss over the last year, your reduced appetite, and your increased need for assistance at home, I think you have already made the transition down the Cancer trajectory cliff and are part of the way down that hill. That and the fact that your cancer has spread beyond the organ of origin, you currently technically meet hospice criteria. That means you are at a point in your journey where I would start to worry that your time might be limited."

- "I am very happy to learn that you feel good enough to continue treatment and have been feeling well over the last several months."
- "Because decline at the end of life with a cancer journey can happen rapidly, it will be important for us to watch for changes you may experience going forward. This could include additional weight loss, a further decline in your energy or ability to participate in your life, an increase in your need for assistance across the day, an increase in the number of hours you spend sleeping each day, mobility issues or falls, or hospitalizations for things like infections, side effects of your cancer medications, or new symptoms caused by your cancer's progression."
- "Once people reach the bottom of the Cancer trajectory cliff, their time is usually very limited, and it can be very difficult for the medical community to help other than to control symptoms enough to keep them comfortable. When patients get that far into their journey, they are at an increased risk of experiencing invasive interventions in the hospital. For instance, an infection can become so severe that it can lead to organ failure. If the lungs were to fail, the patient might need intubation and mechanical ventilation to survive."
- "Because a person's body is so declined by that point, so diminished by cancer, they may not be able to survive without such invasive support, leaving their loved ones faced with the decision to withdraw treatment in the ICU, at a point that is often too late for the patient to say their goodbyes. For patients with advancing cancer who would prefer to pass away at home at the end of their lives, they will need to choose to transition to hospice care before getting to that point. Part of my job is to monitor any progression and to make space for us to talk about your wishes if things change."
- "How does that sound?"

Note that this approach gently introduces the idea that the patient "technically" meets hospice criteria without telling them that their time is definitely limited. Patients at this point may respond to the mention of the hospice criteria by stating that, "I am not ready to give up," "I am not ready for hospice care," or "I wouldn't want that." Provide reassurance, offering a response that aligns with their wishes, such as,

- "Very good. That's important information for me to hear. Part of my role is to learn what your medical wishes are and to help align your wishes with your medical care."

To these replies, it can also be helpful to encourage patients to "Tell me more" to allow them to express any fears or misconceptions about hospice care, which can be corrected later in the conversation during the Hospice Care Arc. Supporting patients with advanced cancer can be a delicate balance of supporting their wishes for continued treatment while gently expressing concerns about their risk for advanced interventions, escalations of care, and rapid progression leading to terminal decline. Provide the reassurance early and often that,

- "There is no right answer, only the answer that is right for you and your family."

This is a loving and kind way of acknowledging the inherent challenges at this point of life and expressing support for patients' wishes of any kind.

Dementia

For those with dementia, the approach to this part of the conversation depends on where the patient is in their dementia journey, the patient's capacity for medical decision making (i.e., their ability to participate in complicated conversations about medical matters), and their sensitivity to discussion about their diagnosis. Remember that patients with dementia tend to either have insight into their decline or not. Those with insight can feel embarrassed and worried by their disease but may be willing and able to participate in their end-of-life planning, particularly if they are early in their journey. Those without insight may be equally distressed by but lack insight into their decline, so they may adamantly refuse to participate in any discussion regarding their diagnosis, need for help, or anticipated medical care. This latter group can be challenging to help directly. For these patients, much of my care focuses on supporting the family.

For patients who are early in their dementia journey, including those in the Recent Memory or Cognitive Function stage, who are able and willing to participate, goals of care conversations are important to have with family members present, particularly spouses and children, who will face decisions about the patient's medical care at some point in the future. It is vital for these family members to hear the patient's articulated wishes about the time in their journey when they will need assistance with all ADLs and, later, when they reach the point of meeting hospice criteria. Hearing a person with dementia say that they would not want a feeding tube, for instance, when they reach the point of metabolic decline when their body is not interested in eating, and when their brain is losing the ability to carefully coordinate their chewing and swallowing, empowers family members to forego such treatments more readily when the time comes.

The goal for patients still early in their dementia journey, who are willing and capable of participating in conversations about their disease, is to provide:

- A detailed description of the dementia journey,
- Reassurance that they are early in their journey,
- Education about what to expect as disease progresses, and
- Education about what to expect when they reach the final stage of their journey.

With this information, patients can articulate their preferences for end-of-life medical care, which will be accomplished during the next part of the conversation in the End-of-Life Wishes Arc. Ideally, this conversation would occur for all patients with dementia early in the course of disease when their cognitive function remains intact.

Consider a patient newly diagnosed with Alzheimer's disease, early in the Cognitive Function stage, who has significant problems with recent memory, who needs assistance with some IADLs, who is aware of their diagnosis and who is willing to learn about their disease so that they can help their family plan for the future. While providing a detailed description of the dementia journey (see Chap. 15), upon reaching the description of the Cognitive Function stage, it would be appropriate to say, with a great deal of compassion and care,

- "I think you are somewhere in this stage of your journey because you are starting to show the need for assistance with some of the tasks around the house, like driving and cooking and finances. In the coming years, it will be my job to keep a close eye on you and your family to make sure you are doing well. By providing your family with the support they need to support you, I can reassure you that both you and your family can have a loving and positive experience on this journey."

As long as the patient and family accept your assessment, it would be appropriate to describe the remaining stages of the dementia journey and then transition the conversation into the next part of the conversation, the End-of-Life Wishes Arc, where the patient will be given the opportunity to articulate their medical wishes for care for their current stage of disease and the point in their journey when they meet hospice criteria.

For all patients on the dementia journey, education about the expected stages of decline is very beneficial for family members, as it normalizes and validates their experiences and prepares them for the changes ahead. For patients who are early in their journey but do not have insight into their decline and who are sensitive about any discussion of their disease, this education may need to be provided to the family without the patient present. Although providing care to family members without the patient present may feel antithetical to patient-centered care, dementia deserves special consideration in terms of the provision of appropriate support to patients and their caregivers because of the expected loss of the patient's cognitive capacity. Anytime care is provided for a patient to family members without the patient present, the rules of HIPAA and the patient rights guidelines of your institution should be followed.

Patients who are further into their dementia journey, including those who have reached the Personal Care or Physical Function stages, are typically not able to participate in their medical decision making because cognitive losses in the prefrontal cortex have impaired their ability to process abstract and new information. For these patients, it is important to determine whether conversations about their disease are distressing for the patient to hear. If it is, to preserve the patient's dignity, this conversation should be held without the patient present.

A special consideration is the patient in the Personal Care stage who has significant cognitive reserve and *appears* to be able to participate in conversations about their care. It can be difficult for family members not to involve such patients in medical decisions. However, it is important to share the concern with family members that by this point in their journey, the patient is likely unable to manage the cognitive skill required to process the information being discussed. Family members who have intimate experience dealing with the patient on a day-to-day basis will often readily agree with this assessment. Acknowledging the personal ethical dilemma family members can experience when managing care for patients with advanced dementia is a validating and loving way of enabling them to do the difficult work of supporting patients on this challenging journey when necessary.

For patients with advanced dementia who are very close to meeting hospice criteria, it is essential to share this information with family members, particularly those responsible for making medical decisions for the patient, and to provide a landmark for when the patient will meet hospice criteria. This information prepares healthcare agents for the oncoming need to make decisions about end-of-life care.

Consider a patient with dementia who has reached the Personal Care stage and needs help with bathing and toileting. Following the detailed description of the entire dementia journey (see Chap. 15), it would be appropriate to share,

- "Currently, the patient is at the end of the Personal Care stage. We can anticipate that the patient will, at some point, begin to experience bladder and bowel incontinence. When this happens, switching from regular underwear to adult diapers would be appropriate."
- "As your loved one continues to progress and move into the final stage of dementia, the Physical Function stage, they will start to show the metabolic decline that I discussed earlier, and at some point, will also begin to have issues with walking, transferring, and swallowing."
- "Patients with dementia can meet hospice criteria in two ways, either with a significant enough amount of weight loss, or when they lose their ability to transfer themselves or to walk without assistance. When the patient develops swallowing issues, they will be at increased risk of aspiration pneumonia and additional hospitalizations."
- "I will keep a close eye on the patient going forward so that I can try to identify as early as possible the moment that they meet hospice criteria so that we can revisit your wishes for their care."
- "How does that sound?"

Frailty

Unlike patients following the other terminal trajectories, those with frailty do not typically receive a formal diagnosis of "age-related decline." However, "protein-calorie malnutrition" and "failure to thrive" often serve as reasonable proxies. Because this terminal trajectory is usually not formally acknowledged or named by the medical community, the most pressing component of helping patients and families understand the Frailty trajectory is to recognize that it is happening to patients. Thus, a review of functional status, weight and appetite changes, mobility issues, and falls should be a routine part of patient care for patients of advanced age or increasing frailty.

For patients of advanced age who are beginning to show signs of weight loss, reduced appetite, mobility issues, or loss of strength, stamina, or speed, the goal of this part of the conversation is to provide:

- A general overview of the trajectory,
- Offer of interventions to try to halt weight loss, and
- Education about what to expect as decline continues.

For example, an 80-year-old patient who is increasingly less interested in eating, who has lost 10% of their body weight over the previous five years, but who has appropriate mealtime support at the facility where they live, would be positioned at the earliest point of the Frailty trajectory.

Following the general description of the Frailty trajectory (see Chap. 15), it would be appropriate to say,

- "Given your weight loss over the last several years and that you're beginning to slow down and are less interested in eating, I think your body has begun to make the metabolic shift I described earlier. I would like to try to interrupt the weight loss you've been experiencing recently because you're starting to get to the point where I worry about how much reserve you have left to tolerate any insult or injury you might experience. I know you have appropriate mealtime support living here at this facility, so what I would like to suggest is a medication that carries the good side effect of weight gain and which we often use in patients with this concern."

Although occasionally a patient's weight will be stabilized by such an intervention, this will not happen for many others, providing support for the assessment that the patient is, indeed, following the expected trajectory of Frailty. This type of confirmation helps patients and family members accept the reality of end-of-life decline on this trajectory as an expected and natural part of life.

For patients of advanced age much further into the Frailty trajectory, who are close to losing a clinically significant amount of weight (5% to 10% in the previous 6 to 12 months), a discussion should include the following:

- A general overview of this type of decline,
- An assessment of where the patient is in the Frailty trajectory,
- Education about what to expect as decline progresses,
- The expectation that, at some point, the patient will meet hospice criteria, as well as a description of the criteria so that the patient and family know what to watch for, and
- A discussion of medical care that the patient and family should consider as that point approaches.

For example, for a patient who has lost 4% of their body weight in the previous six months and who is starting to have significant mobility issues and repeated falls, following the general description of the Frailty trajectory (see Chap. 15), it would be appropriate to say,

- "I worry, with the amount of weight you have lost in recent months and the fact that you are now having mobility issues and falls, that your decline is becoming significant. If your weight loss reaches 5% to 10% of your body weight in a period of 6 to 12 months, you will meet what we call hospice criteria, and at that point, I would worry that your time is limited."
- "The physical decline you've been experiencing is robbing your body of reserve to recover from any significant insult or injury. For instance, if you were to fall and break your hip, the fall and fracture would be one major insult that might be difficult for your body to recover from. But should you need surgery to repair your hip, that would entail two additional major insults—the surgery and the anesthesia—which may prove too much for your body to be able to handle."
- "Now is the perfect time for you and your family to think about what you would want for yourself should something like that happen."
- "Does that make sense?"

~~~

When providing education to patients and families about the disease driving patient decline, the goal is to:

- Provide an accurate assessment,
- Position the patient on the appropriate disease trajectory,
- Prepare the patient and family for what is ahead, and to
- Help anticipate medical considerations the patient or family may be faced with in the future.

Most people will appreciate clear communication regarding what to expect going forward as helpful preparation for making choices that reflect their priorities and values. Remember that most patients want to avoid distressing end-of-life hospitalizations and invasive medical care, if possible, and prefer to experience a soft landing at the end of life in a setting that allows them to focus on what matters most—expressing and experiencing love. Providing patients and families the opportunity to consider and articulate their wishes ahead of time is a compassionate and appropriate focus of patient-centered care.

During the next part of the conversation, the End-of-Life Wishes Arc, we will explore the patient's and family's wishes for their current stage of disease and the end of life more fully.

The End-of-Life Wishes Arc: Exploring End-of-Life, Advance Directive, and Code Status Wishes with Patients and Families

11

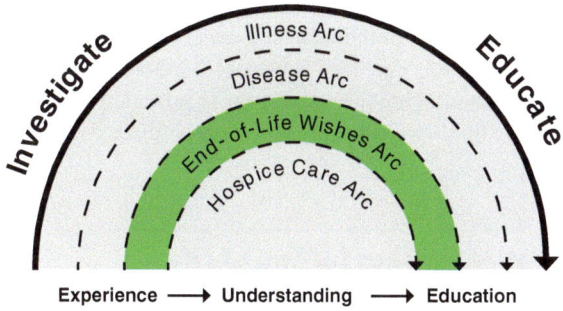

Fig. 11.1 The End-of-Life Wishes Arc

Objectives During the End-of-Life Wishes Arc (Fig. 11.1)

- Investigate patient wishes for the end of life, including:
  - What the patient is hoping for going forward
  - Where the patient wants to be when they die
  - What a good death would be like for the patient
- Investigate patient and family hospice mindedness, including:
  - Whether they are ready to allow nature to take its course
  - Whether they want to avoid returning to the hospital
  - Whether they are ready to focus on quality of life and comfort
- Investigate advance directive and code status wishes, including* the following:
  - Surrogate medical decision maker
  - Advance directive (living will) wishes
  - Code status wishes
  - Wishes for approach to medical care and specific medical interventions

© The Author(s), under exclusive license to Springer Nature Switzerland AG 2024
A. Shaw, PA, *The Arc of Conversation*,
https://doi.org/10.1007/978-3-031-70495-6_11

- Using the **investigate-then-educate** technique, educate the patient and family about the following:
  - Any topic for which the patient or family has a question or concern
  - Advance directive and code status considerations*
- Next steps:
  - Offer a palliative (supportive) care referral when appropriate

*Chapter 16 provides template language for this part of the conversation.

Having established that the patient and family understand that the patient has arrived at the end of their journey or that they will arrive at that point in the future, we can safely transition the conversation into the End-of-Life Wishes Arc. The over-arching objective of this part of the conversation is to investigate patients' and families' wishes for end-of-life care and advance directive considerations. Using the investigate-then-educate technique, education is provided whenever the patient or family has a question or concern and when discussing advance directive considerations.

Investigate Patient Wishes for End of Life

Questions:
- Given what we've just discussed and what you can expect with your disease going forward, what are you hoping for in the time you have left?
- Where would you like to be at the end of your life?
- What would a good death be like for you?

For patients who meet hospice criteria, start to **investigate** the patient's wishes for the end of life by asking the patient to think about what they want their life to be like in the time they have remaining by asking,

- "Given what we've just discussed and what you can expect with your disease going forward, what are you hoping for in the time you have left?"

For those who do not yet meet hospice criteria, this question can be adjusted,

- "Given what we've discussed about what can be expected with your disease going forward, what would you want for yourself when you get to the point in your journey when your time is limited?"

This gentle inquiry invites the patient to think about what matters most to them and articulate their priorities during this period. For many people, this will be the first oppor-tunity the medical community has provided to consider and express these desires.

Typical answers to this question include desires to:

- – Remain at home,
- – Spend time with their family, close friends, and pets,
- – Enjoy their routine, and
- – Avoid a return to the hospital.

Typically, patients will answer with one response. Encourage their continued consideration by asking,

- • "What else are you hoping for?"

Repeat this inquiry or a shortened version of this question, such as "What else?" until the patient has exhausted their replies.

Next, ask,

- • "Where would you like to be at the end of your life?"

For many patients, this is a straightforward question that will be answered by "at home." For patients who are confused by this question, clarify by asking,

- • "Where do you want to be when you pass away?"

If a patient yet remains confused, ask directly,

- • "Would you prefer to pass away at home?" and "What are your feelings about passing away in the hospital?"

Although most people will state a preference to be at home at the end of their lives, some patients will say that they don't care if they die in the hospital. Inquire further about their wishes by asking these patients to "Tell me more" and listen for more specific preferences, such as, "I just want to be somewhere that my family won't have to worry about taking care of me," or "I want to be somewhere that someone can help keep me comfortable." What at first may sound like a preference regarding the location of death often turns out to be a preference regarding the experience of death. Know that many people assume that enrolling in hospice care means that they will need to leave their house, which most prefer not to do. Others want to ensure they are not a "burden to their families" at the end of life.

Next, ask,

- • "What would a good death be like for you?"

This question is very clear, allowing patients to explore their expectations and preferences for the death experience. Many people will express a desire to pass away in their sleep, while others will articulate a hope for comfort at the end of life and a wish to pass away without fear, pain, or other symptoms. Some will have a difficult time answering this question and can be helped by the gentle inquiry,

- "Would you hope to pass peacefully and without pain or other symptoms?"

For those who are unable to answer this question, provide reassurance,

- "That's okay. I know this is a hard question."

Evaluate Patient and Family Hospice Mindedness

Questions:
- Are you at the point in your journey where you are ready to allow nature to take its course?
- How do you feel about returning to the hospital for care?
- Are you at the point in your journey where you are ready to focus on quality of life and comfort?

The questions in the next part of the conversation explore patient and family hospice mindedness. Recall that to receive hospice care, in addition to meeting hospice criteria, patients must also be willing to enroll in hospice care or be "hospice minded" (see Chap. 5). The following questions are appropriate for patients who meet hospice criteria.

The first question is an existential probe of whether the patient is ready to die when their time comes, which is the essence of hospice mindedness.

- "Are you at the point in your journey where you are ready to allow nature to take its course?"

This question also indirectly asks about the patient's willingness to forego further medical interventions, particularly treatment intended to prolong life. Patients who have shared their belief that their time is limited and who have expressed agreement with the assessment that they meet hospice criteria will typically answer in the affirmative to this question, with many adding commentary such as, "I have lived a good long life," or "I'm ready to go."

The next question is a gentle way of investigating a patient's willingness to forego treatment intended to prolong life.

- "How do you feel about returning to the hospital for care?"

This question need not be asked if the patient has already expressed a desire to avoid a return to the hospital, but for those who have yet to articulate this desire specifically, it is necessary to ask directly. The patient's answers to this question are especially helpful for family members to hear. Most patients who have successfully been ushered through the conversation to this point, who meet hospice criteria, and who have acknowledged their belief that their time is limited will express a desire to avoid returning to the hospital.

Some patients, despite meeting hospice criteria and acknowledging their own belief that their time is limited, will have a hard time with the idea of *not* returning to the hospital if the need should arise. This difficulty is based on the assumption that the hospital is the de facto place to go when you are sick, and some people are challenged to imagine a point in their lives when the medical community cannot help them recover. To the question, "How do you feel about going back to the hospital for care?" these patients may reply, "But what if I need to go?"

An effective response to this question engages the **investigate-then-educate** technique to first learn patient or family expectations about hospital care and interventions at the end of life before filling in the gaps to paint a picture of what might happen at this point in the patient's life should they return to the hospital. Most people, when educated about the burdens of advanced interventions in the setting of terminal decline, will express a desire to avoid such treatment.

Begin to **investigate** the patient and family's understanding of potential medical needs during the terminal phase of disease by asking,

- "Can you tell me what you understand about why a person at this point in their journey might need to go back to the hospital?"

This question allows patients and families to imagine a specific reason (or reasons) for a return to the hospital. Answers vary and may include pain, infections, falls, fractures, dehydration, etc.

The effort for patients and families to imagine scenarios that would necessitate a return to the hospital is time well spent, as it often prompts consideration of whether the patient could then tolerate the anticipated treatment. It also allows families to consider a patient's experience of returning to the hospital. For example, families of patients with advanced dementia often quickly articulate a wish to avoid a return to the hospital or a rehabilitation setting once they imagine how distressing such a drastic change in routine would be for the patient. This also provides the opportunity to gently introduce the alternative treatment option to returning to the hospital: comfort-focused therapy, or hospice care.

Consider the example of a family that is concerned about their loved one's need to return to the hospital following a fall, a common event at the end of life. It would first be appropriate to reassure the family that their concern is well warranted by offering,

- "That is an excellent example and something that happens to many patients at this stage of decline. Let's talk about what might happen, for instance, if your loved one falls and breaks their hip. If they were taken to the hospital, chances are that after finding the hip fracture on CT scan, the surgeon would be consulted, who might then offer surgical repair."

At this point, many families will interject to share their concern that their loved one would not be able to survive surgery. It is important to validate this concern by saying,

- "I agree. I think surgery and anesthesia would be very challenging for your loved one. I, too, would worry that they might not survive."

Next, **educate** the patient and family on why the patient might not survive surgery by relating the patient's advanced disease state to the inherent burdens of interventions. This can be done by referencing the patient's metabolic decline, advanced organ failure and risk for invasive procedures, or irreversibility of brainstem degradation at the end of the dementia journey, whichever scenario most appropriately applies.

Continuing our example of a patient with frailty, it would be appropriate to say,

- "When a person's body has moved into a state of metabolic decline, their body is breaking down more tissue than it is building, and it can no longer adequately translate the products of nutrition into bone, muscle, and skin. It can be difficult for the body to heal a fracture or a major surgical wound. Subjecting a person in that state to such major interventions can be life-limiting because these interventions may be too stressful for the body to handle."

Watching for family agreement, again engage the **investigate-then-educate** technique to inquire about their knowledge of the alternative form of treatment that would be appropriate for a patient in this situation by asking,

- "Do you know the alternative to surgery in this circumstance?"

Many people will not know how to answer this question and will say, "No." Others may express worries that their loved one would suffer after such an event by sharing, "But I wouldn't want my mom to be left to die in pain in a hospital bed," or "But what would happen to her? I wouldn't want her to suffer if she needed surgery to take care of the pain."

Most importantly, these responses convey dedication, love, and advocacy by family members for a loved one, providing an opportunity to honor and praise their efforts by offering,

- "These are terrific questions. You are doing an amazing job of caring for and thinking about the experience you want your loved one to have going forward. They are so lucky to have you caring for them in this way."

Such responses also provide the opportunity to gently introduce hospice care as a legitimate form of treatment and to give an introductory bit of education about hospice care. Continuing with our conversation, it would be appropriate to say,

- "If your loved one were to fall and break their hip, given where they are in their journey, and the concern that they either might not tolerate surgery or might not be a candidate for surgery, the alternative treatment option would be comfort-focused care, or what we call hospice care. This type of care focuses entirely on keeping patients comfortable so they can pass peacefully without pain or other symptoms when their time comes. We can talk more about hospice care in a bit, but I wanted to introduce the idea that there is an alternative form of treatment to the interventions that are typically offered for such medical issues, but that may not be beneficial or even survivable at this point in your loved one's life."

When considering reasons a patient may need to return to the hospital for care, families may bring up any number of other scenarios, including urinary tract infections (UTIs), a bout of pneumonia, or even a heart attack. Effective responses pair the current (or expected future) state of the patient's health with the interventions that might be offered, providing the opportunity to explore the patient's candidacy, survivability, and preferences for such care. Not only does this effort empower patients and families to make choices that align with their values, but it also supports their confidence in their choices.

The final question in this part of the conversation applies primarily to patients who meet hospice criteria:

- "Are you at the point in your journey where you want to focus on quality of life and comfort?"

However, this question can be appropriate for patients with advanced disease who do not yet meet hospice criteria, who have limited quality of life, and who experience distress while hospitalized. For example, family members of patients with advanced dementia who do not yet meet hospice criteria often become hospice minded for their loved ones well before their loved ones meet hospice criteria.

The question of whether a patient or family is ready to focus on comfort and quality of life places a direct focus on the primary purpose of hospice care, further refining the evaluation of hospice mindedness of the patient and family. As can easily be imagined, hearing the patient answer this question is incredibly helpful for loved ones.

For those who have previously articulated their desire to focus on comfort and quality of life, it is unnecessary to ask this question. However, for those who meet hospice criteria or are close to meeting hospice criteria who have yet to specify this wish, it is necessary to provide patients and family members the opportunity to respond directly to this question.

Hearing "No" to this question is as important as hearing "Yes." Remember that the primary purpose of pursuing goals of care conversations with patients and families is to align the patient's medical care to their wishes. Therefore, learning that patients who meet hospice criteria are not hospice minded is just as important as learning that they are.

An appropriate and supportive response to hearing that a patient is not yet ready to focus on comfort and quality of life would be,

- "Very good. Because you presently meet hospice criteria, you can choose hospice care at any point in the future, but that is a very personal choice that can only be made by you and your family. There's no right answer to this question, only the answer that is right for you and your loved ones. I will keep a close eye on how you're doing, and if things change or if you go back to the hospital, that would be a good time to revisit your wishes. And if you decide at any point that you are ready for hospice, all you need to do is let us know. Does that sound good?"

As stated earlier, patients and families can also become hospice minded before the patient meets hospice criteria. Patients with advanced disease who do not yet meet hospice criteria but who have expressed hospice mindedness can be provided the reassurance that a transition to hospice care can be made as soon as they meet criteria. That effort can focus on a smooth transition once that time comes, with the goal of avoiding ER visits or hospital admissions in the meantime.

For these patients, it would be appropriate to say,

- "Although you don't meet hospice criteria at this moment, we can work together to help you avoid returning to the hospital for care. Should you develop symptoms or an issue that we cannot manage at home, and should you need to be seen in the ER, you can inform the medical team at the hospital that you prefer to be stabilized and to be evaluated for hospice care. They can work with our team to transition you to hospice care if you meet criteria at that point, sometimes even without admitting you to the hospital overnight. I hope that by keeping a close eye on you to watch for any continued decline, I can identify the exact moment you meet hospice criteria so that we can transition you to hospice care smoothly and hopefully *before* any additional ER visits or future hospital admissions. How does that sound?"

Most patients and families will appreciate this advocacy in helping to achieve their goals.

Investigate Advance Directive and Code Status Wishes

The next objective is to discuss the patient and family's wishes for medical care at the patient's present state of decline and end of life. Because patient choice is best supported from a vantage point of accurate understanding of health status and what can be expected on the horizon, it is best to wait until this point of the conversation to discuss advance directives and code status wishes.

The approach to walking patients through this part of the conversation depends on whether the patient meets hospice criteria and whether those who meet hospice criteria are hospice minded.

For patients who meet hospice criteria and who are hospice minded, a discussion of advance directive and code status wishes does not always need to be held, and because a decision to choose hospice care typically represents an immense emotional and spiritual effort, discussion of code status and advanced directive considerations at this point can muddy the waters and confuse the situation. Because a comprehensive discussion of hospice care will explain that hospice care precludes resuscitation attempts, hospitalizations, ER visits, and escalations of care, patients who both meet hospice criteria and who are hospice minded can be transitioned directly into the Hospice Care Arc (see Chap. 12) without a complete discussion of code status and advance directive wishes.

For patients who meet hospice criteria but who are not hospice minded, discussing advance directive and code status wishes is critically important because these patients carry a significant risk of recurrent admissions, invasive interventions, escalations of care, and death in the hospital. Because patient experience of illness informs patient preferences, it is imperative to revisit advance directive and code status wishes with these patients whenever they experience an admission or their health status changes. Patient and family preferences typically evolve with time, especially with increased healthcare utilization, reflecting a value system responsive to quality of life. (See Chap. 16 for guidance and template language to discuss the patient's preferences for surrogate medical decision makers, living will and code status considerations, and advanced medical interventions.)

It is equally important that patients who do not meet hospice criteria but are hospice minded are allowed to articulate their advance directive and code status preferences, to help them avoid unwanted medical interventions. Again, it is a common occurrence that families of those with advanced dementia become hospice minded well before patients meet hospice criteria.

For patients who do not meet hospice criteria, a conversation about advance directive and code status wishes can be held during a separate appointment, as the conversation to this point can be lengthy. When discussing advance directive and code status considerations at a later time, begin the discussion with a review of the patient's personal experience of illness, understanding of disease, and where the patient is in their journey. Again, patient choice is always best supported by an accurate understanding of health status and what can be expected ahead.

When it is appropriate to discuss advance directive and code status wishes at this point in the conversation, follow the guidance in Chap. 16 before moving patients into the Hospice Care, where we will investigate patient and family experience and understanding of hospice care and provide education about this important form of treatment.

Patients not yet supported by palliative care who are close to meeting hospice criteria, who meet hospice criteria but are not hospice minded, or who are hospice minded but do not yet meet hospice criteria should be offered a referral to palliative care.

Next Steps

Offer a Palliative (Supportive) Care Referral when Appropriate

The clinical framework and technique taught in *The Arc of Conversation*, which is rooted in compassionate, collaborative care, is the essence of palliative care. At its heart, palliative care seeks to improve patient and family quality of life by supporting the physical, spiritual, and psychosocial aspects of living. It does so by investigating and prioritizing patient and family values, wishes, and concerns. Supported by a team that often includes a provider (MD, PA, or NP), social worker, chaplain, and financial navigator, palliative care considers the whole patient, including the spouse, other caregivers, children, and even pets. Palliative care teams work to reduce distress in any of the domains of a patient's life and, by extension, that of their caregivers and family members. At the end of life, hospice care does the same.

Whereas palliative care can support patients at any stage of a disease, terminal or not, hospice care is intended to provide support at the very end of life. Unfortunately, many patients and members of the medical community remain confused about this important distinction between palliative and hospice care, believing them to be synonymous. To address this common misconception, following the lead of the MD Anderson Cancer Center [1], the palliative care department at my institution changed its name to "supportive care." Most patients and families experiencing a chronic or terminal disease intuitively understand how they could use "an extra layer of support," our informal tagline. Importantly, patients and families tend to welcome, rather than shun, an offer of "extra support."

Because disease can ripple through patient and family lives like the stressors calving a glacier, often turning their lives on end, it is important that the medical community think early and often of palliative care to assist the mental, emotional, physical, and spiritual health and well-being of patients and families experiencing any challenging medical journey. Additionally, because any patient with a terminal disease will need to prepare for the end of life, such patients should be referred early to palliative (supportive) care, particularly before decision-making capacity is lost.

Ideally, all patients with chronic and terminal disease would be offered community-based palliative (supportive) care early in their journeys to provide support and symptom management and to ensure that goals of care conversations are held in advance of disease progression, medical crises, loss of medical decision-making capacity, and end-of-life decline. Patients who prefer to avoid returning to the hospital should be offered palliative (supportive) care, which can provide support at home until the time that the patient meets hospice criteria and becomes hospice minded and can be enrolled in hospice care.

It is important to appreciate that palliative (supportive) care is not exclusively warranted for patients with disease expected to be terminal. While it is easy to appreciate that patients with curable cancer could benefit from palliative (supportive) care, so could patients with chronic mental disease, for example. Recall the patient and family vignettes contrasting the illness experience of two young patients and their families in Chap. 6. Whereas the patient and family with the cancer diagnosis experienced robust, comprehensive, ongoing support that helped preserve their family during a very stressful time, the patient and family with the mental disease experienced a dramatically different journey, ultimately ending in divorce. The latter family certainly could have benefitted from comprehensive and ongoing palliative (supportive) care rooted in whole-person care, helping them navigate a very stressful journey and recognizing and addressing the parents' severe caregiver strain. The behavioral health community has a long way to go in recognizing the need to provide the kind of comprehensive, ongoing whole-person support that patients and their families need.

Some neurology clinics offer comprehensive palliative (supportive) care for specific, often very challenging diagnoses, such as Parkinson's disease and amyotrophic lateral sclerosis (ALS). The Alzheimer's and Dementia Care Program I run is a palliative (supportive) care program designed specifically for the complicated and challenging dementia journey. Oncology clinics sometimes have palliative (supportive) care providers embedded within their departments. Whenever such comprehensive support is available, patients and their families should be referred.

Though still mostly targeting patients with terminal diseases or those reaching the very end of their lives, there is increasing recognition in the greater medical community that palliative (supportive) care is a vitally important form of support for patients and their families experiencing any stage or type of disease. I am a strong proponent of palliative (supportive) care being a standard part of patient care throughout the healthcare continuum and of having providers trained in the palliative (supportive) care approach being embedded wherever patients are seen, such as in emergency rooms (ER), care facilities, and in clinics seeing patients with chronic and terminal diseases [2]. Additionally, I strongly believe that every provider should be familiar with the palliative (supportive) care approach, including awareness of how palliative (supportive) care can support patients and families across a medical journey; the knowledge presented in this textbook about disease progression, assessment using hospice criteria, and the skills to navigate patients and families compassionately and collaboratively through goals of care conversations; and the ability to appropriately represent palliative (supportive) and hospice care. In hindsight, I realize how beneficial it would have been for my cardiology patients to have been supported by a palliative (supportive) care provider working in my clinic, and better yet, had I been armed with this knowledge and set of skills.

Although the following list is not exhaustive, when the provision of comprehensive, ongoing palliative (supportive) care is beyond a provider's capacity or scope, a referral to palliative (supportive) care should be offered to patients with:

- A high symptom burden
- Cognitive decline or a diagnosis of dementia

- Difficulty handling instrumental activities of daily living (IADLs) or activities of daily living (ADLs)
- Physical decline
- A change in living circumstance due to the need for additional support (e.g., a move to be closer to family support or a move to a facility offering a higher level of care, such as from independent living to assisted living, memory care, or skilled nursing)
- Curable disease undergoing challenging treatment, especially those who live alone
- Advancing or terminal disease, especially those who live alone
- Advancing or terminal disease who want to avoid returning to the hospital
- Chronic or terminal disease with caregiver(s) experiencing strain
- Chronic or terminal disease with a primary caregiver with chronic or terminal disease
- Chronic or terminal disease characterized by occasional-to-frequent exacerbations or flare-ups that have resulted in hospitalizations, ER visits, or trips to rehabilitation
- Cancer with poor prognosis (e.g., brain cancer, pancreatic cancer, or small cell lung cancer) or that is aggressive, advanced stage, metastatic, or progressing despite treatment
- Cancer who have declined curative or palliative treatment
- Terminal disease who are close to meeting hospice criteria, especially those wishing to avoid future hospitalizations
- Terminal disease who meet hospice criteria and are not yet hospice minded
- Terminal disease who are hospice minded but do not yet meet hospice criteria

Because "palliative care" is so often misunderstood, a gentle and supportive way to offer a referral to palliative care is to talk about "supportive care" instead. The following introduction can be helpful:

- "I think you and your family would benefit from some additional support from our supportive care team. They provide an extra layer of support to patients with chronic or terminal disease."
- "Because each patient and family is unique, that support can look different for everyone. They will get to know you and will work to support you and your family based on your wishes and goals."
- "In addition to helping with symptom management, they can provide support to caregivers, help anticipate future needs, and connect you to resources. Part of their job is to continue the conversations we've started about your wishes."
- "If that sounds good, I'll place a referral."

For patients and families who proactively ask about "palliative care" and seem to have a positive impression of it, it is okay to talk about "palliative care" rather than "supportive care." To clarify any confusion that may arise between palliative and hospice care, the following brief statement can be helpful:

- "You may have heard of 'palliative care.' Many people think palliative care means hospice care. For that reason, we've started calling 'palliative care' 'supportive care' to help clarify that palliative or supportive care can help patients and families at any point in a disease journey, whereas hospice care is there to help at the end of life."
- "Does that make sense?"

It is important to reassure patients that palliative (supportive) care is provided in addition to the support they will continue to receive from their primary care and specialty providers.

- "Your primary care provider and other specialists will continue to follow you. Supportive care provides an additional layer of support."

Finally, reassure patients and families that supportive care is covered by most health insurance plans.

- "Supportive care is covered by Medicare, Medicaid, and most health insurance plans."

References

1. Dalal S, Palla S, Hui D, Nguyen L, Chacko R, Li Z, Fadul N, Scott C, Thornton V, Coldman B, Amin Y, Bruera E. Association between a name change from palliative to supportive care and the timing of patient referrals at a comprehensive cancer center. Oncologist. 2011;16(1):105–11. https://doi.org/10.1634/theoncologist.2010-0161. Epub 2011 Jan 6. PMID: 21212438; PMCID: PMC3228056.)
2. Shaw A. Palliative care has a branding problem—changing how it's perceived can break down silos. In: MedPageToday. 2024. https://www.medpagetoday.com/opinion/second-opinions/108848. Accessed 30 March 2024

The Hospice Care Arc: Exploring Hospice Care with Patients and Families

12

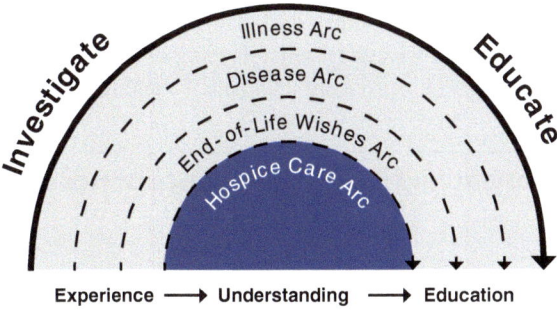

Fig. 12.1 The Hospice Care Arc

Objectives During the Hospice Care Arc (Fig. 12.1)
- Investigate patient and family experience of hospice care
- Investigate patient and family understanding of hospice care
- Educate patient and family about hospice care, including*:
    - Hospice care facts (correcting any misconceptions)
    - Hospice philosophy
    - Approach to hospice care
    - Location options and cost of hospice care
- Next steps:
    - Help patients and families transition to hospice care, or
    - Help patients determine their threshold for transitioning to hospice care.

*Chapter 17 provides template language for this part of the conversation.

© The Author(s), under exclusive license to Springer Nature Switzerland AG 2024 255
A. Shaw, PA, *The Arc of Conversation*,
https://doi.org/10.1007/978-3-031-70495-6_12

For patients who meet hospice criteria, the primary goal of the Arc of Conversation is to transition the conversation into the Hospice Care Arc so that hospice care can be offered as an appropriate treatment option for those wanting a soft landing at the end of life. Recall that many people want to pass away at home, focus on comfort and quality of life, and avoid unwanted escalations of care or life-prolonging interventions at the end of their lives. When patients and families are guided to this point in the conversation patiently, kindly, and compassionately, most will recognize hospice care as the treatment option that best meets their end-of-life goals. Ultimately, the Arc of Conversation is an approach to patient-centered care that compassionately and collaboratively supports patient autonomy.

Spending time with patients and families in the Hospice Care Arc is never a waste of time and should be offered to anyone with a chronic, terminal, or life-threatening diagnosis. Truthfully, an accurate understanding of hospice care benefits everyone; sooner or later, we will all be faced with these considerations, either for ourselves or a loved one. Normalizing the discussion of hospice care should be a goal of modern medicine, and providers and clinical staff at every level of the healthcare system should be equipped with an accurate understanding of hospice care and the training and permission to discuss hospice care with patients and families.

Investigate Patient and Family Experience of Hospice Care

Questions:
- Do you have any experience with hospice care?
- Do you know anyone who received hospice care?

Start to **investigate** the patient and family **experience** of hospice care by asking the following questions,

- "Do you have any experience with hospice care?"
- "Do you know anyone who received hospice care?"

Many people will mention a family member or friend who received hospice care. Follow up by asking,

- "Can you tell me about that experience?"

When listening to patients and family members share their experiences with hospice care, listen for indications of whether their loved one received hospice care in their own home, whether they died in a hospital, or whether they passed away in a care facility, such as a nursing home or assisted living facility.

Many patients and family members will share positive experiences with hospice care, for example, "My mother had a lovely experience here at our hospice center. Everyone took such good care of her." or "I appreciated the amazing support the hospice nurse and team provided when I cared for my dad at home at the end of his life." Positive experiences, including the relief of suffering, the helpful support of caregivers, and the peaceful passing of patients at the end of life, tend to lend a helping hand in the conversation and should be noted. Patients and families may even name a specific agency or facility they would prefer to provide hospice care, providing an opportunity to continue their positive experience of this stage of life.

It is important to listen for indications that the experience with end-of-life care was unsettling, disturbing, overwhelming, poorly timed, or stressful to the family in any way. Learning the pain points for patients and families at the end of life provides an opportunity to explain hospice care in a way that settles fears and concerns by correcting misperceptions about hospice care, addressing missteps in the timing of the start of hospice care, and attending to misguided medical care.

Sadly, the medical community's lack of training in end-of-life care leads many patients and families to report on experiences of "hospice care" that were rife with undertreated or mismanaged symptoms, distressing hospitalizations, or even escalations of care that are antithetical to the fundamental philosophy of hospice care. Delivering high-quality, end-of-life care requires a rich understanding that the purpose of hospice care is to enable patients to experience a soft landing at the end of life while avoiding unwanted escalations of care. This is accomplished by teams with special training and experience in the use of medications that are often used in creative and innovative ways to treat symptoms that can change or escalate quickly and by staff with the skills and availability to usher patients and families through spiritual and bereavement-related distress delicately. Teams with untrained, inexperienced, and inadequate staff can easily mismanage patients at this point in life. Hospitals, home care agencies, care facilities, and primary care providers without extensive experience and expertise in providing high-quality, comfort-focused hospice care put patients and families at risk of negative and misleading experiences with end-of-life care.

For example, many nursing facilities offer "end-of-life care" or "comfort care" programs that are represented to patients and families as the equivalent of hospice care. Despite telling families that their loved ones are on "hospice care," however, many facilities make no real change to patient care, do not provide clinical staff experienced with the unique needs of patients at the end of life, and do not provide social work, chaplain, or bereavement support to patients and families. Many of these facilities continue to bill Medicare for general medical care rather than engaging the Medicare Hospice Election, which provides a per diem reimbursement payment to cover end-of-life care.

Misleading patients and families about the care they are receiving and not adequately equipped to provide high-quality, comfort-focused care, these facilities frequently send patients back to the hospital whenever symptoms outpace the ability of their staff and providers to manage competently. Unaware that hospice care is the mechanism that enables patients to avoid such escalations of care at a time when such escalations are otherwise expected to occur, patients on these "end-of-life care" programs continue to experience healthcare system utilization that is entirely inconsistent with the philosophy of hospice care. Moreover, the spiritual and emotional lives of the patients and families are often neglected at a time when these dimensions can easily contribute to patient and family suffering.

Unfortunately, institutions that support patients in this way poorly represent hospice care, mislead the public, and frequently leave patients and families with negative experiences of, and a bad taste for, hospice care. It is critical to know whether patients and families have been affected by such mislabeled "hospice care" and to appropriately refer to hospice care teams and facilities that genuinely understand the requirements and purpose of hospice care.

Investigate Patient and Family Understanding of Hospice Care

Questions:
- Have you ever heard of hospice care?
- Can you tell me what the word 'hospice' means to you?

Depending on the flow of the conversation, it sometimes makes better sense to ease into the Hospice Care Arc by **investigating** patients' and families' **understanding** of hospice care before asking about their experiences with hospice care. This can be accomplished by asking two simple questions that allow people to summarize their conception of hospice care.

First, ask,

- "Have you ever heard of hospice care?"

Although rare, some patients and families have not heard the word "hospice" before, which is important to know. Patients and families who have not heard of hospice previously may have no preformed conceptions of end-of-life care, which can be beneficial, leaving them open-minded to learning about this treatment option without negative perceptions. At the same time, not having heard of hospice before can be unsettling to patients and families, who might be suspicious of the suggestion of a shift from conceiving of medicine as a tool for curing illness to one that treats symptoms while not attempting to cure or forestall disease. These patients and families frequently require additional time to contemplate and decide about hospice care.

For those who have heard of hospice care, next ask,

- "Can you tell me what the word 'hospice' means to you?"

Answers to this question vary and can reflect an understanding of the treatment approach, location of care, or the expected timeframe to death.

Commenting on treatment approach, answers may run the gamut, from "Hospice is a way of keeping people comfortable when they're dying" to "They stop your medications, so you die," or even, "They use morphine to help you pass." The last two comments reflect common hospice misconceptions that should be noted for gentle correction later in the conversation. (See Chap. 17 for template language for addressing common hospice misconceptions.)

Commenting on the location of care, patients and families will often respond by saying, "Hospice is a place you go to die," conveying the assumption that the patient must leave their home to receive end-of-life care at a hospice facility. Many patients will initially be offended by the mere mention of hospice care simply because they prefer to remain at home. This, too, is a common misconception that should be gently corrected later in the conversation. Fortunately, many patients and families will have experience with a family member or friend who passed away at home with the support of hospice care, providing them special insight for their decision making.

Finally, commenting on the expected timeframe to death, many people will share a belief that hospice care means the patient is expected to die relatively soon, saying something like, "Hospice is for people who are just about to die." It can be helpful to follow up this type of reply with the question,

- "When you think of hospice care, what kind of timeframe do you generally think of a person having?"

This question can reveal yet another misconception about hospice care. Many people will answer this question with a timeframe reflecting the medical community's unfortunate record for referring patients to hospice care when patients have precious little time remaining, "A couple of weeks or less." A compassionate response to this and other common hospice misconceptions is presented in Chap. 17.

Often, I will pose the question of what the word "hospice" means to a patient or family member somewhat differently, to target the emotional weight of the word, by asking,

- "Can you tell me what comes up for you—how you feel inside—when you hear the word 'hospice'?"

This question allows people to reflect internally on the emotional toll that facing the question of hospice care demands. Responses often convey the emotional impact of this consideration, such as, "I thought I would have more time," "I'm not ready to go," "I never thought this point would arrive," "I'm sad that I'll never get to meet my grandchildren or watch them grow up and get married," or "I can't just give up!" Share in the patient's emotional burden by validating and soothing their sorrow, offering, "I'm so sorry," "This must be very difficult," or a tissue for their tears.

Educate Patient and Family About Hospice Care

The next objective is to **educate** the patient and family about hospice philosophy, approach to care, location, and cost and correct common misconceptions. (Chapter 17 provides a primer on these topics and template language to use with patients and families).

While providing education about hospice philosophy, approach to care, location, and cost, address patient and family concerns, fears, and misperceptions by gently referencing their comments and articulating how hospice care differs from their assumptions. Patients and families will appreciate kind and compassionate education, particularly when the correct information alleviates their fears and concerns.

For example, many people assume that hospice care is available for just the last week or two of life. A compassionate approach to correcting this misperception is to share,

- "Actually, the hospice benefit through Medicare was built to give people at least six months of comfort and quality of life at the end of life, but there is no absolute time limit for staying on hospice care. Patients who live longer than six months can continue to receive hospice care as long as they continue to qualify for hospice care by continuing to show some observable decline, with worsening symptoms, progression of disease, weight loss, increasing fatigue, etc. Continuing to qualify for hospice care is typically not an issue for patients."

Refer to Chap. 17 for template language to use when providing education about hospice care to patients and families. After providing this education, it is appropriate to pause, allowing patients and families to process what they've just heard and ask any questions. Check in by saying,

- "'I know that was a lot of information. How are you feeling about what we just discussed?' and 'Do you have any questions for me?'"

It is important to be patient as patients and family members consider a decision about hospice care, recognizing that a choice to transition to hospice care often entails a reimagining of their lives and an acceptance of a new reality, one that is often sad and disappointing to both patients and family members.

Patients and families often indicate their willingness to transition to hospice care by saying, "That sounds like what we want," or asking, "How do we get started?" Others may start troubleshooting the logistics of hospice care at home, for instance, trying to determine where the patient's hospital bed should go in the house.

It is okay to ask patients and family members directly,

- "Do you think you are ready to start hospice care?"

Direct but gentle communication allows patients and families to ponder and answer this important question. Those who appear to be struggling with the question should be provided with the reassurance that,

- "There is no right answer, only the answer that is right for you and your family. There is also no urgency or pressure to make this decision. Take all the time you need."

Sometimes, patients and families will ask for your guidance, such as, "What do you think would be best?" or "What do you think we should do?" The appropriate response would be to suggest the medical option that best aligns with the patient's and family's needs, wishes, and values. Those who have articulated their hospice mindedness, a desire to be at home or in a place where they can focus on comfort and quality of life, and who wish to avoid future hospitalizations should be reassured that hospice care is the treatment option that would meet these needs. Allowing patients to "see" how hospice care can meet their expressed needs is excellent patient-centered care.

For instance, explaining that,

- "You mentioned earlier that you are at the point where you would prefer not to return to the hospital for care, that you want to stay home and experience time with your friends and family. Because your heart failure is so advanced, you run the risk of experiencing symptoms that can change quickly, which could lead to a great deal of discomfort. You also mentioned worrying about your wife's ability to care for you at home."
- "Hospice care would help with both concerns because should you have a crisis or rapid escalation in symptoms, your wife would have the extra support she needs to help keep you comfortable. She will be backed up by the hospice team's support 24/7 and can call anytime, day or night, with questions or concerns. The hospice will triage the call and try to help out over the phone, but, if need be, will send a nurse to the house to help get things situated, no matter what time of day or night. Additionally, because the hospice nurse will be visiting weekly, and more frequently if needed, they can often prevent a worsening of symptoms by treating changing symptoms before they reach a crisis level, allowing you to experience a smoother journey with more comfort."

Patients and families appreciate the help in understanding how hospice care can support their comfort and achieve their priorities at the end of life.

Next Steps

Help Patients Transition to Hospice Care

Patients and families ready to transition to hospice care should next be informed about the process for this transition. Excellent customer service at this point in a patient's journey relieves the patient and family from worrying about anything other than preparing their home to receive the patient in hospice care, for example, preparing the room for the hospital bed delivery. The medical team should handle everything else, allowing the patient and family to focus on their time together.

Transition to hospice care typically involves a selection of the hospice team the patient and family prefer to work with, followed by communication with the selected hospice team that the patient is ready and willing to start hospice care, after which point the hospice team will communicate with the patient's family to schedule an appointment for enrollment.

Patients who are hospitalized and will be transitioning to hospice care at their place of residence[1] should not be discharged until the hospice care team can arrange to meet the patient there, minimizing the time that patients and families are without the support of hospice care. Hospital providers in haste to discharge patients should be aware of the high risk of a quick return to the hospital for patients who meet hospice criteria but who do not yet have the support of hospice care at home, particularly those with moderate to severe symptom burden.

To provide a smooth and timely transition to hospice care, providers must know the names of the local hospice care agencies and establish a prompt means of communicating a patient's readiness for hospice care enrollment. Delays in the start of hospice care risk escalations of care and non-beneficial or unwanted medical treatment, not to mention further distress to patients and families.

Help Patients Determine Their Threshold for Transitioning to Hospice Care

Patients who are not yet ready to transition to hospice care should be encouraged to think about their threshold for enrolling in hospice care. This is time well spent and essential to providing patient-centered, collaborative care.

Unfortunately, many patients who meet hospice criteria but who are not yet ready to transition to hospice care pick up on the not-so-subtle messaging that the healthcare system is "pushing them" into hospice care, making them feel frustrated, angry, and resentful of a medical system that appears to be "giving up" on them. Providers with limited options to "cure" advanced disease can readily communicate their frustration to patients. This is inappropriate and reflects poor training in patient-centered communication and collaborative care. Instead, the goal should be to arrive at a treatment plan that appropriately aligns the patient's wishes and values with the options for care appropriate to the patient's stage of disease.

A patient feeling "pushed" toward hospice care may share their experience that, "Everyone is telling me I should go on hospice care," or "I feel like I'm being forced into choosing hospice care." This is not the experience patients should have at the end of life. Damage control requires apologizing for the patient and family's experience and providing reassurance that a decision about hospice care is the patient's to make, not the medical community's.

For instance, it would be appropriate to say in this situation,

- "I'm so sorry that has been your experience. That is not what we want for you. A decision about hospice care is a very personal decision and one that only

---

[1] Hospice care can be delivered anywhere a patient lives, including at residential care facilities, such as independent living residences, assisted living homes, or skilled nursing and memory care facilities.

you and your family can make. There is no right answer, only the answer that is right for you. Our job is to learn your wishes and, to the extent that we can, help align your medical wishes with your care. That is why we need to ask what you want, but ultimately, a decision about hospice care is yours to make."

For patients who meet hospice criteria but who are not yet ready to transition to hospice care, it would be appropriate to suggest,

- "It might be a good idea for us to have a conversation about what your threshold would be for starting hospice care. That way, we can monitor any changes and revisit the conversation as needed in the future."

Provide the patient the opportunity to specify their threshold for starting hospice care by asking,

- "When do you think you might be ready to transition to hospice care?"

Patients with an appropriate understanding of their disease, its expected decline, and the possibility of escalations of care and who understand the kind of support that hospice care can provide will often answer this question with some consideration. For example, a patient with frailty who met hospice criteria, who experienced frequent UTIs that were mostly managed at home but who occasionally required treatment in the hospital, was able to articulate a threshold for hospice care at a time when hospitalizations became too frequent or exhausting, or no longer provided comfort and support. Another patient, with metastatic colon cancer and abdominal ascites that required routine paracentesis but who still enjoyed swimming and using the hot tub, was able to articulate a desire to wait until they no longer had the energy to swim to have an abdominal drain placed and to enroll in hospice care.

These examples illustrate the reality that respect for patient autonomy at the end of life requires that patients have an accurate understanding of disease, where they are in their journey, what is expected ahead, and the purpose and approach to hospice care.

Supporting Patients Who Meet Hospice Criteria but Who Are Not Ready to Transition to Hospice Care

Some patients and family members, when asked if they are ready to transition to hospice care, may circle back to questions about symptoms, disease progression, and treatment options, and their facial expressions may communicate fear or weighty concern. After addressing their concerns and answering any questions, it is okay to ask again whether they are ready to transition to hospice care. For those who express hesitation or unwillingness to make a transition to hospice care, provide reassurance that,

- "That is perfectly okay. There is no urgency to decide on hospice care, and there is also no pressure to choose one path over the other. There is no right answer, only the answer that is right for you. It's okay to take whatever time you need to make this decision; only you will know when you are ready to make that decision. We can revisit this question in the future. Does that sound okay?"

Patients who are not ready to transition to hospice care but who meet hospice criteria are at significant risk of rapidly evolving symptoms, ER visits or hospitalizations, and escalations of care. These patients should be supported by palliative (supportive) care, which can closely monitor symptom and disease progression and compassionately reengage patients in conversations about medical preferences as circumstances evolve. For template language to use when discussing palliative (supportive) care with patients and families, see Chap. 11.

Regardless of a patient's decision about hospice care, it is important to compassionately, kindly, and gently usher patients with chronic, terminal, or advanced disease through the Arc of Conversation to learn and support their wishes and values. Patient-centered care that appropriately respects patient autonomy requires skillful, effective, compassionate, and collaborative communication.

Part IV

Aligning Patient Wishes with Care

Aligning Patient Wishes with Care: The Goal of Patient-Centered Care

13

Recall John, the first patient we met in Chaps. 2 and 3, who lay in his hospital bed following a bout of aspiration pneumonia at the end of his decade-long dementia journey. His son, busy installing an expensive walk-in bathtub that his father would never use, had no idea that his father had dementia, let alone how little time his father had left. Neither did the hospitalist caring for John, who, in failing to inquire about John's at-home need for assistance, missed both the patient's dementia and the fact that his disease had reached end stage.

Working from a place of ignorance, the hospitalist had failed to offer hospice care to John's son, instead narrowly focusing on treating John's pneumonia with the goal of discharging him to a rehabilitation facility. John's son, left in the dark about how little time his father had left, was unprepared and confused by the sudden change in course when the subject of hospice care was finally introduced.

For John and his son, both the proverbial forest and the elephant had been ignored, leading to treatment recommendations that were inappropriate given the advanced nature of John's disease. Sadly, John's story is not unique.

Recall that Medicare spends a significant portion of its annual expenditure on patients in the last year of life, a statistic that reflects a medical community that is busy swimming upstream against the inevitability of patient death, ignoring disease progression and terminal decline and offering treatment options at a time in patients' lives when those treatments are often nonbeneficial.

Ignoring the forest and the elephant impacts people's lives. A colleague of mine learned that her father was sick with heart failure but didn't have an accurate evaluation of his disease. She left her job, sold her house, and moved across the country to care for him, only to witness her father die a month after her arrival. She realizes now that her father had likely met hospice criteria for many months, and she laments her ignorance of that critical piece of information. Had she known, she would have visited her father more frequently during that year, and instead of altering her life so dramatically before he died, she would have taken leave from her job to stay with him in his final months.

Patients and families deserve better.

A. Shaw, PA, *The Arc of Conversation*,
https://doi.org/10.1007/978-3-031-70495-6_13

They deserve accurate and timely information delivered by providers trained to discuss delicate news gently and compassionately. They deserve a medical system that acknowledges that death is not the surprise ending at the end of a human life, but rather a moment with potential for deep spiritual and family connection, a milestone of life worthy of our outstanding experience and expertise. Patients and families deserve a medical system that honors and embraces every moment of human life, especially the end.

The healthcare system must shift from a narrow focus on acute stabilization—both in the hospital and the clinic—to a holistic approach that considers the patient's overall medical trajectory. Identifying the disease driving a patient's decline and assessing where a patient is in their disease trajectory must become a priority for every provider for every seriously ill patient. At the same time, the medical system must come to terms with the fact that every patient is eventually going to die. That death is inevitable despite our best medical efforts and scientific advances must be a guiding principle in the era of patient-centered medical care.

The disease as journey metaphor is an excellent framework to support this new medical paradigm. Just as you wouldn't drive away from your house without knowing your destination, we should not practice medicine without keeping the ultimate end goal for patients in mind. Eventually, most patients will prioritize a focus on quality of life over a desire for increased longevity at any cost, with most patients preferring to pass away at home, surrounded by their family, friends, and pets. Every provider should be taught how to compassionately lead patients and families through this final leg of their journey.

Although there are ugly sides to the reality that medicine is a business, with its bottom lines and increasing pressure on providers to see more patients on any given day, the truth is that medicine is always an act of customer service. Medicine is about providing care that adds to people's experience and quality of life. Because patient choice reflects a complex system of cultural, spiritual, medical, and personal values, there truly is no right answer, only the answer that is right for each patient and their family.

To respect patient autonomy—to enable patients to arrive at a place where they can determine what is right for them, particularly at the end of life—we must learn to assess disease progression and decline accurately, and we must learn to usher patients and families gently and compassionately through collaborative conversations.

By incorporating the material and techniques taught in *The Arc of Conversation* into everyday practice, providers can better guide patients and families to a point where medical decisions arise authentically from a place of accurate understanding of health status. To empower patients and families, particularly at the end of life, to make choices that are right for them is the ultimate goal of patient-centered care.

Part V
Supplemental Materials

The Arc of Conversation Guide

14

The following table provides a quick reference of the questions to ask and educational tasks to complete during each of the four conversational arcs. It can be copied to use as a road map when practicing the technique with patients and families (Table 14.1).

Table 14.1 The Arc of Conversation guide

	Investigation		Education
	Experience	Understanding	
Illness Arc	• Can you paint a picture of how things have been going?	• How are you making sense of the changes you just described? • Do you know what diagnosis is responsible for these changes?	No education—patients and families are the experts in their own personal experience of illness
Disease Arc	• Have you seen anyone go through the [diagnosis] journey?	• Can you tell me what you understand about your [diagnosis] journey? • Where do you think you are in your overall journey with your health? • What are you expecting ahead?	• Introduce the disease trajectories, including the trajectory the patient is following • Explain where the patient is in their journey • Explain what is ahead • Explain that the patient meets hospice criteria

(continued)

© The Author(s), under exclusive license to Springer Nature Switzerland AG 2024
A. Shaw, PA, *The Arc of Conversation*,
https://doi.org/10.1007/978-3-031-70495-6_14

Table 14.1 (continued)

	Investigation		Education
	Experience	Understanding	

End-of-Life Wishes Arc	***Wishes for End-of-Life Experience***
	• Given what we've just discussed and what you can expect with your disease going forward, what are you hoping for in the time you have left?
	• Where would you like to be at the end of your life?
	• What would a good death be like for you?
	Hospice Mindedness
	• Are you at the point in your journey where you are ready to allow nature to take its course?
	• How do you feel about returning to the hospital for care?
	• Are you at the point in your journey where you are ready to focus on quality of life and comfort?
	Advance Directive and Code Status Wishes
	• Surrogate medical decision maker
	• Advance directive or living will
	• POLST:
	  – Code status
	  – Approach to medical care
	  – Artificial nutrition by tube
			Using the **investigate-then-educate** technique, educate the patient and family about:
			• Any topic for which the patient or family has a question or concern
			Advance directive and code status considerations

	Next Steps: Offer a palliative (supportive) care referral when appropriate		
Hospice Care Arc	• Do you have any experience with hospice care? • Do you know anyone who received hospice care?	• Have you ever heard of hospice? • Can you tell me what the word "hospice" means to you?	• Explain hospice care facts (correcting any misconceptions) • Explain hospice philosophy • Explain approach to hospice care • Explain location options and cost of hospice care
	Next Steps: • Help transition patient and families to hospice care, or • Help patients determine their threshold for transitioning to hospice care		

Disease Trajectory Education for Patients and Families

15

Objectives When Providing Disease Trajectory Education to Patients and Families

- Introduce the idea of the disease trajectory.
- Provide a brief description of each disease trajectory.
- Provide both a brief and detailed description of the disease trajectory the patient is following.
- Explain that terminal disease eventually progresses to the point of meeting hospice criteria.
- Explain what it means to meet hospice criteria.
- Describe the hospice criteria for the disease trajectory driving patient decline.
- Connect the patient's history to the trajectory driving patient decline (See Chap. 10 for examples of how to accomplish this important task).

All the text in this chapter is sample language that can be adopted for use in conversations with patients and families.

Introduce the Idea of the Disease Trajectory

We know what it looks like as patients approach the end of their lives. It might be surprising to learn that in the United States, patients die from a limited set of diagnoses, and that these diseases can be organized into just five general patterns of decline. Most of us will follow just one of three patterns at the end of our lives.

As I describe these patterns, think about the stories of people you have known or heard about who have passed away. You will likely recognize each of the patterns that I describe in their stories.

Provide an Overview of Each Disease Trajectory

Sudden Death

Some patients will die suddenly, following a major acute medical issue or accident, such as a massive heart attack, car accident, or other trauma. These patients are alive, and then they suddenly aren't, which can be very traumatic for loved ones left behind.

Catastrophic Event

Brief Description

Discuss If the Patient Is Not Following this Trajectory

Others will pass away following some type of catastrophic event, such as a heart attack, stroke, or traumatic accident, in which the medical community saves their lives, but often leaves them at a greatly diminished capacity to live on their own. Sometimes, the person is dependent on medical technology to live, for instance, a breathing machine or feeding tube, with limited quality of life. Family is then often faced with the decision to withdraw treatment, after which the patient typically passes away in the intensive care unit or ICU.

Provide an Example, Such as the Following

My uncle suffered a traumatic road bicycle accident. Nobody knows exactly what happened, but tourists found him down on the ground in the state park where he'd been riding. They called 911, and he was taken by ambulance to the emergency room and then promptly life-flighted to a trauma hospital, where he was rushed to the operating room. He underwent emergency surgery to remove a portion of his skull to relieve the pressure on his brain from the bleeding, but although the doctors saved his life, he needed a feeding tube and mechanical ventilation to remain alive. After several days, the team reduced his sedation to see whether his brainstem was healthy enough to allow him to breathe on his own, but they found that it was too damaged from the trauma. My aunt and her children then made the very difficult decision to withdraw treatment for him in the ICU, and he passed away several hours later.

In the United States, most patients follow one of the three remaining patterns of decline at the end of their lives.

Extended Description

Coma: Discuss If the Patient Is Expected to Pass Away from Brain Death

The brain is the most important organ in the human body. It controls everything about us, from the way we walk and talk to how we learn and solve problems to how we heal. It also controls the other organs in the body.

The brain is organized into three major regions. The largest part is called the cerebrum, and its outer shell is called the cortex, or "gray matter." The cortex is the processing center of the human brain and gives us the ability to think, walk, talk, ride a bike, pay bills, see, hear, relate to other human beings, and experience emotions like love and sadness. The large area of the cerebrum under the cortex, the "white matter," is made up of nerve tracks that connect different parts of the brain.

The cerebellum, sometimes called the "little brain," coordinates movement and balance and is located at the back of the brain. The brainstem, which leads from the cerebrum down through the skull to the spinal cord, controls many of the body's life-preserving functions, including breathing, heart rate, swallowing, coughing, and vomiting.

Responsiveness and arousal exist on a continuum that ranges from a fully intact and normally functioning healthy brain to a brain that has experienced "brain death"—the complete and irreversible loss of brain function. At the healthy extreme, among other things, patients can respond to conversations, follow commands, breathe independently, swallow normally, and exhibit a healthy arousal system with a sleep-wake cycle easily disturbed by painful or bothersome stimuli, such as when we gently pinch a person's skin or speak loudly in their presence. At the other end of the continuum, brain death represents the absence of these functions due to widespread damage to the brainstem, cerebellum, and cerebrum, particularly the cerebral cortex. Between these two endpoints exists a range of disordered expressions of consciousness and responsiveness, including concussion, dementia, delirium, minimally responsive state, persistent vegetative state, and coma. These reflect the wide variation and severity of brain injury.

We evaluate a patient's consciousness using a clinical scale called the Glasgow Coma Scale or GCS, which assesses brainstem, cerebellum, and cortical function by evaluating eye-opening and verbal and motor responses to stimuli (pain, sound, and command). We use this scale in the emergency room and afterward to monitor a patient's response to treatment. Patients are given a score between 3 (low) and 15 (high), with 3 representing the absence of all responses and 15 representing a patient with no deficits. Scores in the range of 3–8 signify severe head injury with profoundly impaired consciousness. These patients typically require intubation (a tube that keeps their airway open) and mechanical ventilation (a machine to breathe for them). Scores of less than 5 are associated with an 80% risk of death or remaining in a persistent vegetative state.

Brain death can result from any number of physical or metabolic causes, including heart attack, seizure, stroke, hemorrhage, infection, trauma, tumor, or experiencing time without oxygen. Brain cells are very sensitive to a reduction in blood flow and are unable to tolerate even a short time without oxygen. Within several seconds of a lack of oxygen, brain cell activity becomes impaired, and patients quickly lose consciousness.

Brain death is the irreversible loss of brain function in which blood flow is absent, and the cells are no longer functioning. Patients remain unconscious, show no brainstem reflexes, are unable to breathe on their own, and do not follow commands, verbalize, or respond to pain or sound. A diagnosis of brain death is determined by hospital policy which usually includes a neurologic exam that reveals an absence of voluntary movement, purposeful motor response to deep painful and verbal stimuli, and all brainstem reflexes. These include the pupil response to light, cough and gag reflexes, and the very important respiratory reflex, which allows us to breathe on our own. To evaluate whether patients can breathe on their own, they are temporarily removed from ventilator support to see whether their brainstem can spontaneously resume breathing control.

Brain death is different from coma. A coma is not a specific diagnosis. Rather, it is an umbrella term for cerebral, cortical, and brainstem dysfunction in which the patient remains unconscious and doesn't show willful verbal or motor response but can show abnormal brainstem reflexes and may be able to breathe on their own. Brain metabolism is usually reduced in a coma, and brain activity, evaluated with an EEG or electroencephalogram, is usually abnormal. Comas typically resolve in one way or another within two to four weeks, as patients either improve—moving into a vegetative state, minimally unconscious state, or recovering more fully—or deteriorate further, with many going on to a diagnosis of brain death.

Coma is not a cause of the unconscious state. In your loved one's case, the coma was caused by X. *(Provide a description of the medical situation leading to the coma.)*

As stated earlier, the brainstem controls the body's important automatic and life-preserving reflexes for heartbeat, breathing, coughing, vomiting, and swallowing. The swallow reflex is critical in protecting our lungs. When we swallow, a little flap of skin called the epiglottis moves over the airway to protect our lungs from aspirating or inhaling food or liquid. Patients unable to eat on their own in a coma are provided with nutrition by a feeding tube. It is important to understand that the liquid food from the feeding tube delivered to the gut, which is continuous with the throat, can regurgitate up the esophagus into the back of the throat and then down into the lungs, causing aspiration pneumonia. In fact, in patients with swallowing dysfunction, aspiration pneumonia is the most common side effect of a feeding tube and a common cause of death. This is something that is likely to continue to occur and that cannot be prevented. *(Certainly, if this has happened to the patient, it is important to point out that this is likely to continue and cannot be prevented.)* Patients unable to coordinate the swallow of food or liquid will also have issues with the saliva that builds up in the mouth and can develop aspiration pneumonia from that as well.

Patients who experience a coma and recover to a minimally conscious or persistent vegetative state can be supported with a feeding tube or mechanical ventilation. Over time, these patients may show signs of metabolic decline. The metabolism is the body's energy system, a constant balance of building and breaking down tissue. Across the lifespan, the metabolism shifts a couple of times. From the time we are born until a bit past our adolescence, we're building more tissue than we're breaking down; we're growing. As adults, we roughly maintain about the same, keeping a steady balance between building and breaking down tissue. And at the end of life, regardless of what disease trajectory we might follow, our metabolism shifts again as we start breaking down more tissue than we're building. This is an expected part of the end of every terminal disease we follow as we approach the end of life, including organ failure, cancer, age-related decline, and dementia. Patients with brain injury supported by feeding tubes and breathing machines can also start to exhibit metabolic decline as they approach the end of life.

When the metabolism shifts toward the end of life, the body is not as efficient at translating the products of its nutrition into the body components—muscle, bone, skin, blood vessel walls, parts of the immune system, etc. Organs and systems function less effectively, and as a patient's metabolism declines, we will see a constellation of related physical symptoms, including weight loss, loss of muscle mass, recurrent infections, and wounds that have a difficult time healing.

Patients who have lost 5% to 10% of their total body weight in a short amount of time—6 to 12 months—in a situation where they have appropriate nutritional support, can be said to have moved into a state of frailty, or cachexia. This is clinically significant, dramatically increasing their risk of passing away in subsequent months.

If the body has made the metabolic shift, the medical community has not found any treatment to successfully reverse that trend. At that point, in patients who are able to eat on their own, even forcing nutrition on the body, such as with a feeding tube, cannot make the body translate the nutrition it receives into new muscle, bone, and skin. Moreover, feeding tubes that introduce liquid food into a patient's body experiencing end-stage decline can overwhelm the heart and kidneys, whose job is maintaining the appropriate fluid balance. *(If this is starting to happen with the patient, connect this information with their medical experience.)* This extra fluid can build up in the legs, causing swelling, weeping skin, and infections. As explained earlier, feeding tubes can also lead to aspiration pneumonia if the fluid regurgitates up the esophagus into the back of the throat and passes down the windpipe into the lungs.

Just like we have criteria to diagnose and stage disease, we also have criteria to evaluate when a patient gets to the point when their condition is beyond the medical community's ability to provide support other than to manage symptoms. At that point, the patient is said to meet what we call "hospice criteria," and we worry that their time is limited. Patients with a coma meet hospice criteria after three days in a coma if they exhibit any three of the following: abnormal brainstem responses, no verbalization, no response to pain, and a serum creatinine level higher than 1.5, which indicates that their kidneys have been injured. Kidney injury in the setting of traumatic brain injury often occurs early and is a sign of poor prognosis; when the kidneys cannot filter toxins, toxins build up and damage the organs.

When a patient meets hospice criteria, any subsequent insult, injury, or infection could be too much for their body to recover from. *(For patients not supported with mechanical ventilation, add the following.)* At that point, if their lungs fail, such as in the setting of pneumonia, they are much more likely to require invasive procedures to support their life, such as intubation and mechanical ventilation, from which they may not recover. Families who would like their loved one to experience a soft landing and pass peacefully without distressing symptoms will need to choose to transition the patient to hospice care before their condition becomes so advanced.

Stroke: Discuss If the Patient Is Expected to Pass Following a Stroke or If a Stroke Is Contributing to Overall Patient Decline

Having a stroke is like having a heart attack in your brain. Strokes are most commonly caused by the same process that leads to a heart attack, called atherosclerosis, in which cholesterol plaque blocks the blood flow of an artery supplying oxygen to the brain. This type of stroke is called an "ischemic" stroke; the word ischemia means damage due to a lack of oxygen.

A stroke can also be caused by a blood clot that cuts off the blood supply to brain tissue; this is called a "thrombotic" stroke. Patients can also experience a stroke following a hemorrhage, in which a blood vessel ruptures and blood leaks into the area surrounding the brain instead of flowing appropriately to the healthy brain tissue. This is called a "hemorrhagic" or "bleeding" stroke. Because there is a limited amount of space inside the skull, the extra blood volume from a hemorrhage can put pressure on the brain tissue, leading to a herniation, in which brain tissue shifts due to the pressure from the bleed. This shift can damage any area of the brain, but the brainstem is particularly at risk of damage due to herniation downward through the opening where the brainstem leaves the skull and becomes the spinal cord.

Brain cells are very sensitive to a reduction in blood flow and are unable to tolerate even a short time without oxygen. Within several seconds of a lack of oxygen, brain cell activity becomes impaired, and patients quickly lose consciousness.

The brain is organized into three major regions. The largest part is called the cerebrum, and its outer shell is called the cortex, or "gray matter." The cortex is the processing center of the human brain and gives us the ability to think, walk, talk, ride a bike, pay bills, see, hear, relate to other human beings, and experience emotions like love and sadness. The large area of the cerebrum under the cortex, the "white matter," is made up of nerve tracks that connect different parts of the brain. The cerebrum also contains areas called "ventricles," in which the cerebrospinal fluid is found.

The cerebellum, sometimes called the "little brain," coordinates movement and balance and is located at the back of the brain. The brainstem, which leads from the cerebrum down through the skull to the spinal cord, controls many of the body's life-preserving functions, including breathing, heart rate, swallowing, coughing, and vomiting. Three protective membranes surround the brain and spinal cord; hemorrhages can occur between any of these layers.

Ischemic and thrombotic strokes that affect the front part of the cortex and subcortical regions, both sides of the brain, or the brainstem, carry a very poor prognosis. Hemorrhagic strokes that are large in volume, extend into the ventricles, cover 30% or more of the cerebrum, shift the brain more than 1.5 cm across the midline, or block the cerebrospinal fluid from leaving the brain, which can result in a dangerous buildup of the cerebrospinal fluid, also carry a very poor prognosis.

Following a stroke, patients can experience a profound functional and nutritional decline. For patients with an intact arousal system who can follow commands and breathe independently, a swallow study will be completed to evaluate their ability to swallow safely without aspiration. Patients unable to swallow safely will first be offered a nasogastric feeding tube, which will be inserted through the nose and into the stomach to provide nutrition. This also protects their lungs from aspirating during a time of recovery when the patient will work with speech and language therapy to hopefully recover their swallow function.

A nasogastric feeding tube can be left in place for only a short time, typically no longer than four to six weeks, because it can erode the inside of the nasal passage. After this time, patients unable to swallow safely on their own will be offered a permanent feeding tube, which will be inserted surgically into the abdomen.

It is important to consider what it is like for a patient to experience a permanent feeding tube if they are not able to swallow safely after a stroke. If the patient can't swallow safely enough to eat or drink by mouth, they also cannot swallow their saliva safely. Saliva continually builds up in the mouth, collecting at the back of the throat, and not only can this saliva leak down into their lungs, causing aspiration pneumonia, but the build-up of saliva in the back of the throat can cause patients to feel incredible anxiety and panic from the sensation that they are suffocating. A stroke also often damages the diaphragm and chest muscles and reduces the strength of the patient's cough, which can also impact their ability to clear saliva from the back of their throat.

Also, consider what happens when we introduce liquid food into the gut of a patient whose swallow function isn't reliable. If that patient were to lean over at just the right time, or if the patient is lying down and some of the liquid food regurgitates up the esophagus into the back of the mouth, in a throat that cannot swallow properly, that liquid can very easily leak down the trachea, or windpipe, into the right lung, leading to aspiration pneumonia. Aspiration pneumonia is the most common side effect of a feeding tube and the most common cause of death for patients with a feeding tube. Developing aspiration pneumonia leads to hospitalizations, and if pneumonia leads to respiratory failure, the patient may need to be supported with intubation and mechanical ventilation in the ICU.

Many patients will make a full to partial recovery following a stroke, but many will not. Of those who survive a stroke and go on to make a partial recovery, many will go on to pass in the following weeks, months, or years. Stroke is currently the fifth leading cause of death in the United States.

Just like we have criteria to diagnose and stage disease, we also have criteria to evaluate when a patient gets to the point when their condition is beyond the medical community's ability to provide support other than to manage symptoms. At that point, the patient is said to meet what we call "hospice criteria," and we worry that their time is limited. Patients with any type of stroke meet hospice criteria if they are bedbound, unable to walk on their own, need assistance with most aspects of daily living, decline or discontinue a feeding tube, or show signs of clinically significant metabolic decline.

Following a stroke, patients who remain bedbound, are unable to walk, and need assistance with most aspects of daily living, likely suffered a significant stroke that dramatically impacted their quality of life. However, some patients will recover to a certain point but will go on to experience physical, functional, and metabolic decline.

The metabolism is the body's energy system, a constant balance of building and breaking down tissue. Across the lifespan, the metabolism shifts a couple of times. From the time we are born until a bit past our adolescence, we're building more tissue than we're breaking down; we're growing. As adults, we roughly maintain about the same, keeping a steady balance between building and breaking down tissue. And at the end of life, regardless of what disease trajectory we might follow, our metabolism shifts again as we start breaking down more tissue than we're building. This is an expected part of the end of every terminal disease we follow as we approach the end of life, including organ failure, cancer, age-related decline, and dementia. Following a stroke, patients can also start to exhibit metabolic decline as they approach the end of life.

When the metabolism shifts toward the end of life, the body is not as efficient at translating the products of its nutrition into the body components—muscle, bone, skin, blood vessel walls, parts of the immune system, etc. Organs and systems function less effectively, and as a patient's metabolism declines, we will see a constellation of related physical symptoms, including weight loss, loss of muscle mass, recurrent infections, and wounds that have a difficult time healing.

Patients who have lost 5% to 10% of their total body weight in a short amount of time—6 to 12 months—in a situation where they have appropriate nutritional support, can be said to have moved into a state of frailty, or cachexia. This is clinically significant, dramatically increasing their risk of passing away in subsequent months.

If the body has made the metabolic shift, the medical community has not found any treatment to successfully reverse that trend. At that point, in patients who are able to eat on their own, even forcing nutrition on the body, such as with a feeding tube, cannot make the body translate the nutrition it receives into new muscle, bone, and skin. Moreover, feeding tubes that introduce liquid food into a patient's body experiencing end-stage decline can overwhelm the heart and kidneys, whose job is maintaining the appropriate fluid balance. This extra fluid can build up in the legs, causing swelling, weeping skin, and infections. As explained earlier, feeding tubes can also lead to aspiration pneumonia if the fluid regurgitates up the esophagus into the back of the throat and passes down the windpipe into the lungs.

When a patient meets hospice criteria, any subsequent insult, injury, or infection could be too much for their body to recover from. At that point, they are much more likely to require invasive procedures to support their life, such as intubation and mechanical ventilation, for example, if their lungs were to fail. Those wishing to pass away at home at the end of their lives will need to choose to transition to home hospice care before getting to the point that their disease is so advanced.

Organ Failure

Brief Description
Approximately 1 in 3 patients who pass away each year in the United States die of some type of organ failure, with heart and lung failure accounting for the majority of those deaths. In 2020, heart failure was the leading cause of death for patients in

the United States. Any of the major organs can fail, including the heart, lungs, liver, or kidneys.

Patients following the organ failure journey will experience progressive decline over a number of years, with worsening physical stamina, more limiting symptoms, and an increasing need for support to make it through the day. This decline is punctuated by acute (or sudden) periods of worsening symptoms when the organ struggles to do its job and keep itself in balance. During these episodes, which we call "exacerbations" or "flare-ups," symptoms often become severe enough that patients need to go to the hospital to be helped to feel better. Often, it is during one of these exacerbations that the patients' organ failure is initially diagnosed.

Exacerbations are an expected part of the organ failure journey. Eventually, patients with organ failure will get to a point in their journey where the next exacerbation and hospitalization may be the last time they leave their house.

Extended Description

Heart Failure: Discuss If the Patient Is Expected to Pass from Heart Failure or If Heart Failure Is Contributing to Overall Patient Decline

Like a house, the heart has rooms—upper chambers called "atria" and lower chambers called "ventricles." It has doors—the valves between the chambers—that keep the blood flowing in one direction and prevent it from flowing in reverse. It has an electrical system that creates the heartbeat, starting in a bundle of tissue in the upper right chamber called the "pacemaker," whose job is to create an electrical impulse 60 to 100 or more times a minute throughout our lives. That signal travels down the wall between the right and left sides of the heart to the bottom chambers, where it stimulates both ventricles to squeeze in a coordinated fashion. The heart also has a plumbing system made up of arteries that travel on the outside of the heart to supply the heart muscle with oxygen. Any of these systems can develop problems leading to failure of the heart pump to pump blood throughout the body, which is the heart's job.

The heart has two pumps: the right side of the heart pumps blood to the lungs, where it picks up oxygen, and back to the left side of the heart; the left side of the heart is the stronger pump, responsible for pumping blood to the brain, arms, and legs, and back again to the right side of the heart. The heart relaxes to fill with blood and then squeezes or "ejects" a portion of that blood forward with each heartbeat. The percentage of the blood pumped forward with each heartbeat is called the "ejection fraction" or EF. Healthy hearts pump 55% or more of the blood that fills the left ventricle forward with each squeeze.

When the heart pump fails, the ejection fraction declines, and fluid collects upstream. When the left side of the heart fails, blood builds up in the lungs, the right side of the heart, and in the limbs. When the right side of the heart fails, blood builds up primarily in the limbs. Excess blood increases the pressure in the blood vessels, causing water molecules to leak from the vessels into the surrounding tissue. This accumulation of fluid, called "edema" when it occurs in the limbs or lungs, can lead to uncomfortable swelling, weight gain, or shortness of breath. Extra fluid in the system, either in the blood vessels or in the heart itself, increases the effort of the heart to pump the excess blood against elevated pressure in the system, which can cause the heart pump to fail.

Water is very heavy, so a person's weight will increase noticeably and quickly if they begin to accumulate extra fluid in their body because of heart failure. They will often gain weight before they notice the fluid buildup in their legs or develop a cough or shortness of breath due to extra fluid in their lungs. This is why patients with heart failure are encouraged to monitor their weight daily. An increase in body weight of 3 to 5 pounds overnight or in just a couple of days is concerning and can indicate that a person is beginning to experience an exacerbation, in which the heart fails to pump effectively.

Diuretic medications are often required to eliminate the extra fluid. Patients are encouraged to contact their cardiologist if they notice a rapid increase in weight, and often, patients are instructed to increase their at-home diuretic medication to attempt to get rid of the excess fluid before it builds up to the point where they need to return to the hospital for care.

When a heart remains constantly in fluid overload, the extra fluid stretches the thin-walled upper chambers, and this stretching, called "remodeling," can become permanent. Remodeled atrial tissue is electrically excitable and often creates extra electrical impulses. When these impulses get transmitted down the electrical wiring system in the heart, they can frequently, erratically, trigger the ventricles to squeeze. As one squeeze interrupts the prior squeeze, forward blood flow is diminished. This erratic heartbeat, called "atrial fibrillation," can lead to symptoms of heart failure, including edema in the legs as well as chest pain and light-headedness as the heart and brain suffer from insufficient blood flow.

Heart valves can also develop problems, becoming too loose or too tight. If the upper chambers become remodeled or permanently stretched, the valves between the atria and the ventricles also become stretched. Think of a doorway that has been stretched, with the door remaining the same size. When the heart squeezes, the value is no longer the correct size to prevent the blood from flowing backward through the heart. Not all of the blood that should move forward or out of the heart does, and some of it moves in the wrong direction, contributing to the heart being overloaded with fluid and forming clots which can cause stroke.

Tightening of the valves can happen because of different processes called "stenosis" or "sclerosis." This typically affects the valves controlling blood flow out of the ventricles. Tightening of these valves can lead to extra fluid building up in the heart and upstream because the blood doesn't move out of the heart properly. Patients with stenosis or sclerosis often experience shortness of breath and chest pain and can even pass out if too little blood flows from the heart to the brain. Many patients with severe enough valve problems receive a new value during a surgical procedure.

When patients experience ongoing heart failure and chronic fluid overload, the excess fluid in the blood vessels of the lungs can lead to damage to those vessels. That excess fluid also increases the pressure against which the weaker right side of the heart must pump to move the blood through the lungs to the left side of the heart.

This condition is called "pulmonary hypertension," which means elevated blood pressure in the lungs. Forced to pump against higher pressure than it was designed for, the thin-walled muscle of the right side of the heart can also begin to fail.

Heart failure is often initially caused by a heart attack in which blood flow in the arteries supplying the heart muscle gets blocked by cholesterol plaque, damaging the heart muscle to the point that the heart fails to pump a normal amount of blood forward. Of course, a heart attack can be very painful or even fatal. Heart failure often recovers following heart catheterization, a procedure in which a thin metal tube called a "stent" is placed inside the artery to keep it open where the blockage occurred. Other patients may need open heart surgery, a procedure called "CABG," which stands for coronary artery bypass graft, in which veins from the legs are taken and sewn into the heart to replace the arteries that were blocked by plaque. Many patients can do very well for many years after these procedures. However, some patients experience permanent damage to their heart muscle following a heart attack, or slowly develop any number of problems in the heart, resulting in worsening heart failure over time.

Patients whose ejection fraction does not recover to a normal percentage are sometimes offered a device called an implantable cardioverter-defibrillator (ICD). The ICD monitors the heart's electrical signal and delivers a strong electrical impulse if it detects a dangerous or deadly heart rhythm, which can occur after heart tissue is scarred following a heart attack.

When medications fail to control the heart's electrical rhythm, patients with electrical system heart disease can benefit from a procedure called an "ablation," in which tissue that is creating erratic or dangerous electrical impulses is burned with radio waves. Patients with atrial fibrillation often undergo this procedure several times before the decision is made to permanently ablate the bundle of tissue that transmits the electrical signal from the atria to the ventricles so that the extra impulses of atrial fibrillation cannot be communicated to the ventricles. At the same time, a device called a pacemaker is implanted. An implanted pacemaker monitors and delivers an electrical signal to stimulate the heart muscle to squeeze if the heart's own pacemaker fails to deliver an impulse. Patients with atrial fibrillation who have undergone the ablation procedure to cut the electrical connection between their upper and lower chambers are then fully dependent on their implanted pacemaker to deliver the electrical signal for their heartbeat going forward.

Sometimes electrical disease leads to the ventricles squeezing at slightly different times. Patients with this problem can develop heart failure symptoms because the blood does not flow through or out of the heart normally. A device called a cardiac resynchronization device or CRT, which is like a pacemaker, can be implanted with electrical leads placed in both ventricles to stimulate them to squeeze at the same time. Often, this therapy will help a heart in heart failure recover to normal function.

Patients with worsening heart failure experience physical and functional decline over a number of years as their heart failure worsens. Any of the issues I've described can occur in patients with heart disease, and often, patients experience a pattern in which one problem leads to another, causing issues in multiple systems of the heart.

When a patient experiences an exacerbation, they can experience shortness of breath, chest pain, palpitations, light-headedness, less tolerance for walking or exerting themselves, and an increasing need for support to make it through the day.

Over time, as the heart continues to fail, the support patients need in the hospital to recover from an exacerbation tends to become increasingly invasive. Initially, patients may need just oral diuretics or other medications, but over time, as their heart failure worsens, they may need IV diuretics or medications called "pressors" that force the heart to pump. Patients with heart disease can also develop lung failure or kidney failure, since these organs work so closely together. Eventually, patients with terminal heart disease will get to a point where any next exacerbation may be the last time they've left their home.

Just like we have criteria to diagnose and stage disease, we also have criteria to evaluate when a patient gets to the point where their disease is beyond the medical community's ability to provide support other than to manage their symptoms.[1] At that point, the patient is said to meet what we call "hospice criteria," and we worry that their time is limited. Patients with heart failure meet hospice criteria when they experience untreatable disease that is expected to get worse to the point of death, when they have symptoms even at rest despite our best medical treatment, or when they have symptoms that limit their exertion to the point that they are spending most of their day in their bed or chair.

When a patient meets hospice criteria, it is typically only a matter of time before the patient will need to return to the hospital for care. However, their disease may be beyond the medical community's ability to do more than keep them comfortable. At that point, they are much more likely to require invasive procedures to support their life, such as intubation and mechanical ventilation, for example, if their lungs fail in line with their heart. Those wishing to pass away at home at the end of their lives will need to choose to transition to home hospice care before getting to the point that their disease is so advanced.[2]

Lung Failure: Discuss If the Patient Is Expected to Pass from Lung Failure or If Lung Failure Is Contributing to Overall Patient Decline

Think of the lungs like a tree turned upside down. The trunk is the trachea or windpipe, and the branches are the bronchi, which become smaller and smaller like tree branches. At the end of the branches, instead of leaves, are hundreds of millions of

---

[1] Note that many patients with advanced disease who do not yet meet hospice criteria will progress to a point in their disease journey when the medical community can offer little aside from symptom management. These patients should be offered palliative (supportive) care to address symptoms and ensure a smooth transition to hospice care when patients become hospice minded and meet hospice criteria. Ideally, all patients with a chronic and potentially terminal disease will be supported from the time of diagnosis with comprehensive disease management that prioritizes whole-person care and the compassionate, collaborative approach detailed in this book. For a thorough discussion of palliative (supportive) care and template language that can be used to discuss palliative (supportive) care with patients and families, see Chap. 11.

[2] For template language to use when discussing ICD and pacemaker therapies in patients reaching the end of life, see Chap. 16.

tiny "alveoli," tiny, balloon-shaped structures that bring air into the lungs from the atmosphere. The alveoli are covered with flat lung cells whose job is to exchange gases across their surface—carbon dioxide and oxygen. A network of tiny blood vessels called capillaries surrounds the alveolar cells, releasing carbon dioxide and capturing oxygen molecules on hemoglobin molecules inside red blood cells.

Patients with lung disease experience damage in the branches or tiny air sacs of their lungs, most commonly from smoking. The chemicals in cigarettes cause inflammation, leading to scar tissue formation and the loss of alveolar cells for exchanging gases. Patients with a significant enough smoking history to develop COPD (chronic obstructive pulmonary disease), have lost enough alveolar cells to impact their lungs' ability to exchange gases appropriately. Patients with COPD frequently require supplemental oxygen by nasal cannula to make up the difference from what their lungs can do.

Smoking also damages the cells lining the lung branches, which are covered with tiny, finger-like structures called "cilia" that together, in a wave-like motion, move foreign particles, germs, or mucus up and out of the lungs. Patients with lung failure who develop a "cold" are at increased risk of developing a serious infection like pneumonia more quickly than patients with healthy lungs due to the loss of cilia to move viral particles and bacteria out of their lungs.

Patients with various lung diseases experience hyperinflation of their lungs due to the loss of lung recoil. Air gets trapped in the lungs, compressing the capillaries, and reducing blood flow through the lungs. Air trapping leads to chronic expansion of the lungs beyond a comfortable point, with patients having to force air out of their lungs with effort, often with pursed lips.

If you inhale a deep breath and then hold that expanded lung position as your new baseline, never allowing your lungs to recoil to a smaller diameter after an exhale, you can experience the exhaustion that accompanies the work of breathing by patients with advanced COPD and other forms of lung failure. Much of their daily energy allowance and caloric intake is dedicated to breathing, an effort most of us take for granted. This is very tiring and can lead to fatigue and weight loss. The patient's inability to exercise can further decrease muscle mass and strength, and depression can worsen all of these.

Patients with lung failure will experience episodes called "exacerbations," in which the lungs are unable to function properly. Patients can develop symptoms including shortness of breath, cough, wheezing, intolerance for exertion, and fatigue. Patients with COPD or other lung diseases who develop symptoms of a cold or respiratory virus should contact their pulmonologist or primary care provider within the first day or two so that they can be started on antibiotics and steroids to prevent them from developing pneumonia. Often, patients experiencing a lung failure exacerbation will need to be treated in the hospital because their lungs are unable to recover without IV antibiotics or steroids, or higher capacity oxygen delivery than they can receive from their at-home oxygen concentrator.

As lung failure progresses, the support patients need in the hospital to recover from an exacerbation tends to become increasingly invasive. For instance, early on in a patient's journey with lung failure, they may only need oral medications and oxygen support by nasal cannula. Later, they may need IV medications and more forceful oxygen delivery in the form of a CPAP or BiPAP mask, which forces air into the lungs. Later still, they may need to be intubated and mechanically ventilated. Because the heart and lungs work together to deliver oxygen to the body, as one organ fails, the other organ often develops problems and can fail as well.

Just like we have criteria to diagnose and stage disease, we also have criteria to evaluate when a patient gets to the point where their disease is beyond the medical community's ability to provide support other than to manage their symptoms. At that point, the patient is said to meet what we call "hospice criteria," and we worry that their time is limited. Patients with lung failure meet hospice criteria when they experience untreatable disease that is expected to get worse to the point of death, when they have symptoms even at rest despite our best medical treatment, or when they have symptoms that limit their exertion to the point that they are spending most of their day in their bed or chair.

When a patient meets hospice criteria, it is typically only a matter of time before the patient will need to return to the hospital for care. However, their disease may be beyond the medical community's ability to do more than keep them comfortable. At that point, the only treatments likely to help are invasive procedures such as BIPAP or intubation and mechanical ventilation, from which patients may not be able to recover. Those wishing to pass away at home at the end of their lives will need to choose to transition to home hospice care before the point that their disease is so advanced.

Liver Failure: Discuss If the Patient Is Expected to Pass from Liver Failure or If Liver Failure Is Contributing to Overall Patient Decline

Approximately half of patient deaths in the United States from liver failure are due to alcohol intake, but many patients will develop liver failure because of non-alcoholic fatty liver disease. In both situations, healthy liver tissue becomes increasingly replaced by nodules and fibrous tissue (similar to scar tissue) that interfere with the liver's function. Although the liver is an amazing organ with the ability to regenerate itself, once enough healthy tissue is replaced in this way, the liver is said to have developed cirrhosis, which is irreversible. Patients with cirrhosis who are not candidates for a liver transplant can be expected to die from liver failure.

As liver failure worsens, patients can experience a multitude of symptoms because the liver does so many jobs. One of its essential jobs is to remove toxins from the blood. As healthy liver tissue is increasingly replaced by cirrhotic tissue (again, think scar tissue), the liver can't detoxify the blood as well. A patient's skin can turn yellow because of the buildup of bilirubin, which comes from the breakdown of old red blood cells. Patients can also experience severe itching as bile salts build up in the skin. Patients with severe disease can experience a buildup of toxins, which affects brain function and can become severe enough to cause a coma that leads to death. It is not uncommon for patients with liver disease to become confused.

A symptom that frequently occurs with a liver failure exacerbation (in the case of the liver, we call an exacerbation a "decompensation" event) is that fluid can build up in the abdomen. In a healthy body, blood vessels carry the products of digestion from the digestive tract to the liver, which detoxifies the blood. As the liver gets replaced with cirrhotic tissue, blood has difficulty flowing from the digestive tract through the tiny blood vessels in the liver. This increases the blood pressure inside the liver system, a condition called "portal hypertension." Portal hypertension, which is irreversible, causes the blood to back up in the abdomen, where water molecules in the blood vessels then leak out into the surrounding tissue. This buildup of fluid in the abdomen is called "ascites."

Patients with ascites often require a procedure called "paracentesis" to remove the fluid from their abdomen with a large needle. When ascites repeatedly occurs despite paracentesis, it is said to be "refractory," a sign that the patient's liver disease is very advanced. Over time, ascites tends to return more quickly following paracentesis. When this happens, the patient's time is typically very limited. Patients who would prefer to stay at home at the end of their lives can be supported with an abdominal drain, which allows the fluid to be removed comfortably without the need to return to the hospital for paracentesis.

Patients with severe disease are at risk of developing a life-threatening infection of the ascitic fluid, called "spontaneous bacterial peritonitis." Patients typically have a very limited number of weeks left to live if this occurs.

Another place that blood congests in the digestive system is in the veins of the esophagus, creating what are called "esophageal varices," which are like varicose veins in the esophagus. These carry a risk of life-threatening rupture, which can lead to sudden death. As part of routine monitoring of liver failure, a procedure called "endoscopy" is done. A tube with a tiny camera on end is passed down the patient's esophagus to look for varices, which can be treated during the procedure with a rubber band that cuts off blood flow to prevent them from rupturing.

The liver produces many components of the "coagulation system," which controls the healthy balance between bleeding and clotting. Some people have problems with this system and either bleed or clot too easily. Many people are on "blood thinners," medications that impact this system to prevent blood clots. As liver failure advances, the liver's ability to create the components to clot the blood declines, leaving patients at risk of life-threatening bleeding events, including during an endoscopy procedure. We monitor the liver's ability to make the components of the coagulation system with lab values called PT and INR, which stand for "prothrombin time" and "international normalized ratio." Large amounts of blood can be lost due to vomiting blood or gastrointestinal bleeding.

The liver also makes a large protein called "albumin." In a healthy body, albumin is a transport molecule in the blood vessels, holding onto water molecules, electrolytes, and hormones. It is too big to cross the blood vessel walls, but it keeps water molecules in the blood vessels, helping to maintain our blood pressure. As the liver fails to make albumin, water molecules, which are small enough to move across the blood vessel walls, leak out of the blood vessels into the surrounding tissue. This can cause shortness of breath if the fluid collects in the lungs, or discomfort if it collects in the abdomen, arms, or legs.

Just like we have criteria to diagnose and stage disease, we also have criteria to evaluate when a patient gets to the point where their disease is beyond the medical community's ability to provide support other than to manage their symptoms. At that point, the patient is said to meet what we call "hospice criteria," and we worry that their time is limited. Patients with liver failure meet hospice criteria when the PT, INR, and albumin levels get to a certain point, indicating end-stage disease.

When a patient meets hospice criteria, it is typically only a matter of time before the patient will need to return to the hospital for care. However, their disease may be beyond the medical community's ability to do more than keep them comfortable. At that point, they are much more likely to require invasive procedures to support their life, such as paracentesis, which may pose too great a risk. Those wishing to pass away at home at the end of their lives will need to choose to transition to home hospice care before getting to the point that their disease is so advanced. As mentioned before, patients with refractory ascites can be helped to be comfortable at the end of life by having an abdominal drain placed, which allows the ascites to be removed comfortably at home.

Kidney Failure: Discuss If the Patient Is Expected to Pass from Kidney Failure or If Kidney Failure Is Contributing to Overall Patient Decline

Chronic kidney disease, or CKD, is the progressive loss of kidney function that ultimately leads to the failure of the kidneys to excrete toxins, electrolytes, and fluid. The final stage of CKD, stage 5, also called end-stage kidney disease, or ESKD, results in a wide range of abnormalities and symptoms called "uremic syndrome." Without hemodialysis, patients at this stage of kidney failure will typically pass within one to three weeks.

Patients with kidney failure, like with other forms of organ failure, will experience exacerbations in which their kidney failure becomes suddenly worse. Over time, kidney function will decline to the point where the medical team will anticipate the need for dialysis, at stage 5, or ESKD. Although CKD affects millions of Americans and contributes to overall patient decline, ESKD is rarely the primary driver of terminal decline or the primary reason patients with kidney failure elect hospice care. This is because the vast majority (80–90%) of patients with CKD will die of some form of cardiovascular disease—heart failure, stroke, heart attack, or peripheral vascular disease—long before arriving at the point of needing dialysis.

Of those with kidney failure who survive long enough to require dialysis, about half will also die from cardiovascular disease. Others will pass following voluntary discontinuation of dialysis. Patients who qualify for an organ transplant often pass away before a suitable kidney is found.

When patients have arrived at the point of requiring dialysis to survive, many patients will experience a number of quality years. However, the risk of passing away in any given year is relatively high: 1 to 2 out of 10 patients on dialysis pass away each year, and less than half of patients starting dialysis survive to five years. Patients requiring dialysis can receive hospice care if they discontinue dialysis. Patients who discontinue dialysis typically pass away within one to three weeks. Hospice nurses have shared that patients with end-stage kidney disease who discontinue dialysis have a very peaceful passing, as the toxins building up in their system cause them to sleep until they pass peacefully.

Cancer

Brief Description

Approximately 1 in 5 patients who pass away each year in the United States die of some form of cancer. In 2020, cancer was the second leading cause of death in the United States.

While modern medications can help patients with advanced cancer live well for a long time, the end of the cancer journey is best described as a ball rolling off a very steep cliff: a significant amount of decline in a short amount of time.

Extended Description

This happens for one of two reasons: either the cancer outpaces available treatment, or the treatment results in side effects that either limit its effectiveness or make the patient too sick to continue. In either case, the cancer advances to the point of death.

The end of the cancer journey is marked by a change in the patient's metabolism, causing a constellation of symptoms that collectively we refer to as "cachexia." Cancer, for reasons that we don't wholly understand, changes the patient's metabolism, stealing the body's nutrition and energy for itself, leading to loss of weight, appetite, muscle mass, energy, strength, stamina, and speed. In this frail state, patients are much more likely to get infections and often experience sepsis, which is a life-threatening response to an infection. It can be very difficult for patients with cancer to reverse that trend.

Because end-of-life decline can occur very rapidly, it is critical for patients with cancer that is advancing despite treatment to have the chance to think about and articulate their wishes for where they would like to be at the end of their lives. Patients with cancer that is advancing despite treatment, whose disease is very aggressive (including pancreatic cancer, brain cancer, and lung cancer), those with metastatic disease, or those with disease of any kind who chose not to pursue treatment meet what we call "hospice criteria," and we worry that their time is limited.

It is at this point that the medical community is no longer able to change the course of their disease or to provide care beyond keeping them comfortable and managing their symptoms. Patients at this point who return to the hospital for care are much more likely to require invasive procedures to sustain life, such as cardiopulmonary resuscitation (CPR) and mechanical ventilation if their heart or lungs fail. Those who want to be at home in their final days or weeks, who want to be able to spend quality time with their loved ones, and who want to be alert and aware enough to say their goodbyes will need to choose the treatment option we call hospice care before the point that their decline prevents them from making that choice on their own.

Frailty/Age-Related Decline

Brief Description

Approximately 1 in 3 patients who pass away each year in the United States die from age-related decline. This is the journey we describe when we say someone is "dying of old age."

On this journey, patient decline is slow and steady, without many crises, with patients and loved ones incrementally accommodating to the patient's new reality.

Detailed Description

On this journey, the patient's metabolism changes, leading to a condition we call frailty, a state of poor reserve from which it can be challenging to recover from any subsequent insult or injury.

The metabolism is the body's energy system, a constant balance of building and breaking down tissue. Across the lifespan, the metabolism shifts a couple of times. From the time we are born until a bit past our adolescence, we're building more tissue than we're breaking down; we're growing. As adults, we roughly maintain about the same, keeping a steady balance between building and breaking down tissue. And at the end of life, regardless of what disease trajectory we might follow, our metabolism shifts again as we start breaking down more tissue than we're building. This is an expected part of the end of every terminal disease we follow as we approach the end of life, including organ failure, cancer, and dementia, and this is the mechanism by which patients experience age-related decline.

When the metabolism shifts toward the end of life, the body is not as efficient at translating the products of its nutrition into the body components—muscle, bone, skin, blood vessel walls, parts of the immune system, etc. Organs and systems function less effectively, and many older adults experience changes in cognition or thinking, which can lead to depression and less interest in social activities. As a patient's metabolism declines, we will see a constellation of related physical symptoms, including weight loss, loss of appetite, loss of muscle mass, and loss of strength, stamina, and speed. This physical decline leads to mobility issues, balance issues, and falls. Importantly, this is the context in which many patients fall and break a hip. In fact, the bones can become so frail that they break and cause a fall. Although sometimes, it might seem reasonable to think that if only the patient hadn't fallen, they would have been fine, the reality is that many patients fall and experience a fracture because their body was already in the process of declining; it was the metabolic decline that led to the fall and fracture.

Patients who have lost 5% to 10% of their total body weight in a short amount of time—6 to 12 months—in a situation where they have appropriate mealtime support, can be said to have moved into a state of frailty, or cachexia. This is clinically significant, dramatically increasing their risk of passing away in subsequent months. At that point, many patients will meet what we call "hospice criteria," and we worry that their time is limited.

We can try to interrupt the weight loss with a medication that has the desired side effect of weight gain. However, if the body has made the metabolic shift, the medical community has not found any treatment to successfully reverse that trend. Even forcing nutrition on the body, such as with a feeding tube, cannot make the body translate the nutrition it receives into new muscle, bone, and skin. Moreover, feeding tubes that introduce liquid food into a patient's body experiencing end-stage decline can overwhelm the heart and kidneys, whose job is maintaining the appropriate fluid balance. This extra fluid can build up in the legs, causing swelling, weeping skin, and infections. Feeding tubes can also lead to aspiration pneumonia if the fluid regurgitates up the esophagus into the back of the throat and passes down the windpipe into the lungs.

As the metabolism falters at the end of life, organs and systems begin to decline, and patients can experience symptoms related to organ dysfunction, as well as falls and infections. When patients pass the point of meeting hospice criteria with age-related decline, they are much more likely to require invasive procedures to support their prolonged existence, for instance, surgical repair of fractures, mechanical ventilation if they experience respiratory failure, and a feeding tube. These treatments, which might have been beneficial in helping them recover when they were younger and more robust, may not confer the same benefit at this stage and may even be life-limiting.

As patients with age-related decline approach the point of meeting hospice criteria, any next insult or injury may prove too challenging for their body to recover. At that point, any hospitalization may be the last time they've left their home. Those wishing to pass away at home at the end of their lives will need to choose to transition to home hospice care before the point that their decline is so advanced that they are unable to recover with the help of hospital-based treatments.

It is critical for families of patients with age-related decline who meet or who are close to meeting hospice criteria to consider whether their loved one would be able to tolerate or survive hip repair surgery. To heal a bone fracture, a patient needs to be able to translate the products of their nutrition into healthy bone and muscle tissue. This function is in significant decline when a patient with age-related decline meets hospice criteria. The fall and fracture, representing one major insult, may be too challenging for the patient to recover. Surgery to repair a hip fracture, which is highly invasive and traumatic, represents a second major insult. Furthermore, anesthesia, which can be challenging for patients of advanced age who don't yet meet hospice criteria, represents a third major challenge. Together, these three significant insults are often too much for patients with age-related decline who meet or who are close to meeting hospice criteria to tolerate, and many patients are discharged from the hospital following hip repair surgery directly to hospice care.

For families who are worried about their loved one's ability to survive something like hip fracture surgery but who are concerned about the potential pain they may experience, the alternative form of treatment in this circumstance is hospice care. Hospice teams are experts at using medication to treat pain to keep patients comfortable in these circumstances. Patients who have reached the end of their lives with age-related decline, who have experienced a fall and hip fracture, and who would not be a good candidate for surgical repair can be kept comfortable and allowed to pass peacefully when their time comes with the support of hospice care.

Dementia

The following primer is provided to caregivers and family members of patients with dementia. Sometimes, this education, particularly about how to interact with a patient with dementia in a way that supports their dignity, is enough to reduce the distress caregivers experience during interactions, preventing the need to start a medication to address the patient's anxiety and agitation. This primer is lengthy but essential in helping family members understand the why, how, and what of the dementia journey, especially the need for those living alone to, at some point, be moved to a care facility or provided with in-home support appropriate to meet their needs.

Brief Description

Many patients who pass away each year in the United States die from some form of dementia or neurodegenerative disease, such as Parkinson's disease or amyotrophic lateral sclerosis.

For most patients, decline is slow and steady, without many crises. This journey takes its greatest toll on caregivers, who themselves are at risk of physical, emotional, and mental exhaustion.

Detailed Description

Dementia is the general or umbrella term for what we call brain failure. Just like your heart, lungs, liver, and kidneys can fail, so too can the organ of the brain.

Of course, the human brain is the most important organ in the human body, controlling everything about who we are as individuals and everything about our physical bodies, from our personality and laugh to the way we walk or speak, to how we think about and remember people or experiences, to our heartbeat and how we heal.

We can think of the brain as a problem-solving organ whose job is to solve problems in three domains: inside our physical bodies and in our physical and social environments. As dementia progresses, the brain atrophies or shrinks, as brain cells die and neural networks are lost. As brain tissue is lost in different areas of the brain, the functions in those areas become affected, and patients experience changes in thinking, how they navigate their physical and social world, and how their bodies function.

There are many different types or causes of dementia. Alzheimer's disease is the most common type of dementia, affecting 60% to 80% of patients with a diagnosis of dementia. This type of dementia is believed to be caused by an accumulation of abnormal proteins over several decades that eventually cause brain cells to die.

The second most common type of dementia is vascular dementia. This type of dementia results from problems with blood flow to the brain. The word "vascular" means "vessel." Vascular damage can be caused by a stroke, which is like having a heart attack in the brain. Strokes are most commonly caused by the same process that leads to a heart attack, called atherosclerosis, in which cholesterol plaque blocks the blood flow of an artery supplying oxygen to the brain. This type of strike is called an "ischemic stroke"; the word ischemia means damage due to a lack of oxygen.

A stroke can also be caused by a blood clot that cuts off the blood supply to brain tissue; this is called a "thrombotic" stroke. Patients can also experience a stroke following a hemorrhage, in which a blood vessel ruptures and blood leaks into the area surrounding the brain instead of flowing appropriately to the healthy brain tissue. This is called a "hemorrhagic" or "bleeding" stroke. Because there is a limited amount of space inside the skull, the extra blood volume from a hemorrhage can put pressure on the brain tissue, leading to a herniation, in which brain tissue shifts due to the pressure from the bleed. This shift can damage any area of the brain.

People can also have ministrokes or transient ischemic attacks (TIAs), blockages of much smaller vessels in the brain that can nevertheless impact blood flow. Finally, patients can experience changes in the walls of the blood vessels because of diabetes or high blood pressure, in which blood vessels can become twisted or hard, making it difficult for the blood to flow properly to nourish the brain tissue. Approximately 30% of patients with a stroke will go on to develop generalized brain failure.

Brain cells are not resilient when the oxygen supply is reduced. Even though the brain is only about 2% of the body's total mass, it consumes approximately 20% of its oxygen supply at rest. Brain cells do not have an internal storage system for fuel, so when blood flow to brain cells stops, the cells can be damaged very quickly.

Patients with traumatic brain injury (TBI), including those with a single event or multiple injuries (such as concussions), can also go on to develop generalized brain failure. This can be seen in patients who participated in contact sports like football or in those who suffered trauma to the head while serving in the military.

Other causes of dementia include Lewy body dementia and frontotemporal lobe dementia. These types of dementia are much less common, each affecting approximately 3% to 5% of patients with dementia. Both types show up with more dramatic presentations. Lewy body dementia typically presents with robust hallucinations and delusions in which patients frequently see people or animals or believe that other people are trying to harm them in some way. Frontotemporal lobe dementia often presents with unpredictable personality shifts and socially inappropriate behaviors resulting from a lack of social impulse control or poor judgment. These two dementias can result in dramatic behavioral challenges, and they often involve patients or family members calling the police for help in the weeks or months before a formal diagnosis is made.

Patients with progressive neurodegenerative diseases like Parkinson's disease, amyotrophic lateral sclerosis (ALS), or Huntington's disease can also experience general dementia. Many patients will first display motor issues with these disorders, with many progressing to show general brain failure.

Currently, there is no widely available technology to definitively diagnose the specific type of dementia a patient has. Although a definitive diagnosis of dementia can be accomplished with a brain biopsy and examination of the brain tissue under a microscope, we do not do that on living people.[3] When we examine the brain tissue of deceased patients who were known to have had dementia, what we almost always find is what we call a "mixed picture," with evidence of some of the plaques and tangles that we believe cause Alzheimer's disease, some evidence of "ischemia" (damage due to poor blood flow caused by vascular disease), some of the Lewy body proteins that cause Lewy body dementia, and some of the proteins involved in frontotemporal lobe dementia.

In clinical practice, it is often the case that patients have a range of symptoms alongside the changes in thinking expected with dementia, pointing to a less-than-clear diagnosis. Many patients exhibit personality changes and hallucinations but do not appear to have a clear picture of Lewy body dementia or frontotemporal lobe dementia. Many patients with straightforward Alzheimer's disease show several of the symptoms commonly seen in Parkinson's disease—shuffling gait, slow initiation of movement, tremor, flat facial expression, and low voice volume—but don't ever receive a formal diagnosis of Parkinson's disease.

The reality is that for almost all patients, dementia is, at best, an indefinite and indirect diagnosis. Dementia is a "clinical diagnosis," meaning the diagnosis is primarily made in the clinical setting by talking with the person who most closely witnesses the patient making it through their day. This person's report is then corroborated with a cognitive screening assessment and imaging studies; however, while imaging studies can show blood flow issues and volume loss, imaging can only *support* a diagnosis of dementia, rather than *definitively point* to a specific cause. That is because the brain is a complicated organ, and we currently do not have any imaging technology sophisticated enough to show exactly which neural networks are being lost over time. The use of imaging to diagnose dementia is not at all like the use of an X-ray to diagnose a bone fracture. Whereas an X-ray can show precisely where a bone is broken, brain images are indistinct and cannot show detail at the level of neural networks and specific brain function. Especially in the early stages of dementia, imaging is usually not diagnostic.

Perhaps in a few years, the amyloid PET scan technology currently being introduced will help to definitively diagnose Alzheimer's disease for many patients with dementia, but even that technology will not reveal exactly which neural networks for each brain function are being lost. Presently, amyloid PET scan technology is not widely available to patients. Blood and cerebrospinal fluid markers are also being developed, but are also not widely available to all patients.

The important thing to understand about diagnosing dementia is that it is done primarily through conversation with the caregiver or family member who most closely sees and helps to navigate the patient through their day; that is, the person who can report on exactly which activities of daily living the patient needs assistance with. If other potential causes of cognitive decline have been ruled out, such as infections and electrolyte and hormone disturbances, then a diagnosis of dementia can reliably be made by talking with caregivers.

---

[3] People often laugh at this comment, which is an excellent way of reducing the weight of this heavy conversation.

Regardless of the type of dementia a patient has, there is a unifying story that is common across the spectrum of dementia: a story of progressive loss in the ability to make it through the day without help. Patients lose the skills they gained growing up in approximately the reverse order of acquisition. Again, if we think of the brain as a problem-solving organ, as patients progress through the dementia journey, their problem-solving skills diminish in a way that mimics the reverse of developmental aging, and their cognitive sophistication and skill to solve problems inside the body, and in the physical and social environments decline.

As we grow, our brain develops from the brainstem to the cortex—what we call "grey matter"—and on the dementia journey, neural networks are lost in approximately the reverse order. The cortex, particularly the prefrontal cortex, the part of the brain that serves as the processing center, matures when we reach early adulthood, by our early to mid-20s. As a person goes through the dementia journey, their cognitive sophistication declines so that by the end of the journey, they will have approximately the cognitive sophistication of an infant. A helpful way to describe the dementia journey is that it is the journey of going from infancy to adulthood, in reverse.[4]

This doesn't mean that the patient *becomes* a child. But as the patient's cognitive sophistication declines, so does their problem-solving and thinking ability, and it becomes increasingly important to manage the patient's physical and social environment to keep them safe.

To evaluate where a patient is in their dementia journey, we use a clinical staging system called the FAST scale (Functional Assessment Staging of Dementia). The FAST scale was designed to describe the patient's progression through the journey of Alzheimer's disease; however, it very well describes the unifying, overall story of the "loss of capacity to make it through the day without help," as seen in the other types of dementia as well. The FAST scale describes seven stages, which is a lot for people to remember. These seven stages can be collapsed into four major stages, making it easier to remember the different types of memory and skills that are affected as dementia progresses.

Before I describe the four major stages of the dementia journey, I want to take a minute to describe two fundamental aspects of human nature and human development. Keeping these two aspects in mind when interacting with someone with dementia will help ensure that they can experience love, joy, and contentment no matter their capacity as they progress through their journey.

First, it is a fundamental aspect of human nature that each of us wants to feel competent, capable, and in control. We all, no matter how old we are—two or ninety-two—and no matter whether we have dementia or not, want to perceive ourselves as being competent, capable, and in control. More importantly, we want to perceive that other people perceive us to be competent, capable, and in control.

Second, one of the very first things we learn as infants is how to be an emotionally relatable member of our social group. At two months, babies learn to smile.

---

[4]Caregivers often nod in agreement with this statement or chime in with a comment confirming their observation of this reality, expressing relief at the acknowledgment of their experience.

Shortly after that, they learn to giggle and coo back and forth with their parents, which is the underpinning of language. These skills develop many months before babies learn to comprehend or produce words. At four months, babies can pair their mother's facial expression with the appropriate tone of her voice, meaning her happy face with her happy voice and her sad face with her sad voice. Shortly after that, babies can do that with everyone else in the room.

That means, long before we learn to use language to communicate concepts or ideas in any meaningful way, we learn to mine an incredible amount of information from our social environment by paying attention to tone of voice, facial expression, body language, and the energy of the communications happening between those around us.

This is one of the first things we learn as infants and one of the last things that leaves us on the dementia journey.

These two aspects of human nature and development play a critical role in every interaction with a patient with dementia. If we're not careful, our tone of voice, body language, and the words we use can convey judgment, nagging, condescension, or the impression that the patient with dementia is wrong, which can insult their sense of competence, capability, and control, triggering embarrassment, shame, frustration, anger, or agitation. Thus, it becomes essential to manage how we speak to someone with dementia. Likewise, as a patient's capacity changes over the course of their journey, it is important to manage our expectations of their communication capacity by adjusting our demands in conversation.

As I describe the stages of dementia and the cognitive losses at each stage, I will teach four pillars of support for patients on this journey. These pillars include, *first*, managing our expectations of the patient's changing cognitive, physical, and social skills; *second*, managing our communications, including our tone of voice, body language, facial expression, and the words we say; *third*, managing the patient's physical and social environment to keep them safe; and *fourth*, self-care to ensure that as caregivers, we can remain loving and patient. I will tie the specific cognitive functions of the brain being affected at each stage to strategies for managing the first three pillars. Because the dementia journey eventually becomes primarily a caregiver journey, prioritizing time for self-care is not only important; it is essential. By doing these things, it is possible for everyone on the dementia journey—patients and caregivers alike—to have a positive, loving, and dignified experience.

Recent Memory Stage

The first major stage of dementia, called the **Recent Memory** stage, affects a part of the brain called the hippocampus. The hippocampus resides in the cortex deep in the temporal lobes, the part of the outer shell of the brain that wraps up under the ears. The hippocampus is responsible for a type of memory storage that most of us call "short-term memory," but is actually a type of long-term memory storage called "recent memory." Recent memory allows us to store and later retrieve new pieces of information about our world or personal experience: what I had for breakfast, who visited yesterday, what appointment my wife told me I have coming up later today, what was just talked about in conversation, whether I took my morning medications, etc.

The loss of the recent memory system makes people very poor historians of their own experiences very early in the dementia journey. Because patients at this stage do not reliably store new pieces of information, when asked a question, they may not provide an accurate answer.

Think about how you feel when someone asks you a question, and you can't remember the answer. Or how you feel when you forget someone's name or an appointment. Or worse, how you feel when someone asks you a question or responds to you in a way that implies that you should have remembered what they're asking, such as, "You can't remember that? I just told you where we were going two minutes ago." Most people would feel bad in any of these situations.

Anytime we ask someone a question, they must go into their brain to find the answer. Because the storage system for new pieces of information is not reliable early in the dementia journey, asking questions of people with dementia forces a potential confrontation with their internal cognitive deficits, which can leave them feeling bad about themselves.

Thinking about our pillars of support, we want to remember to expect that patients with dementia may have problems remembering new pieces of information. Our communication strategy, therefore, is to ask fewer questions for information finding. If you need to know something, go and look for yourself. For instance, did the patient eat the sandwich you left them for lunch? Go and look in the fridge. Did they take their morning medications? Go and look in their pill box.

If you ask a question, let it be for human connection. Regardless of the answer, respond in a way that promotes love and connection with enthusiasm, engagement, excitement, and support. For instance, if you ask a patient with dementia what they had for lunch, and they answer, "prime rib," even though you suspect they had a peanut butter and jelly sandwich, respond in a way that shows excitement, pleasant surprise, or joy, such as, "Wow, that sounds delicious!"

Most of us know that if a friend calls and tells us that they're getting divorced, we shouldn't respond by saying, "Well, I could see that coming. Your spouse was a jerk. I don't know why you married them in the first place." In the same vein, we want to be supportive, kind, and loving with a patient with dementia, no matter what they say.

Unless the next thing the person is about to do will result in harm to themselves or someone else, there is no benefit in correcting a person with dementia. Corrections, arguments, and coercion will leave them feeling incompetent, incapable, and as though things are not in their control. Distraction or changing the topic might be a better option.

Sometimes, caregivers of patients with recent memory loss think that trying to task a patient's memory through repetitive practice can help. For example, a caregiver may tell a patient with dementia a new piece of information, instructing the patient to focus on what they're being told so they can remember it, and then quizzing the patient about the information later. Although this might have worked when the patient's brain was healthier and younger, when patients have dementia, this is cruel and can leave them feeling incompetent, incapable, and like their experiences are no longer in their control.

I like to compare a person with dementia and a person with a broken arm. We would not ask someone with a broken arm to help carry the groceries. It's the same thing on the dementia journey. As brain cells are dying, and the skills stored in those cells are lost, it is no longer appropriate to expect the person to be able to do those skills.

To help manage the person's physical or social environment at this stage, attending important appointments to keep track of what is being said becomes necessary. It is also important to understand that because patients with dementia readily answer questions in a way that maintains their competence, capability, and control, they may answer questions in a way that communicates that nothing is wrong. This leads patients with dementia who attend doctor appointments on their own to frequently answer questions inaccurately. Therefore, it is important to have a reliable historian present who can gently provide accurate answers to the provider so that appropriate care can be delivered. When patients are sensitive to other people answering for them, speaking separately to the physician may be necessary.

The fact that patients with dementia frequently attend doctor appointments on their own, answering questions in a way that makes it sound as though they are reporting reliably, is part of the reason that the dementia journey goes undiagnosed for so long for so many patients.

Cognitive Function Stage

In the second major stage, called the **Cognitive Function** stage, patients experience further loss in the cerebral cortex. The cerebral cortex is the outer shell of the human brain—the gray matter and powerful processing center. Particularly the prefrontal cortex, the part of the brain right behind the forehead, is what makes humans unique in the animal kingdom, giving our species the ability to develop cultural wonders such as math, science, religion, politics, medicine, and art. On an individual level, our prefrontal cortex gives us high-level cognitive skills, including logic, reason, abstract thinking, computation, anticipation, planning, and judgment. It also gives us our social impulse control (our ability to behave appropriately in social situations) and our internal self-awareness (knowing if we are tired, hungry, thirsty, cold, angry, sad, or need to go to the bathroom). This area is sometimes referred to as the "executive function" center.

Also in the cortex resides our semantic memory, which is our memory for words or concepts—our *conceptual inventory*—that we manipulate when communicating with written or spoken language. On the left hemisphere are two language centers that allow us to read, write, and pronounce words. Above our ears are the auditory cortexes, and at the back of our brain are the visual cortexes. Adjacent to these sensory cortex regions are association cortex areas, which are responsible for making sense of what our eyes and ears perceive through connections to our prefrontal cortex, semantic memory, emotion center, and long-term memory storage. We have myriad connections between these areas.

In this way, our brain acts a lot like a computer. We take in information with our eyes and ears, like typing on a keyboard or downloading information from the internet. Our prefrontal cortex, which acts like the computer's central processing unit, or CPU, processes that information. We have both short- and long-term memory storage, like working RAM and an internal disc drive, and we have cognitive and physical skills like logical thinking and the ability to ride a bike, just like a computer has various programs or applications that it runs. And just like a computer, our brain, which is continuously processing our internal and external worlds, essentially plays a movie in our minds, like the image a computer displays on its monitor, that each of us inherently trusts as real, from the moment we are born until the moment we die. In this way, our brain, like a computer, continuously constructs our reality, and each of us believes the movie playing in our mind to accurately represent the truth.

As patients progress through the dementia journey, losing brain mass in the different cortex regions affects the programming and processing so that the movie that plays in their minds can be wildly different from the movie that plays in ours, even when we are all standing in the "same" room, seeing and hearing the "same" things. If you've ever experienced a difficult time trying to change the mind of someone with dementia, this is why. Although we may call a misperception a "hallucination" or "delusion," it is real to the patient.

Thinking about the pillars of support, first, we need to manage our expectations to understand that this is how the human mind works and to expect that the movie playing in the patient's mind can be very different from ours, and yet they trust that truth just as we trust ours.

Second, the communication strategy at this stage is to stop using logic and reason to explain things to patients or convince them that what they believe or remember is incorrect. The corollary is to stop asking "Why?" questions because "Why" questions require the person to first go into their brain to recall the experience, and then use logic and reason to explain it.

Because logic and reason are skills stored in the prefrontal cortex, once the region responsible for logic and reason is lost, those skills are no longer available to the patient. Using logic and reason in conversation can force a confrontation with a patient's internal cognitive capacity, being more complex than the patient can manage, and any communication that tells a person with dementia that they are not correct is a second confrontation—one that ultimately insults their sense of competence, capability, and control. These confrontations can offend a patient's dignity, leaving them feeling angry, insulted, or useless.

Instead of disagreeing with a patient with dementia or trying to change their mind, it can be more effective to provide reassurance, step into their reality, adjust their environment to change their perception of reality, attempt to change the subject, or offer an innocuous "white lie" that supports the approach of "kindness over truth." Learning what works for a particular patient can require a lot of trial and error, and the same response may not work for two different people. You will know which response is appropriate by how they react—do they appear content or express frustration or anger?

As an example, I take care of two women with dementia who live at the same care facility. Both of their husbands have died. Whenever the first patient asked about her husband, the staff would share the news that her husband had died, and she would experience that trauma over again each time. The staff reached out to me to ask how to help her. After explaining the loss in her Recent Memory system, I helped the staff understand that it was kinder to tell this patient that her husband had stepped out for an appointment, reassuring her that he would be back shortly. Because of her loss of Recent Memory, she would quickly forget the interaction but remain content. In this way, their response supported the reality in her mind, a world in which her husband was still alive.

The other woman, when learning that her husband had died, wanted to know how his funeral was, who attended, and most importantly, if she had been there. The staff lovingly reassured her that she had indeed been present at his funeral, where she sat in the front row and was surrounded by their children and grandchildren. This information equally reassured her, and although she quickly forgot, she also remained content until she thought to ask about her husband again. For these women, two very different movies were playing in their minds, and following the guidance of "kindness over truth," the staff responded in a way that upheld the world in which each of them lived.

A different example illustrates how adjusting the patient's environment can often help resolve the distress a patient can experience due to how their brain makes sense of their physical world. A patient of mine routinely experienced visual hallucinations and the distressing belief that a disco was being held in her bedroom each night. Upon visiting her house, I asked to see her room, where it was easy to spot the culprit: a prism hanging outside of her window that was no doubt casting a colorful spectrum on her walls, making good use of the streetlight nearby. Once the prism was removed, the nightly disco ceased, along with the patient's hallucinations and distress.

Sometimes, it can be most kind and supportive to move into the patient's reality with them. For reasons that we don't entirely understand, long-term memories from decades earlier tend to be preserved in Alzheimer's dementia, and patients who have a difficult time answering questions about what they had for breakfast can relay stories from their youth as though it was yesterday. A patient of mine who was unable to answer my questions at the beginning of our visits about his symptoms and recent experiences (his wife provided answers) always ended our visits by retrieving his photo album from the submarine he served on during the Korean War some 70 years ago. Taking me through the pages of the album, he would report on the experiences from his years of service, and knowing how competent, capable, and in control this exchange made him feel, I always responded with enthusiasm and interest by remaining engaged, asking questions, and sharing in the wonder of his stories. "Reminiscing" is a valuable technique. Photo albums, stories, and songs can be therapeutic and comforting.

As patients experience losses in their cerebral cortex, in addition to experiencing a changing sense of reality, they lose their ability to manage an important set of tasks that the medical world refers to as instrumental activities of daily living, or

IADLs. These tasks allow adults to live independently in their homes and interact successfully with society, and include cooking, cleaning, driving, shopping, and managing appointments, medications, mealtime, finances, the house, and pets. Each task relies heavily on logic, reason, abstract thinking, computation, anticipation, planning, and judgment.

Losses in these cognitive skills make the stakes very high for mistakes that patients can make in managing their IADLs. People can forget to pay bills, be victims of financial fraud when they answer the phone and give out their Social Security number, have accidents while driving, get lost while shopping, wander outside their homes and get lost, take the wrong medication or the wrong dose, lose weight when they forget to eat or prepare meals, or risk starting a fire by leaving something on the stove.

Because eventually, patients in this stage will lose their ability to manage all of their IADLs, this stage at some point becomes what I call the "just do it" stage, when caregivers will need to just step in and manage these tasks to ensure that their loved ones can safely make it through the day. Sometimes, this involves removing the car keys or even the car from the premises, removing the patient's access to their debit or credit cards, or removing their phone to keep them safe from spam callers.

As patient competence for managing IADLs deteriorates, so too does their capacity for participating in complicated conversations about those matters. Most patients with dementia will lose their ability to make complex medical, legal, and financial decisions at some point in the second major stage. When it becomes evident that discussions about medical, legal, financial, and IADL-related topics primarily frustrate the patient, it is better to support patients by avoiding such conversations altogether.

When patients need assistance with medication management, patients are appropriate for an assisted living level of care because these facilities often include nursing staff to manage medications and appointments. In addition, these facilities may offer a dining plan to provide mealtime support, a driver and van to take patients to appointments, and their apartments typically have a limited kitchen to help keep them safe. Although not every patient will need to move to an assisted living facility, I like to point out the level of care that would be appropriate for a patient by the end of this stage to validate caregivers who, by this point, often begin to experience significant caregiver strain.

The reality is that it is an incredible amount of work to get a patient with dementia through their day, and by the end of the Cognitive Function stage, caregivers are essentially providing an assisted living level of care. At a care facility, staff members work 8 to 10 hours, but they can go home at the end of their shifts. Caregivers rarely get a break, which can lead to caregiver strain, which can impact the caregivers' health, well-being, and longevity.

Therefore, it is crucial that caregivers find ways to have breaks or respite and prioritize taking good care of themselves. If it is too much effort—physically or mentally—to get a spouse or loved one with dementia through the day, considering a move to a care facility can be an important and effective way of meeting the needs of both the caregiver and the patient. There are no medals for martyrdom in caring for patients with dementia, and there is no shame in seeking additional help. When we think about the importance of managing a patient's environment to help keep them safe, this can mean a move to a care facility for some patients.

If caregivers are willing and able, it is possible to keep a loved one at home during their dementia journey. Families that need extra support in the home can hire home care agency support to assist with getting patients through their day. Often, just hiring in help a few hours a week to give caregivers respite and move some items off their to-do lists is all that is needed. There is no right answer, only the answer that is right for the patient and family.

Personal Care Stage

The third stage of dementia, called the **Personal Care** stage, affects a type of long-term memory storage called "procedural knowledge," which allows us to learn physical tasks that require a sequence of steps to be completed in the correct order. Procedural knowledge underlies an important set of tasks that the medical community calls the basic activities of daily living, or ADLs. These tasks, which allow us to take care of our personal, physical selves, took a lot of practice to learn, roughly between the ages of two and eight, and include feeding ourselves, tying our shoes, getting dressed, learning to take a bath or shower safely on our own, and toileting ourselves.

Toward the beginning of the Personal Care stage, families often need to remind their loved ones to change their clothes or take a bath or shower. As patients progress further into this stage, they will have problems with the mechanics of dressing, bathing, and toileting and will need increasing assistance with these tasks. The stakes at this stage can be very high for patients who live alone, who can go entirely without bathing or appropriately toileting themselves. Patients can also burn themselves in the shower as they forget how to adjust the knobs to control the water temperature.

Because the entire brain is involved in toileting, the toileting habit can become disordered in various ways. Our prefrontal cortex gives us our self-awareness, which integrates a signal from the brainstem that comes from the organs of the bladder and bowel, letting us know that they're full. That signal gets sent to the prefrontal association cortex for processing, where the decision to head to the bathroom is made. That center controls the motor cortex and cerebellum, which enable us to walk to the bathroom. We must have the geographic information stored in our cortex to tell us where the bathroom is and the procedural knowledge of what to do when we arrive. We must have a healthy visual cortex to make sense of the toilet and a healthy brainstem, which signals to the organs to allow us to evacuate voluntarily.

As such, this system can start unraveling in a variety of ways. Patients can soil themselves where they sit, unaware of their need to go. They may decide too late to start heading to the bathroom or miss making it in time. They may forget where the bathroom is and go outside or in a closet. They may forget what to do when they get there, failing to wipe or pulling up their pants before they're finished. One of my patients mistook his kitchen chair for the toilet, struggling to lift the seat.

During the Personal Care stage, patients often forget where the bathroom is and what to do when they get there. As they head into the final stage, toileting reminders become essential to helping patients avoid accidents that can be challenging for family members to clean up. Patients may become angry and resist toileting, hygiene, and other tasks, which can be challenging for the caregiver.

Because thinking about the past and future relies on abstract thinking, which is lost during the second stage, patients in the Personal Care stage are essentially in the here and now. Thinking about the past to figure out the present, or thinking about the past and present to anticipate the future can be very challenging for patients at this stage. Conversations about things that are abstract, that aren't concrete or right there in front of them, can also be very difficult.

Consider the question, "What do you want for lunch?" This question tasks the prefrontal cortex by asking the patient to go into their brain and pull up a selection of possible food items that are not right there in front of them, which requires abstract thinking and then choosing. Rather than asking the question like this, it is more supportive of a patient at this stage to provide what we might call the "illusion of choice" by providing two concrete options that the patient can see, such as strawberry yogurt or blueberry yogurt, which can be placed in front of them. By the end of this stage, it is more helpful to provide one option and the suggestion, "Let's eat."

Considering the pillars of support, it is appropriate at this stage to expect that patients will have problems doing physical tasks such as getting dressed, bathing, toileting, and using a telephone, microwave, or remote control. They will have significant difficulty thinking about things that are not concrete or very simple and right there in front of them. They will also have challenges learning new skills, such as how to use a walker or cane, and activities that were once enjoyable, like reading, watching television, or playing games, are often far too cognitively difficult by this stage. Upgraded technology, such as a new phone, can be overwhelming.

The communication strategy at this stage is to narrate the present and to keep instructions or requests very simple. By the end of this stage, patients will often only be able to handle one simple piece of information or directive at a time. For instance, the request, "Let's put our shoes on so we can go for a ride. I want to drop some books off at the library before we have lunch," is a rather complicated description of a series of activities, which can be cognitively overwhelming to patients at this stage. It is better to keep things simple by offering one instruction at a time, "Let's put our shoes on," and when that task is accomplished, "Let's go for a ride." While this oversimplification would be more appropriate for a patient at the end of the Personal Care stage, caregivers will learn through trial and error how much information a patient can handle at a given instance.

Another critical aspect of cognition that changes across the dementia journey is that processing speed slows way down. Using the computer metaphor again, it is as though we are moving backward in computer generations to slower and slower processors. As patients progress through their journey, particularly during the Personal Care stage, it is important to provide plenty of time to complete tasks and answer questions. Something that might have previously taken 20 seconds might now take 20 minutes to complete. Simplifying the day to one rather than six errands or spacing out appointments and activities across the week to provide plenty of preparation or recovery time is also important. These adjustments can reduce overall stress, improving the caregiver-patient relationship.

In terms of managing their environment, it is vital to understand that at this stage, patients with dementia are unsafe to be left home alone. Because the cognitive sophistication of a patient with dementia is significantly diminished by this point in their journey, leaving a patient at home alone carries a significant risk of injury due to issues they would not be able to safely navigate, for instance, a fire or a fall.

Although patients at the beginning of the Personal Care stage can succeed in an assisted living facility, by the end of this stage, when they require assistance with all aspects of personal care, including bathing and toileting, they are more appropriate for memory care or nursing home support. Caregivers providing full-time support for patients during the personal care stage are at significant risk of caregiver strain, as they essentially provide a nursing home level of support 24 hours a day.

Physical Function Stage

The final stage of the dementia journey, called the **Physical Function** stage, showcases the comprehensive nature of brain failure that is the dementia journey. Of course, our brain controls everything about our physical body, including our heartbeat, blood pressure, organ function, the healing process, the way we chew food and swallow, etc. As patients reach the end of the dementia journey, they will lose the ability to walk, chew food, swallow safely, speak, and smile. Eventually, they will become entirely bedbound, needing care around the clock.

The leading edge of the Physical Function stage is frank bladder and bowel incontinence, as the brainstem begins to degrade, and patients experience leak or urge incontinence, bladder retention, or bowel frequency or constipation. Patients with white matter vascular disease, evident on brain imaging studies, often exhibit bladder incontinence earlier in the journey than one would expect with the typical Alzheimer's course.

After incontinence, the next thing we typically see is the type of decline that is captured in the phrase "dying of old age."[5] What is happening in the body is that the metabolism is shifting. The metabolism is the body's energy system, a continual balance between building and breaking down tissue. Across the lifespan, the metabolism shifts a couple of times. From the time we are born until a bit past our adolescence, we're building more tissue than we're breaking down; we're growing. As adults, we roughly maintain the same, and at the end of life, regardless of what disease trajectory we are following, our metabolism shifts again, and we start breaking down more tissue than we build. Commonly, patients die of heart disease, cancer, lung disease, dementia, and age-related decline. Metabolic decline is an expected part of the end of each of these journeys.

As metabolic decline advances, we see a constellation of symptoms. Patients experience a diminished appetite. They eat less and lose weight, especially in their arms and legs, which leads to mobility and balance issues, which in turn, can lead to falls. Importantly, this is the context in which many patients fall and break a hip.

---

[5] I will typically ask family members if they have ever seen someone "die of old age" at this point.

Only about 40% of patients who fall and break a hip are alive a year later. That is because the fall and fracture are a symptom or result of this ongoing metabolic decline, not the cause of it.

As the metabolism shifts, the body is not as efficient at translating the products of its nutrition into healthy tissue—muscle, skin, bone, blood vessel walls, parts of the immune system, etc. As a patient's metabolism declines, patients move into a state of frailty or poor reserve, from which recovery from any subsequent insult or injury can be difficult. Patients with dementia are at particular risk of recurrent infections—a hallmark of end-stage dementia—including urinary tract infections and pneumonia.

The cause of pneumonia in end-stage dementia often relates to brainstem degradation. Along with the bladder and bowel reflexes, the brainstem controls the body's important automatic and life-preserving reflexes for heartbeat, breathing, coughing, vomiting, and swallowing. The swallow reflex is critical in protecting our lungs. When we swallow, a little flap of skin called the epiglottis moves over the airway to protect our lungs from aspirating or inhaling food or liquid. As the brainstem degrades at the end of the dementia journey, this reflex begins to falter, and patients are at risk of aspiration pneumonia, the most common cause of death for patients with Alzheimer's dementia.

Although antibiotics can treat a lung infection, we cannot fix the underlying problem of the swallow reflex failing, so patients will continue to be at risk of developing aspiration pneumonia.

Sometimes, people wonder if a feeding tube might solve the problem of helping people with advanced dementia survive when their body is losing its impulse to eat and the ability to swallow. If the body has naturally made its transition into metabolic terminal decline, the medical community has not found any effective approach to reverse that trend. After attempting to interrupt the weight-loss cycle with medication and ensuring that mealtime support is appropriate, if, despite these interventions, we see the constellation of signs, including weight loss, appetite loss, mobility issues, falls, and loss of strength, stamina, and speed, we can be pretty sure that patients with advanced dementia are moving into the final stage of their journey. In that circumstance, even forcing nutrition on the body, in the form of liquid food delivered by a feeding tube directly to the gut, will **not** effectively enable the body to translate that nutrition into healthy body tissue.

Introducing liquid food into the gut of a patient whose swallow system is degrading introduces a new layer of problems. Should that food regurgitate up the esophagus into the back of the throat, it can easily pass down the windpipe into the lungs, leading to aspiration pneumonia. Aspiration pneumonia is a very common side effect of a feeding tube, particularly in a patient with end-stage dementia or swallowing issues. The reality is that a feeding tube is **never a good idea** for a patient with end-stage dementia, who will not be able to remember from minute to minute why they have the tube and may pull it out, chew through it, or otherwise become distressed by it.

Patients with dementia will eventually get to a point in their journey where they meet what we call "hospice criteria," when we worry that their time is limited. This point occurs for patients with dementia either when they become too weak to transfer or walk without assistance or when they lose a clinically significant amount of body weight in the setting of bowel and bladder incontinence, each situation indicating that the patient has progressed into the final stage of their journey. That is the point where hospitalizations are increasingly likely, as their body is declining, and families are faced with decisions about the type of care they would want for their loved ones.

For those wishing to support the comfort, contentment, and dignity of their loved ones and who prefer to avoid hospitalizations, which can represent a dramatic and distressing change of routine and scenery for patients with dementia, hospice care is available to help support patient dignity, to allow the patient to pass peacefully and without distressing symptoms, and to have a soft landing when their time comes.

Psychiatric Symptoms

The final thing I need to mention about the dementia journey is that there is a set of mood and behavior-related symptoms that patients with dementia can experience at any stage of their journey. These are called **psychiatric symptoms** because they relate to the brain; they are expected and possible with brain failure, just like shortness of breath and leg swelling are among the expected and possible symptoms with heart failure.

Although not everyone with dementia will have these symptoms, most patients will have one or more, with symptoms ranging from mild to severe or even crisis level. Unlike the previously described changes in cognitive and physical capacity, these symptoms do not typically correlate with the stage of disease. There are a few exceptions, such as Lewy body dementia, which tends to show up initially with very robust hallucinations, or frontotemporal dementia, which can show up with dramatic personality changes. Many people worry about symptoms like agitation and anger as dementia progresses. I like to provide the reassurance that patients whose symptoms are mild tend to remain that way. Severe symptoms are often unmanaged, and unmanaged symptoms tend to worsen. Psychiatric symptoms that worsen abruptly can be a sign of an underlying problem, such as constipation or an infection, such as a urinary tract infection or pneumonia.

The psychiatric symptoms can include any of the following:

Anxiety is the sensation of things not feeling right or in our control, which can feel like panic, stress, or discomfort.

Agitation is often a manifestation of anxiety, showing up physically, verbally, or cognitively. **Physical agitation** can range from mild pacing to picking skin and causing skin wounds, to hoarding things like toilet paper in pockets (used or unused), to walking so much that weight is lost, to more severe forms that can include pushing, hitting, or even trying to strangle someone. **Verbal agitation** can range from repeatedly asking the same question to angry outbursts, including cussing, yelling, or calling people names. **Cognitive agitation** can also show up as preoccupation with tasks, conversations, or thoughts. Often, patients become fixated or obsessed with finances, medications, or doctor appointments.

Although people usually think of anger or aggression when hearing the word "agitation," that is not always how agitation appears.

Depression is quite common and often appears in the years before a diagnosis of dementia is made. Depression can show up as tearfulness, sadness, or a general "down in the dumps" presentation. Patients with insight into their cognitive decline often experience depression as a sense of "loss" or personal failure to manage the tasks they could once so easily perform.

Apathy can also occur with dementia, in which people lose all interest in participating in life, including in both physical and social activities, where they don't seem to care about anything or anyone. Apathy can be challenging to manage, and it can also be difficult to differentiate from the natural changes that happen with dementia in which activities or social settings that make people feel less competent often become situations that they want to avoid.

Hallucinations are the experience of seeing people, insects, animals, or objects that other people don't see. These can be distressing but aren't always. Often, patients see little children in their homes and don't seem bothered by their presence. Of course, if symptoms are distressing to the patient or caregiver, we consider treating them with medications if an adjustment to the environment, as discussed earlier, doesn't suffice.

Delusions are beliefs that other people don't share and are often paranoid, such as the belief that a spouse is cheating on or trying to divorce the patient or that people are stealing the patient's things. Not all delusions are distressing. One patient of mine was convinced her husband had divorced her yet remained available every day to help support her, for which she remained grateful. Sometimes, delusions can become severe enough that patients call 911 for support or become physically or verbally agitated or even aggressive. A patient who believed she had killed several people, which caused the patient significant distress, required urgent hospital admission for medication management.

It can sometimes be challenging to differentiate a hallucination from a delusion because, to do so, we must rely on the patient's reporting, which can be problematic. An example is a patient who reported seeing pictures of a party that included people they knew, including the neurologist who had recently performed a cognitive assessment of the patient. The patient believed the party attendees were working collaboratively to move the patient from home to a care facility. It is hard to know if the patient saw and misinterpreted an actual photograph, hallucinated images in their mind, or if their recent neurological assessment created fears about their potential loss of independence that resulted in this delusional and paranoid belief. Either way, hallucinations or delusions that are severe enough to cause the patient or caregiver distress are worthy of medical management.

Because the brain controls our sleep–wake cycle, patients can also experience **insomnia**, which can present as trouble falling asleep, staying asleep, or returning to sleep after waking in the middle of the night. Patients can also confuse their sense of time, mixing up the days and nights, so they sleep during the day and remain awake at night. It is important to treat these symptoms so everyone in the house can get a good night's sleep.

Patients can also become more confused as the day progresses, what we call **sundowning**, with increased agitation and confusion as the sun goes down.

Finally, patients often bring people or objects they were dreaming about into their waking state immediately after waking. This **sleep confusion**[6] can almost seem like a hallucination or delusion, as patients can start looking for a parent or loved one they are convinced had just visited.

Part of our support to patients and families is to ensure that patients and caregivers are not suffering because of any of these symptoms, which can make caregiver support to patients on this journey very difficult. Mild symptoms often resolve with changes in how the caregiver interacts with the patient or with adjustments to the patient's environment, but more significant symptoms often require medication management.

---

[6] I try to avoid using the words hypnopompic or hypnogogic when speaking with caregivers and refer to hypnopompic hallucinations as "sleep confusion."

Advance Directive and Code Status Discussions

16

Advance directive conversations should be included as a routine part of patient health care, initiated when patients reach adulthood and revisited with any change of health status or major life circumstance such as marriage, divorce, having a child, losing a parent, etc. For patients with dementia who have not previously completed advance directives, the best time to pursue this conversation is early in disease course, when their cognitive capacity is still robust.

Objectives During the Advance Directive and Code Status Discussion
- Investigate preferences for:
  - Surrogate medical decision maker
  - Advance directive or living will
  - POLST:
    - Code status
    - Approach to medical care
    - Artificial nutrition by tube
- Legal considerations:
  - Durable power of attorney
  - Guardianship and conservatorship
  - Competence and capacity

© The Author(s), under exclusive license to Springer Nature Switzerland AG 2024
A. Shaw, PA, *The Arc of Conversation*,
https://doi.org/10.1007/978-3-031-70495-6_16

Investigate Patient Preferences for Surrogate Medical Decision Maker

Questions:
- Who would you want to make medical decisions for you if you could not make them yourself?
- Do you have a document specifying who you would want to make medical decisions for you if you could not make them yourself?

Helping patients anticipate when they will lose the ability to make medical decisions for themselves is an essential aspect of patient-centered care that keeps patient values center stage, supporting patient autonomy across the lifespan. This is important for all patients but must be prioritized for those with chronic or terminal disease or disease that robs patients of their cognitive capacity.

A surrogate decision maker (sometimes called a "proxy") is a person who has the authority to make decisions for a patient when the patient is unable to do so themselves. The responsibility of a surrogate medical decision maker starts when a provider deems a patient incompetent to make decisions or when a legal document is signed that transfers responsibility to a surrogate.

The responsibility of a surrogate medical decision maker is to make decisions for the patient *as though they are the patient*, according to the patient's values, wishes, and preferences. Thus, patients should be encouraged to choose a surrogate medical decision maker who can make decisions objectively, without bias or prejudice, and keep the patient's values and preferences front and center even during great emotional or spiritual distress. Patients should also be encouraged to talk openly and often with their chosen surrogate about their values, wishes, and preferences so the surrogate will know how to decide.

Begin a conversation about the patient's surrogate medical decision maker by asking,

- "Who would you want to make medical decisions for you if you could not make them yourself?"

Most people will identify a spouse, child, or parent as the person they would want to serve as their surrogate medical decision maker. Those who have difficulty answering this question should be provided with reassurance and compassion, as this can reflect relationships gone awry, estrangement from family, experiences with the legal or penal system, or tragic loss of loved ones.

Follow up this initial question by asking,

- "Do you have a document specifying who you would want to make medical decisions for you if you could not make them yourself?"

Many patients and families will reference documents such as a durable power of attorney for health care (DPOA-HC), medical durable power of attorney (MDPOA), advance directive, or living will. Patients may also mention a trust, which may contain one or more of these documents.

DPOA-HCs, MDPOAs, or advance directives can specify a variety of preferences, including **who** the patient wants to serve as their primary (and alternate) surrogate medical decision maker, **when** the surrogate's responsibility will begin, **what** that responsibility will entail, and **specific preferences for care,** including, but not limited to, preferences for resuscitation, nutrition and hydration by tube, organ donation, pain control at end-of-life, and advanced interventions such as mechanical ventilation and hemodialysis. Living wills, per se, also specify preferences for care, particularly when patients are terminally ill or permanently incapacitated, but they do not appoint or identify surrogate decision makers. In many states, a DPOA-HC/MDPOA and a living will are combined into a single "omnibus" advance directive.

Because these documents are often completed with attorneys instead of healthcare providers, reviewing the patient's preferences with the patient and their surrogates present is important to ensure everyone has a similar understanding. Copies of the documents should be scanned and stored in the patient's electronic medical record with the local healthcare system. A hard or electronic copy should also be maintained by the family in case the patient receives care in another health system.

Some patients will be unable or unwilling to address questions related to their surrogate medical decision maker. This may be because the patient has lost cognitive capacity or the emotional task is too great. Provide reassurance, explaining that in the United States, almost every state has a legal statute to help determine who can fulfill that role for patients who have become incapacitated and who have not formally specified their choice. U.S. state laws governing these matters can be found online by combining the search term "surrogate medical decision maker law" with the name of the state of interest.

For example, *Wyoming statute 35-22-406. Decisions by Surrogate* specifies that "any member of the following classes of the patient's family who is reasonably available, in descending order of priority, may act as surrogate," including "a spouse, unless legally separated; an adult child; a parent; a grandparent; an adult brother or sister; an adult grandchild; an adult who has exhibited special care or concern for the patient." Additional guidance for specific circumstances, such as a situation in which multiple children are involved who do not agree on medical decisions for the patient, are also addressed in the Wyoming statute. Refer to the statute governing the state where care is provided for further guidance appropriate to a patient's situation.

Those whose choice of surrogate decision maker aligns with state law but who have not formalized that choice in a legal document can be reassured that while a document would be helpful, it is not entirely necessary and certainly not something that would need to be completed should the patient have very limited and precious time remaining. Patients in this situation should be reassured that allowing surrogate decision makers to hear their preferences is more important than completing paperwork.

However, a legal document is crucial for patients whose choice of surrogate medical decision maker does not align with the default specified by state statute and when there is concern about conflict among potential surrogate decision makers. For example, patients with children who do not get along, parents who might not consider the patient's unmarried partner, or a spouse who is estranged but not legally separated should be encouraged to formally specify their surrogate medical decision maker to avoid potential conflict among family members. For similar reasons, patients should also be encouraged to formally document their legal power of attorney—the person they would want to take care of legal and financial matters if incapacitated.

When family members experience conflict regarding medical decisions for a patient, it can be beneficial to usher everyone through the Arc of Conversation together, allowing them to collaborate while hearing each other's concerns, experiences, and insight. Family conflict often arises from an imbalance in caregiving, in which those taking on more caregiving responsibility can experience caregiver strain, leading to resentment of those they feel are contributing less. At the same time, those labeled as contributing less often feel alienated and can develop resentment from feeling "left out" of important decisions. Provide reassurance that not everyone has the capacity, time, financial resources, or ability to contribute equally; if necessary, gently share the observation that some offers of "help" coming from those who are less involved can feel like a further burden to those taking the caregiving lead; and help families to understand that conflict is a normal symptom of family strain when a loved one experiences chronic or terminal decline. These efforts can validate everyone's experience, leading to improved family dynamics.

Family conflict about medical decisions for a loved one can also arise from a lack of clear understanding about the patient's health status and frustration with the medical community for not offering more to help their loved one survive. This incongruity can explain the inability of a family member to "let go" and to allow a parent or spouse to pass peacefully, which can contribute to strained family dynamics. What is often labeled as "denial" is usually a robust expression of advocacy and love, and time spent in helping those who struggle with the disappointment and fear that can result when medical care fails to reverse a loved one's decline is always worthwhile. In addition to helping families come together around medical wishes for a loved one, validating different expressions of love can help those having a hard time "letting go" through the emotional and spiritual labor required to arrive at a point where they can feel more at ease (and even relief) with such difficult decisions. Most importantly, this represents incredible patient-centered care at a challenging time of patients' and families' lives.

Another important expression of patient-centered care is to assist spouses with considerations about surrogate medical decision makers, particularly spouses of those with dementia. Because a diagnosis of dementia is often made well into the journey, many patients with a dementia diagnosis will already be beyond the point of serving reliably as their spouse's medical decision maker. Privately ask the spouse of a patient with dementia,

- "Do you think the patient could make medical decisions for you right now?"

This is a gentle way of encouraging the spouse to consider their needs. If the answer is "No," then it is essential that the spouse formally specifies an alternative surrogate medical decision maker, someone other than the patient with dementia. This is a consideration that many spouses caring for a loved one with dementia don't anticipate on their own, that can be accompanied by an additional layer of grief, and that should be handled with a great deal of compassion.

Investigate Patient Preferences for Advance Directive or Living Will

Questions:
- Do you have a document called an advance directive or living will?
- Let's imagine you are very sick and are hospitalized, likely in the ICU. The medical community has done everything within its power to help you recover, but they do not believe recovery to any meaningful degree is realistic. Interventions such as a breathing machine or feeding tube are being used to maintain your life, without which you would be expected to pass or to remain incapacitated. Would you want to continue to receive those interventions?

People usually think of an advance directive or living will coming into play in the wake of a catastrophic event, when a patient is being kept alive with interventions without which the patient would be expected to pass. Recall the example of my uncle, whose brain injury damaged his brainstem, leaving him dependent on mechanical ventilation. An advance directive or living will communicates a patient's wish about life-prolonging interventions, empowering surrogate decision makers to make the difficult decision to withdraw treatment and to allow the patient to pass, confident that their decision represents what the patient would have wanted.[1]

Start with the inquiry,

---

[1] Legally, a living will is "self-executing," in the sense that medical providers are obligated at least morally to follow the instructions and do not need the consent of a surrogate to do so. In practice, however, medical professionals prefer that decisions to withdraw treatment that will result in patient death be made by surrogates acting to uphold patient values.

- "Do you have a document called an advance directive or living will?"[2]

Many people will have such a document, which can be reviewed, copied, and scanned into the electronic medical record. For those who do not, provide reassurance that,

- "Even without having the document complete, it is important for you to consider your wishes and even more important for loved ones whose responsibility will be to make decisions for you to hear your preferences."

Without a living will, decisions to forgo life-sustaining treatment must be made by a surrogate, either appointed in an MDPOA/DPOA-HC, verbally designated by the patient when they have the capacity to make decisions, or selected by state statute.

Next, introduce the living will document, asking the important question it contains.

- "A living will asks a particular question about a circumstance that most of us hope our loved ones will never face. Let's imagine you are very sick and are hospitalized, likely in the ICU. The medical community has done everything within its power to help you recover, but they do not believe recovery to any meaningful degree is realistic. Interventions such as a breathing machine or feeding tube are being used to maintain your life, without which you would be expected to pass or to remain incapacitated. Would you want to continue to receive those interventions?"

Most people will answer "No" to this inquiry, regardless of age or health status. Some, however, may answer "Yes." Confirm that the answer specified in their advance directive or living will is consistent with their stated response.

The choice made by patients in a living will also applies to the other disease trajectories. However, the connection between life-prolonging interventions at the end of a journey like Organ Failure or Frailty/Dementia can be more challenging for patients and families to appreciate. Helping people understand this connection is an important aspect of supporting patient autonomy.

To help patients and families better appreciate how a living will comes into play on an Organ Failure or Frailty/Dementia journey, it can be helpful to ask the question slightly differently,

- "Let's imagine you are very sick, likely because your disease has progressed beyond the point where the medical community can offer more than symptom management. Despite medical efforts and attempts, the medical team is

---

[2] Even though an advance directive and living will are not the same thing, most people will not know how they differ, so it can be helpful to reference both documents when asking this introductory question.

unable to help you recover to your former state of health, and you require advanced interventions, such as a breathing machine or feeding tube, to remain alive. Would you want to continue to receive those interventions?"

Most patients will readily answer, "No." Some patients, however, will respond by saying, "I would want them to try," meaning they would want efforts to help them recover. Gently point out that embedded in the question is the presumption that the medical team had already done everything possible to help the patient recover. The question is whether the patient would want to be kept alive with advanced interventions, without which they would be expected to pass. This allows patients and families to consider quality of life in the context of such interventions.

Upon hearing this clarification, most people will answer in the negative, offering commentary such as, "I wouldn't want to live like that." Some patients, however, might say something like, "It's not up to me or my doctors when I die; that will be God's choice," or "People wake up from comas all the time; I'd want to be given a chance to get better."

Patients expressing a desire to be kept alive with advanced interventions should be reassured, "Okay, very good," before inquiring further about their wishes,

- "Tell me more. Is there a timeframe or milestone you have in mind to continue receiving life-support treatments?"

Often, patients will offer an experience of a loved one whose extended time on a ventilator resulted in what they perceived to be a miraculous recovery, or they may share doubts about the accuracy of the medical community in pronouncing someone brain dead, expressing frustration with a system that seems all too willing to "give up" on people. They might offer a statement of belief such as "God will take me when it's time" or "There's always hope for a miracle." They may also answer by specifying what they would consider a reasonable amount of time to be kept alive with artificial means, such as "Six weeks. I would just them to make sure I wasn't going to wake up." Such responses provide important insight into patients' medical beliefs and deserve to be handled compassionately, with acceptance and validation.

Patients might also respond in a way that betrays a more profound fear of death or an unwillingness to let go of life by saying something like, "I would want them to keep me around for as long as they can. I'm not ready to go." Such wishes should also be treated compassionately and with reassurance before being investigated further. Appropriate and helpful responses include,

- "Okay, that's understandable," and
- "Can you tell me what you mean when you say you're not ready to go?"

To this inquiry, patients will often share life experiences they are looking forward to. When their wishes significantly misalign with the medical reality, respond compassionately using the "Wish, Worry, Wonder" technique described in Chap. 7.

If, at any point, patients sound defensive or begin to push back forcefully when discussing advance directive decisions, respect their emotional and spiritual boundaries by compassionately pausing the conversation and providing the reassurance that "There is no right answer, only the answer that is right for you and your family." Consider resuming the conversation later.

Investigate Patient Preferences for POLST

Investigate Patient Preferences for Code Status

Questions:
- If you were to die right now, would you want the medical community to undergo efforts to attempt to bring you back to life?
- Do you know what efforts I'm talking about?
- Do you know the percentage of patients who survive a resuscitation attempt?
- Do you know what happens to a person's brain when the heart stops pumping blood forward?
- Do you know what the most common cause of death is for patients who survive a resuscitation attempt?

Having asked the important question in the advance directive or living will, transition the conversation into a discussion about preferences covered by the POLST (Physician/Provider Orders for Life-Sustaining Treatment) form. The POLST form carries different names across the United States, including MOST (Medical Orders for Scope of Treatment), MOLST (Medical Orders for Life-Sustaining Treatment), POST (Physician/Provider Orders for Scope of Treatment), and many more. Nationally, the form and accompanying program are referred to simply as POLST, without spelling it out. Understanding that it may be called something different where you practice, this text will use POLST.

The POLST form allows patients to specify their preferences for code status, approach to medical care, and artificial nutrition by tube; when the form is signed by a physician or (in some states) a nurse practitioner or physician assistant, it becomes a medical order set, which must by law be honored across all healthcare settings.

Introduce the POLST form by saying,

- "The question I just asked relates to a scenario that most of us hope to avoid during our lifetimes. However, many of us will pass away in the hospital because either we suffer a serious and catastrophic event or because our disease has progressed to the point that the medical community cannot support our lives without such interventions. The next questions allow you to specify preferences for medical care well before getting to that point. There is a separate form we can complete to allow you to specify these medical preferences."

The first section (Section A) on the POLST form asks about the patient's preferences for a resuscitation attempt. On the National POLST form, the options are YES CPR: Attempt Resuscitation, including mechanical ventilation, defibrillation, and cardioversion; or NO CPR: Do Not Attempt Resuscitation.[3] **The option of NO CPR will be referred to as DNR in the following text.** Most patients and families understand and may even reference having "a DNR." The purpose of this chapter is to provide patient-friendly language that can be readily adapted in conversations.

Do not start a conversation about resuscitation preferences by referencing "the heart stopping," "restarting the heart," "CPR," or any other related phrases.

Remember that patients need clear language that accurately describes the only circumstance in which CPR is performed—when a person has died. Asking a question about code status by saying, "If your heart stops, do you want us to restart it?" or, "If your heart stops beating and you stop breathing, do you want us to do CPR to resuscitate you?" misleads patients by implying a high likelihood of a successful outcome. Such questions suggest that restarting someone's heart is as easy as restarting a computer, implying that resuscitation attempts are equally successful in all patients when, in reality, the likelihood of success depends on myriad factors, including the patient's age and disease status.

Instead, pose the question in a way that allows patients to focus on their mortality:

- "If you were to die right now, would you want the medical community to undergo efforts to attempt to bring you back to life?"

This question is intended for patients with decisional capacity. A POLST form can also be completed by a surrogate for a patient who does not have decisional capacity. The question can be adjusted to reference the patient's name in that case.

- "If your loved one was to die right now, would you want the medical community to undergo efforts to bring them back to life?"

Many patients of advanced age and declining health will answer this question by saying, "No." Regardless of whether the patient answers in the negative or the affirmative, it is essential to follow up on this question to ensure a clear understanding of the question by asking,

- "Do you know what efforts I'm talking about?"

Many patients will say "Yes," adding some variation of "CPR," "Resuscitation like they do on television," "They push on your chest and breathe into your mouth,"

---

[3] Just as the names of the POLST programs differ from state to state, the forms differ slightly. This text follows the National POLST form.

or "They shock you to get your heart going again." Provide reassurance and some education,

- "Yes, the effort is called cardiopulmonary resuscitation, or CPR, and it follows specific steps that include compressing your chest to force your heart to pump your blood, providing rescue breaths to add air into your lungs, administering medications, and shocking your heart, if necessary."

Because medical decisions that align with patient values are best made from a position of accurate understanding, the next priority is to investigate the patient's assumptions about CPR before providing accurate information about its success rates and outcomes. Begin by asking,

- "Do you know the percentage of patients who survive a resuscitation attempt?"

Many patients and family members will have no idea, or their ideas will be informed only by inaccurate presentations of CPR on television [1, 2]. Common answers range from 10% to 70%. Encourage patients to guess before providing accurate statistics.

- "Many people have only seen CPR performed on television, where most patients survive and recover fully. Whereas on television, as many as 70% of patients survive CPR [1, 2], in the real world, the rate of survival is much more grim. Less than 10% of patients who experience a resuscitation attempt outside of the hospital survive [3]. When CPR is attempted in the hospital, about 25% of patients survive that attempt [4], but only about 10% of patients will survive that hospitalization" [5].

Next, direct the patient and family toward considering the short- and long-term repercussions of a resuscitation attempt aside from mere survival, encouraging them to consider what quality of life means to them. Ask the following questions, providing plenty of time for the patient and family to consider and answer.

- "Do you know what happens to a person's brain when the heart stops pumping blood forward?"
- "Do you know what the most common cause of death is for patients who survive a resuscitation attempt?"

Next, provide education about how brain injury can occur in the setting of a cardiac arrest and resuscitation attempt.

- "The moment the heart stops beating, oxygen delivery to the body's vital organs, including the brain, stops, and brain cells begin to suffer serious injury from a lack of oxygen and glucose. Brain cells do not have a storage system for glucose, which supplies energy to the neurons. Within 4 to 10 seconds of loss of blood flow to the brain, a patient loses consciousness as brain cell function is disrupted. Injury to brain tissue results immediately."

- "Even if high-quality CPR is started right away, blood flow to the brain is only, at best, approximately half of what a normal beating heart delivers. The entire time that even the best quality CPR is being administered, the patient's brain is suffering serious injury [6]. Brain damage in the setting of cardiac arrest is the most common cause of death in patients who survive a resuscitation attempt" [6].
- "Those who don't go on to die after surviving a resuscitation attempt often experience memory, attention, and other cognitive deficits, leading to disability from work and anxiety and depression. Additionally, patients who experience brain injury following a resuscitation attempt have a significantly increased risk of developing dementia [7]. Not surprisingly, the more significant the patient's cognitive dysfunction, the greater the experience of caregiver strain" [8].

This is often enough information for patients and family members to feel informed enough, given the patient's medical status, to make a decision regarding a resuscitation attempt. It can be helpful to restate the original question.

- "I'll ask the original question again. If you were to die right now, would you want the medical community to undergo efforts to bring you back to life?"

Of note, there will be times when it is evident that the patient or family has carefully considered and definitively chosen the option of DNR, rendering the investigation of their understanding of CPR and the provision of education about CPR unnecessary. Because a decision of DNR carries a potentially life-limiting consequence, it is better to err on the side of full investigation and education and to let the patient and family tell you when they've heard enough to be confident in their choice.

The next task during a conversation about code status is to assess whether the patient's preference for resuscitation aligns with their health status, to ensure that patients understand the implications of their choice. If the risks of CPR outweigh the benefits, given the patient's age or health status, or if anything the patient has communicated about their values contradicts their code status wishes, it is usually helpful to paint a clear picture of CPR in their situation.

For instance, for a patient with end-stage disease who wants CPR, it is essential to explain the specific risks of a resuscitation attempt, which would include broken ribs, a punctured lung or heart, and the high likelihood of ending up in the ICU dependent on interventions keeping them alive. An explanation such as the following is often helpful,

- "In your situation, with your lung disease as advanced as it is, where I worry that your time is limited, if your body were to die, there is very little chance of a resuscitation attempt being successful. Even if we were able to bring you back, there is a very high likelihood that your body would then require extra support to remain alive, likely in the form of intubation and mechanical ventilation. Your family would then be faced with the decision to withdraw treatment and allow you to pass, leading back to the consideration we discussed earlier that is covered by your living will."

This type of explanation often provides the reassurance patients and family members need to feel comfortable choosing DNR.

Another example is the patient who wants CPR, who meets or is close to meeting hospice criteria, but who has very clearly specified a wish to pass away at home at the end of their life. This scenario represents a stark contradiction that many patients and families do not immediately understand and that a compassionate explanation can help them better appreciate.

- "With your cancer as advanced as it is, and which is currently not being treated, with your high level of symptoms, and with your stated wish to spend time at home with family and to pass away in your home, I would very much worry that choosing CPR might prevent your wishes from coming true at the moment of greatest importance."
- "As your body continues to decline, your organs, including your heart and lungs, will fail. Eventually, the reason you will die is that your disease has progressed beyond the point where your body can keep itself alive on its own. If, by very slim chance, we were successful in resuscitating you with CPR, there is a very high likelihood that you would require advanced and invasive interventions to remain alive, for instance, a breathing machine, without which you would likely pass away again."
- "You have told me that you want to have a soft landing at the end of life and to pass away peacefully in your sleep and at home. The way to ensure that happens is for you to choose to stay at home with the support of hospice care, where we will use medications to manage any symptoms you have so that you can pass away comfortably in your bed and not in the hospital. Does that make sense?"

It can also be helpful to put in perspective the risk of a patient experiencing the most common cause of death leading to CPR—cardiac arrest. Often, explaining to a patient, for instance, who is dying of cancer or age-related decline, that they are less likely to die from a cardiac arrest than their body's continued decline helps them process the reality of their medical journey, eliminating the false sense of hope that a resuscitation attempt might offer in extending their life.

For patients with advanced age or disease who yet choose CPR, an extra dose of compassion is required, as this level of disconnect between wishes and the medical reality often reflects spiritual or existential distress in the face of their imminent mortality. Provide reassurance to those patients, validating their choice and the effort required to have the conversation,

- "Okay, very good. I know this is such a difficult conversation."

It is important to revisit the conversation about resuscitation with these patients at any evolution of health status or interaction with the healthcare system (i.e., hospital admission, ER visit, or rehabilitation stay).

Sometimes, patients will provide a response indicating that they want CPR but only for a short time, saying, "Well, I would want them to do CPR for five minutes." To this type of response, it is important to explain that the question of a resuscitation attempt is black and white, with no in-between or prespecified time-limit option. For instance, you can explain,

- "The question of CPR is black and white. You can choose YES CPR or NO CPR, meaning 'DNR, or do not resuscitate,' but there is no option for 'Yes, I want CPR but only for a few minutes.' The medical professionals who perform CPR go through a protocol that involves chest compressions, rescue breaths, medications, airway support, and electric shock if required. They follow a step-wise approach until it is determined that pulse and respirations are restored or the patient is not recoverable. It's not possible to tell them to do CPR for only five minutes."

Other patients will respond by saying, "Well, it would depend. If I was going to survive, I would want them to try," or "I would want CPR, at least until they figure out what happened." To this type of response, it is important to help patients and families understand that it is typically not possible to know what happened to cause a patient's death until after the patient is recovered. It can be helpful to explain,

- "The only time we ever do CPR is when a patient has died. Only if we are successful in resuscitating them, can we then investigate the cause of their death. By that point, most patients will experience brain injury, and most of those who survive will go on to pass away from that brain damage."

This explanation helps tie the reality of the impact of going without oxygen delivery to the brain to the event of CPR, allowing patients to consider their mortality, quality of life, and desire for quantity of life in any case.

For patients with dementia, it is imperative to help patients and families appreciate the connection between brain injury that occurs during CPR and the expected subsequent progression of their baseline dementia. Often, a simple explanation is all that is needed to allow families to choose the option of DNR, reflecting their goals for supporting their loved one's long-term quality of life.

- "For patients with dementia, who are already experiencing brain failure resulting from the death of brain cells and neural networks, the brain injury that occurs during a CPR attempt will likely have a significant impact on their disease. It will push them further into the journey and greatly impact their ability to make it through the day without help."

When dementia is advanced, most families, upon hearing this, will choose DNR as a way to ensure their loved one's continued quality of life.

Patients with implantable cardioverter-defibrillators (ICDs) who choose DNR deserve additional conversation that should be guided by the diagnosis leading to the ICD implant and the patient's health status. While many patients receive an ICD in the setting of heart failure, which carries an increased risk of sudden death due to ventricular fibrillation, some patients receive an ICD to prevent sudden death due to ventricular fibrillation caused by hypertrophic cardiomyopathy. This inherited condition is not often terminal, especially if the patient has an ICD. These two patients would need very different explanations to help them make decisions about continuing or discontinuing their ICD therapies to align with their values.

Very frequently, patients and families do not understand the purpose of an ICD or why it was implanted. The first step is to assess the patient and family's understanding of the device by asking,

- "Do you know what the device in your chest is called, its job, and why it was put there?"

After listening to the patient's response, fill in the gaps in their understanding by describing the device and explaining its role in preventing the patient's death by linking its therapies to the patient's diagnosis.

To start, provide a basic description of the device and its purpose,

- "The device is called an ICD, or implantable cardioverter-defibrillator. Its job is to monitor the heart rhythm and deliver an electric shock to the patient's heart if it detects an abnormal rhythm that could cause the patient to die."

Patients who have never been shocked by their ICD should be well informed of the significant pain and emotional trauma that can accompany an ICD shock.

For a patient who received an ICD in the setting of heart failure, it would be appropriate to explain,

- "In your case, after your major heart attack five years ago, your heart function declined. Although you were given medication to support your heart muscle's recovery, your heart function remained low, indicating that your heart muscle was severely injured or even scarred by the damage from the heart attack. Heart muscle that is scarred tends to create abnormal electrical impulses that can disrupt the heart's normal electrical signaling, leading to a dangerous and deadly heart rhythm called ventricular fibrillation. Ventricular fibrillation causes the lower chambers of the heart—the ventricles—to quiver instead of relaxing and squeezing so that no blood is pumped forward, which can lead to sudden death. The ICD's job is to continually monitor the electrical rhythm of the heart muscle, and if it detects this deadly rhythm, to deliver an overwhelming electrical impulse to reset the heart's electrical circuitry so that the heart can resume its healthy heartbeat again. This impulse can be very painful, with patients describing it as getting kicked in the chest by a horse."

- "An ICD functions similarly to CPR, in that if you die because your heart stops, the ICD's job is to try to bring you back to life. For those ready to allow nature to take its course and who want a peaceful passing, it becomes critical to turn off the ICD therapies because a failing heart can trigger a very painful ICD impulse at a time when the patient prefers to be comfortable."

For a patient with hypertrophic cardiomyopathy, who is not expected to die from heart failure, the description would be very different.

- "In your case, your heart muscle is abnormally thick in places, and that can impact the electrical signaling in the heart, leading to a dangerous and deadly rhythm of the lower chambers called ventricular fibrillation. The ICD's job is to continually monitor the electrical rhythm of the heart muscle, and if it detects this deadly rhythm, to deliver an overwhelming electrical shock that resets the heart's electrical circuitry so that the heart can resume its healthy heartbeat again. This impulse can be very painful, with patients describing it as getting kicked in the chest by a horse."
- "An ICD functions similarly to CPR, in that if you die because your heart stops, the ICD's job is to try to bring you back to life. Because patients with hypertrophic cardiomyopathy rarely die from that disease if they have an ICD in place to monitor and respond to their heartbeat, patients who choose DNR may still want to keep their ICD therapies functioning to avoid a preventable death."

This type of commentary provides a foundation for helping patients navigate decisions about ICD therapies that uphold their values for longevity *and* quality of life. Decisions about ICD therapy are always highly personal, and, like the decisions about code status and approach to medical care, tend to shift with advancing age and disease. It is important to help patients understand the implications of their ICD to help them make the complicated decision about whether or not to turn off its therapies.

Patients with early-stage heart failure who have chosen DNR may be reluctant to turn off their ICD therapies. Provide reassurance that although an ICD might cause pain and emotional trauma, it may resuscitate the patient quickly, avoiding the brain injury that can accompany a CPR attempt. Although painful, an ICD shock also does not carry the risk of lung or heart puncture or broken ribs.

For patients with advanced or end-stage disease, including both heart and lung failure, it is crucial to discuss the increased likelihood of the ICD shocking the patient, especially if the patient has residual, untreatable coronary artery disease (CAD), which can lead to another heart attack, precipitating ventricular fibrillation and sudden death. Patients with advanced lung failure should be helped to understand how the heart often fails in the setting of lung failure, which could lead the ICD to shock the patient, especially toward the end of life.

Despite this education, some patients with advanced or end-stage heart failure may choose to continue their ICD therapies despite choosing DNR. A decision to turn off ICD therapies, like a decision to choose DNR, is often fraught and can reflect an existential coming to terms with one's mortality that might need to be accomplished in stages. Provide compassion and whatever time patients and families need to make decisions that align with their values, knowing that a decision to turn off ICD therapies at the end of life can feel tantamount to signing one's own death certificate.

For patients with hypertrophic cardiomyopathy, it might make good sense to keep the ICD therapies active until the patient reaches the end of life and transitions to comfort-focused care, when any ICD therapy would be antithetical to the philosophy of hospice care and patient wishes for a soft landing.

A final note about ICDs: in addition to providing life-preserving therapies, ICDs function as pacemakers. Patients and families must be educated that while the ICD therapies can be turned off, pacemaker function can continue within the same device. Of course, many patients have a pacemaker instead of an ICD, and these patients also frequently remain confused about their pacemaker's function, especially at the moment of death. It is important to help patients and families understand,

- "The job of a pacemaker is to monitor the heart's electrical signaling and to provide an impulse to the heart if the heart's electrical signaling system fails. Whereas an ICD can provide an overwhelming impulse to reset a heart that has experienced a dangerous and deadly heart rhythm, a pacemaker provides a softer intervention. It continually monitors the signaling that causes the ventricles to squeeze. If it notices an impulse is not reaching the ventricle, it can stimulate at just the right moment to cause the ventricles to squeeze together so that the heartbeat (squeeze) is well-coordinated and strong. A pacemaker's impulse is much less invasive, and if the settings are adjusted correctly, the patient should not be aware of its function."
- "The decision to turn off pacemaker therapies typically relates to whether the patient's heart function is dependent on the pacemaker. In patients dependent on their pacemaker therapies, the device can be considered a life-prolonging intervention that the patient or surrogate may discontinue. Stopping pacemaker therapies in this case can lead to patient death, but before death may result in a symptomatic, slow heart rate leading to other issues. This can be very uncomfortable and even cause patients to suffer. Often, pacemaker therapies are not discontinued at the end of life, either in a stand-alone pacemaker or inside an ICD. When patients reach their final seconds of life, the pacemaker will simply stop delivering an impulse when the dead ventricular tissue no longer reacts."

The cardiology team's insight into the pacemaker or ICD function is often helpful and should be integrated into a conversation with the patient and family to help support their careful consideration of therapies, especially when patients choose DNR or get to the point of meeting hospice criteria.[4]

---

[4] Note that decisions to discontinue ICD or pacemaker therapies represent a nexus of ethical and moral decision making impacting patients, families, and healthcare providers. Discussions by Ballentine [9] and Quill et al. [10] nicely capture the complex and nuanced nature of this topic. A

Helping patients and families understand how these therapies function and cease functioning at the end of life is critically important to supporting care decisions that align with their values, alleviating fears, and reassuring them that a peaceful passing is possible.

Investigate Patient Preferences for Approach to Medical Care

Continuing with Section B on the POLST form, transition the conversation into a discussion of patient preferences for *approach to medical care* by saying,

- "The question I just asked was about a situation where you have died. The next question on this form is about a situation in which you are alive but need more medical care than you might typically be able to receive at home."

There are two practical approaches to this part of the conversation based on how advanced the patient's disease is. For patients who do not yet meet hospice criteria, it can be helpful to introduce all three options; however, be aware that if the person has selected YES CRP, then the only possible option they can choose in Section B is the first one—Full Treatments.

- "There are three options to specify your preference for the approach to medi-cal care based on your overarching goal. Patient choice tends to shift across the lifespan, with many patients wanting a less invasive approach to care as they get older or as disease progresses."
- "The first options refer to different approaches to care in the hospital. The first option is called Full Treatments. That means your goal is to prolong life by any medical means available. In other words, you would be open to anything and everything possible to help you recover to your former state of health. That would include escalations of care that typically happen in the ICU and that are often supports for organs that have failed. This includes intubation (a tube to maintain your airway) and mechanical ventilation (a machine that breathes for you) if your lungs fail, dialysis if your kidneys fail, pressor medi-cations that force your heart to pump if your heart fails, a feeding tube, etc."
- "The second option is called Selective Treatments. That means your goal is to attempt to restore function while avoiding intensive care and invasive treatments. In other words, you would prefer to avoid the ICU and the escalations of care that typically occur there and would prefer to be treated on the medical floor, with IV or oral medications and less invasive forms of airway support, such as a nasal cannula or a BIPAP or CPAP machine rather than mechanical ventilation."

---

proposed set of guidelines for the discontinuation of ICD and pacemaker therapies by Quill et al. [10], beyond the scope of this text, accounts for the complexity of decision making, the need to anticipate possible resulting symptoms, and the ethical and moral effort involved in helping patients and families arrive at a decision that aligns with their values.

- "The third option is called Comfort-focused Treatments. That means your goal is to maximize comfort, not prolong life, and allow natural death. Generally, this option is picked by or for people who have enrolled in hospice care, meaning their disease is advanced to the point that we worry their time is limited, and they are ready to allow nature to take its course. However, this option is not limited to people enrolled in hospice."

For patients who meet hospice criteria but are not yet enrolled, an alternative approach is to first start with a general inquiry of the patient's willingness to return to the hospital for care by asking,

- "How do you feel about returning to the hospital again?"

This question allows patients who have arrived at a point in their journey where they would prefer never to return to the hospital again to articulate that wish. Often, patients with advanced age or disease will answer this question definitively and in the negative, "No, I don't want to go back to the hospital ever again."

For patients with advanced disease who meet hospice criteria and who are hospice-minded—who are ready to allow nature to take its course and who have indicated a wish for DNR—this type of response would warrant transitioning the conversation into a discussion of hospice care by moving into the Hospice Arc in the Arc of Conversation (Chap. 12). Make this transition by asking,

- "Do you know what type of treatment option is available to patients with very advanced disease who no longer want to return to the hospital for care?"

Many patients prefer not to return to the hospital but do not yet meet hospice criteria. Selecting Comfort-focused Treatments on their POLST form ensures their goal to avoid hospitalization can be met.

- "It makes sense that you don't want to go back to the hospital again. But right now, you don't meet what we call hospice criteria, meaning your disease is not advanced enough yet that we could enroll you in hospice care. If you were enrolled in hospice care, and if you were to have a crisis, instead of calling 911, you would call the hospice team. They would respond to your crisis, which would be the mechanism by which we could ensure that you could remain at home and not need to go back to the hospital, even if your symptoms changed quickly or became severe. But for people who don't yet meet hospice criteria and are not yet enrolled in hospice care, selecting Comfort-focused Treatments on your POLST form will ensure that even if someone calls 911 or takes you to the ER, you will receive the care you want and no more. Does that make sense?"

Provide patients and families time to process the options for approach to medical care before asking, "What do you think?" Most people who have been successfully led through the Arc of Conversation to this point can easily articulate a preference for the approach to medical care. Usually, their choice will align with what would make sense given their health status.

Some people will need assistance considering the different options. Support their consideration by connecting the patient's disease trajectory and health status with interventions that might be required to help them recover. For instance, patients with heart failure or COPD may not understand why and when they might need to be intubated and mechanically ventilated. Connecting worsening organ failure to the need for increasingly invasive medical care is an important way of empowering patients and families to proactively align their medical care with their values *before* a crisis occurs.

When a patient's choice wildly misaligns with their medical reality, it is especially important to connect their disease and its progression with the possibility of interventions. For example, a patient who meets hospice criteria with COPD who chooses Full Treatments would almost certainly benefit from a more detailed conversation about the high likelihood of their need for intubation and mechanical ventilation, the equally low likelihood of their ability to recover from those interventions, and their significant risk of passing away in the hospital.

To help patients and families through this type of conversation, use the investigate then educate approach, asking,

- "Do you know why you might need to be intubated and mechanically ventilated?"

Then, link their worsening lung failure to the likelihood of needing increasingly invasive airway support in the setting of an exacerbation.

- "As an organ fails, it struggles more and more to perform its primary function, and it's usually only a matter of time until the organ suffers some imbalance from which it cannot recover without help. We call these episodes exacerbations, and with COPD exacerbations, patients are at risk of developing pneumonia and varying degrees of respiratory failure. As the lungs continue to fail, the treatments in the hospital to help the patient recover tend to become increasingly invasive. Whereas early in the disease, a patient may only require a nasal cannula to recover, later, the patient may need the support of a CPAP or BiPAP machine, and later still, they may need to be intubated and mechanically ventilated. Patients with advanced COPD who need that level of support often cannot survive without it, and families are often faced with a decision to withdraw treatment in the hospital, allowing the patient to pass there."

Painting a picture of disease progression by linking treatment options with the stage of disease is a powerful way of supporting patient autonomy by empowering patients and families with accurate understanding. Most patients and families, when thus informed, will be able to make choices for medical care that accurately reflect their values.

Patient preferences for resuscitation and approach to medical care typically evolve with the evolution of disease, reflecting a value system responsive to patient experience and understanding of their medical journey. Patient choice typically shifts across the lifespan and a disease journey, moving from **YES CPR plus Full Treatments** to **NO CPR (DNR) plus Full Treatments** to **NO CPR (DNR) plus Selective Treatments** to **NO CPR (DNR) plus Comfort-focused Treatments**. This evolution underscores the necessity of continual collaboration with patients and families about medical wishes and personal values across a disease trajectory, not only at the end.

If, along the way of this conversation, other preferences emerge around treatments not explicitly mentioned on the POLST form, such as dialysis, transfusions, transplants, extracorporeal mechanical oxygenation (ECMO), etc., you can note them in Section C, Additional Orders or Instructions.

Investigate Patient Preferences for Artificial Nutrition by Tube

Continuing with Section D on the POLST form, start with a general statement investigating the patient or family's preference for a feeding tube, asking,

- "The next section on this form is about artificial nutrition by tube."

Often, this is enough to allow patients and families who oppose such interventions to articulate that wish. Usually, they will shake their head or say something like, "No, I wouldn't want to be alive if I couldn't eat," or "No, that's artificial life support, and I wouldn't want that."

For patients and families who do not offer such a response or who look pensive, explain that,

- "The options are: 'I would be okay with feeding through a new or existing tube surgically inserted into my abdomen'; 'I would be okay with a trial period of feeding through a tube, but not one surgically placed'; or 'I wouldn't want artificial feeding of any kind.'"

Provide time for patients and families to consider these options, knowing this question often reminds people of relatives or national new stories about people who experienced artificial nutrition. Encourage sharing of these experiences, listening for concerns, fears, worries, and preferences in their descriptions. Many people will respond with thoughtful speculation, such as, "Well, I guess it would depend on why I needed it."

Validate this response before investigating the patient or family's understanding of the circumstances in which artificial nutrition is typically offered and providing education to paint a picture of those circumstances.

- "Very good. Do you know the most common reasons a person might need artificial nutrition by tube?"

People commonly answer, "If the person can't eat or swallow."

Supporting their answer, transition the conversation into an explanation of three of the most common circumstances in which a feeding tube is offered, painting a picture of why and when this type of intervention might be offered, allowing patients and families to consider how a feeding tube might align or conflict with their values.

- "Yes. One of the most common reasons people are offered a feeding tube is after a stroke. A stroke, which cuts off blood flow to a portion of the brain, can damage the brainstem, which controls the swallow reflex. The swallow reflex moves the little flap of skin, called the epiglottis, over the airway to protect our lungs from aspirating or inhaling food or liquid when we eat or drink. After a stroke, patients undergo a swallow study to see if their swallow reflex is functioning appropriately, and if it isn't, they aren't allowed to eat or drink by mouth and instead are offered a nasogastric tube for feeding that is inserted into the nasal passage and down into the stomach. That tube can only stay in place for a short time (up to several weeks) because it can erode the inside of the nasal passage. During those weeks, the patient will work with speech and language therapy to hopefully recover their swallow function. If the patient is unable to recover their swallow function, they will be offered a permanent feeding tube that is surgically inserted directly into the abdomen."
- "I want us to think about what it is like for a patient to experience a permanent feeding tube if they are not able to swallow safely after a stroke. If the patient can't swallow safely enough to eat or drink by mouth, they also cannot swallow their saliva safely. Saliva continually builds up in the mouth, collecting at the back of the throat, and not only can this saliva leak down into their lungs, causing aspiration pneumonia, but the build-up of saliva in the back of the throat can cause patients to feel incredible anxiety and panic from the sensation that they are suffocating. A stroke also often damages the diaphragm and chest muscles and reduces the strength of the patient's cough, which can also impact their ability to clear saliva from the back of their throat."
- "Also, imagine what happens when we introduce liquid food into the gut of a patient whose swallow function isn't reliable. If that patient were to lean over at just the right time, or if the patient is lying down and some of the liquid food regurgitates up the esophagus into the back of the mouth, in a throat that cannot swallow properly, where do you think that liquid food is likely to go?"

This provides an opportunity to gauge whether the patient and family are following the explanation and can appreciate the risks of this therapy. Most people will speculate that the liquid food will go into the lungs.

- "Yes, that liquid can very easily leak down the trachea, or windpipe, into the right lung, leading to aspiration pneumonia, which is the most common side effect of a feeding tube and the most common cause of death for patients with a feeding tube. Developing aspiration pneumonia leads to hospitalizations,

and if pneumonia leads to respiratory failure, the patient may need to be supported with intubation and mechanical ventilation in the ICU."
- "One of my patients experienced a stroke, was unable to recover his swallow function, received a feeding tube, and then experienced several hospitalizations for aspiration pneumonia and a number of ER visits for panic attacks because he was unable to swallow his saliva. He and his wife eventually decided to withdraw the feeding tube and enroll in hospice care, and he passed several weeks later."

This very helpful narrative empowers patients and families with an accurate picture of a therapy that most people will want to avoid if made fully aware of the risks.

- "Another reason patients are offered a feeding tube is when they have head or neck cancer. A feeding tube is surgically inserted into the abdomen before the start of radiation therapy. The patient is fed by tube and not allowed to eat by mouth until after the patient has healed from the inflammation caused by the radiation treatments. The expectation is that the patient will recover from the radiation therapy, the tube will be removed, and the patient will be allowed to return to eating by mouth again. I have seen this work successfully to support several patients with head and neck cancer."

This scenario is particularly helpful for patients with advanced age or disease, allowing them to consider two interventions—radiation and a feeding tube—in the context of their values outside a medical crisis.

- "The other reason patients are sometimes offered a feeding tube is when they reach a point in either a Frailty journey or Dementia journey where their body is making a metabolic shift toward breaking down more tissue than it builds."

If the full description of the metabolic shift has not already been provided, it should be provided at this point (see Chap. 15). Assuming it has already been described, continue,

- "If the body has transitioned toward metabolic decline, we, the medical community, have no effective method to reverse that trend. Even forcing nutrition on the body with a feeding tube does not make the body capable of utilizing that nutrition. Furthermore, introducing liquid food into a body that is in decline can overwhelm the heart and lungs, whose job it is to maintain the fluid balance in the body, causing edema (swelling) in the legs, which can lead to weepy skin, skin breakdown, and infection; fluid can overload the lungs leading to shortness of breath and cough; and the excess fluid can worsen heart failure."
- "When patients with advanced dementia get to the point in their journey when their body starts making this metabolic transition, they are also at the point in their journey when their brainstem begins to degrade, and the swallow function starts to decline. A feeding tube in the setting of advanced dementia is

usually not a good idea because patients can't remember why they have it; they chew through it or pull it out; and, of course, the feeding tube increases their risk for aspiration pneumonia, which is the most common cause of death for patients with Alzheimer's disease even without a feeding tube."

- "While it is not possible to cover every condition in which a feeding tube might be offered, it is important to know that anytime the swallow function is impacted, a feeding tube carries a high risk for aspiration pneumonia."

Most people prefer to focus on quality of life over quantity in the setting of advanced age or disease. When provided with a full picture of the risks and potential for negative outcomes of an invasive treatment like a feeding tube, particularly in the setting of advanced age or disease, most patients and families will choose to avoid such interventions.

Completing the Conversation and the POLST Form

Once the selections on a POLST form have been finalized, it must be signed by the patient or the patient's surrogate, and a physician or, in some states, a nurse practitioner or physician assistant. The back side of the form contains some fields that are helpful to complete, including contact information, who was involved in the discussion, and whether advance directives are also available and were consulted.

While most states specify that the most recent form rules, it is important to ensure that POLST forms do not contradict advance directives. Because most advance directives do not cover preferences for code status, this is not typically an issue.

To wrap up a conversation about the medical preferences covered by the POLST form, direct patients to hang the signed form on or near their refrigerator, where emergency medical technicians (EMTs) are trained to look for it.

- "The POLST form should be kept on the front or side of the fridge, where emergency medical technicians (EMTs) know to look for it to quickly understand your wishes. Even though some advance directives can also specify a wish for DNR, EMTs typically do not have time or scope of authority to interpret legal paperwork. Rather, they need to see the easy-to-read check marks on the POLST form."

Particularly when patients specify a wish for DNR, it is crucial that they complete and sign the POLST form with a healthcare provider.

- "It is important to complete this form when your choice evolves from CPR to DNR because EMTs are required to perform CPR unless they see a medical order that refuses it, such as a POLST. EMTs cannot take someone else's word for it, and an advance directive is not a medical order."

Finally, encourage patients to discuss their specified preferences with whoever will be responsible for making medical decisions on their behalf should they become incapacitated.

- "It's important to understand that while completing this form is very important, it is equally important that the loved ones whose job it is to make decisions for you if you become incapacitated are aware of your wishes. Be sure to discuss the choices you have made on this form with your surrogate medical decision maker(s) and other loved ones."

Legal Considerations

Durable Power of Attorney

Just as it is important for patients to specify a medical surrogate decision maker, it is equally important that they specify who they would want to make legal and financial decisions for them if they were to become incapacitated, a decision that can be documented in a Durable Power of Attorney. Typically, the authority to make medical decisions and the authority to make financial decisions are separately documented (in a medical durable power of attorney (MDPOA) and durable power of attorney (DPOA), respectively) and often held by different people close to the patient. The word "durable" in this context indicates that the authority granted to the surrogate to act on the patient's behalf continues even after the patient becomes incapacitated.

For all patients with terminal disease, but especially for those with dementia, specifying a surrogate legal and financial decision maker is critical, as decisions about medical care will often require financial and legal decisions as well. For instance, patients with dementia who live alone will need to be supported either by in-home care or by moving to a care facility, both of which incur financial costs not covered by Medicare or most other health insurance. Someone will need to be empowered to access and utilize the patient's financial and real property (e.g., real estate) resources to support the patient on their journey. Often, patients need to "spend down" resources to qualify for Medicaid, which can cover the cost of support in the home or long-term care. Additionally, because patients with dementia are at increased risk of financial and legal fraud, they will need the protection of someone who can appropriately manage their finances to keep them safe.

All patients should be encouraged to consider the legal and financial impact of their disease and death on their partners, married or unmarried. Partners of patients with terminal disease of any kind should be encouraged to identify an alternative surrogate decision maker for their own legal and financial safekeeping.

Patients whose partners would be at risk of losing their housing or other resources after the patient's death should be encouraged to consider their wishes for their partners, and to specify in a will, who should take control of their assets. Although these matters are beyond the scope of this book, social workers, case managers, elder attorneys, and financial navigators can assist patients and partners with these considerations. Because patient-centered care means caring for loved ones and family members, these considerations are well within the scope of caring for patients, and appropriate referrals should be made.

Guardianship and Conservatorship

Patients without the ability to make medical, legal, or financial decisions, who have not specified who they would want to be their medical, legal, or financial surrogate decision makers, are of particular concern. Guardianship and conservatorship are legal processes conducted by the court system, in which someone is appointed to make decisions for a person who lacks legal or mental capacity to make decisions for themselves.

States can define the terms and the scope of authority differently, but generally speaking, "guardianship" refers to legal responsibility for a minor child or never-competent adult, or specifically health and well-being decision-making authority for an incapacitated adult. "Conservatorship" generally refers to financial authority. Typically, these powers are separately conferred and held by different people.

Both processes are costly and time-intensive and best avoided, if possible. Medical guardianship can be avoided by several mechanisms, most easily by completing a durable power of attorney for health-care or medical durable power of attorney, to specify who should act as the person's medical decision maker if the person becomes incapacitated. Likewise, conservatorship can be avoided by estate planning, including the completion of a durable power of attorney.

Patients who have not specified medical, legal, or financial surrogate decision makers should be encouraged to complete MDPOAs and DPOAs. Those who are without a spouse or other family who are reliable candidates for surrogates should be referred to case management, social work, or financial navigation for referral to appropriate professionals who can assist them.

Competence and Capacity

There is a great deal of confusion in the medical community regarding the terms "competence" and "capacity." It is important to understand the difference so that appropriate support can be provided to patients and their families.

Competence is a legal term referring to a determination made by a court about a person's ability to engage in a specific task, such as standing trial or making medical decisions. A competency judgment involves an evaluation by a medical professional, typically a psychiatrist, but a judge makes the final determination. Competence is not something that medical professionals determine in their day-to-day work with people, outside the exception of psychiatrists specializing in evaluations to support competence decisions by a court.

Capacity, on the other hand, is very much something that medical professionals should feel confident assessing in their day-to-day work with patients, such as in the hospital or in the clinic. Capacity is not a legal determination and is not determined by attorneys or judges. Rather, capacity determinations are made by medical providers. That said, a determination of capacity can have profound effects on legal processes, such as the initiation of a medical durable power of attorney or the validity of a will. Most surrogates' authority only officially begins with a determination of the incapacity of the patient.

A critical misunderstanding about capacity decisions is that many healthcare providers believe that these determinations can only be made by psychiatrists. This is not true. *Any* provider involved in the care of a patient should feel empowered to assess whether the patient has decision-making capacity for medical, legal, and financial matters. For patients with dementia, whose disease will rob them of these essential capacities, it is critical that professionals supporting this patient population develop a rich understanding of the disease, learn when capacity tends to be lost on this journey, and how to appropriately determine capacity in conversations with patients.

Another important misunderstanding about capacity decisions is that many providers believe capacity is an all-or-nothing situation. This is also not true. A patient, for example, may have the capacity to determine what they want to eat but not to determine whether they should have invasive surgery to repair a hip fracture. This is what we mean by "decision-making capacity is decision specific."

Finally, it is important to understand that except for patients on the dementia journey, capacity for medical, legal, and financial decision making can change from day to day or even over the course of a day, depending on many factors, including medication regiments, time of day, disease progression, environmental changes, etc. Patients hospitalized for infections, fractures, and other major health events can experience a loss of capacity in the setting of delirium, which frequently resolves but can often unmask underlying dementia. Delirium that does not resolve with the resolution of the medical issue at hand should prompt concern for dementia, and patients should be referred to neurology or a dementia specialist for further evaluation of their cognitive capacity.

Unfortunately, modern medical practice does not often allow providers the time needed with patients and their families to accurately assess patients' decision-making capacity. This is a real problem that frequently results in providers discussing and offering treatment options to patients who *appear* to have medical decision-making capacity but who do not, leading to treatments that the family would have chosen to avoid had they understood the reality of their loved ones' cognitive deficits.

Patients with dementia, in particular, in their drive to be perceived as competent, capable, and in control, and given their capacity to read social cues from tone of voice, facial expression, and body language, often appear to follow a conversation but struggle, in follow up, to explain what was discussed or the repercussions of a choice. Single, short-duration conversations are typically insufficient to determine whether a patient has medical decision-making capacity, particularly in dementia, which early on robs patients of short- and delayed recall due to the loss of recent memory storage capacity in the hippocampus. Later, patients lose their prefrontal cortex executive functions for logic, reason, anticipation, planning, and judgment, further impacting their decision-making capacity.

Because dementia predictably robs patients of their capacity to make medical, legal, and financial decisions, and because dementia is so prevalent in the population older than 65 (as high as 33% of patients over age 85), there should be a low threshold for performing a cognitive assessment of patients who are hospitalized, and for consulting neurology or a dementia specialist to accurately assess the patient's dementia. Primary care providers and hospitalists should be armed with the knowledge and skills to accurately assess dementia, understanding that loss of complex medical, legal, and financial decision making capacity tends to occur in step with the loss of capacity to handle the instrumental activities of daily living (IADLs), which also rely on prefrontal cortex skills, including logic, reason, abstract thinking, computation, planning, and judgment. These losses occur during the Cognitive Function stage and around an MMSE score of 16/30 for patients with Alzheimer's dementia [11]. Thus, knowing that a patient with dementia needs assistance with managing appointments, medications, and finances should prompt an evaluation of their capacity for complicated medical, legal, and financial decisions.

Because dementia is a leading cause of patient death, palliative care teams and those caring for patients in hospitals, long-term care, and rehabilitation facilities should also be trained to accurately evaluate where a patient is in their dementia journey and empowered with the ability to comment on patient capacity for legal, medical, and financial decision making.

When appropriate, families of patients with dementia should be provided with a letter specifying that their loved one has lost the capacity to make medical, legal, and financial decisions on account of the advanced nature of their disease, so that family members can step in to manage these tasks and keep their loved ones safe. Check with your institution to ensure the Legal and Risk department approves the language. It is not uncommon for Legal and Risk department employees, including attorneys, to also be confused about competence and capacity and to work from the inaccurate assumption that attorneys and not medical providers should make capacity decisions.

Because caring for patients following any terminal trajectory can require medical, legal, and financial support by families, having a healthcare system empowered with the knowledge and confidence to assess and comment on the patients' medical, legal, and financial capacity is a critically important aspect of patient-centered care.

References

1. Diem SJ, Lantos JD, Tulsky JA. Cardiopulmonary resuscitation on television. Miracles and misinformation. N Engl J Med. 1996;334(24):1578–82. https://doi.org/10.1056/NEJM199606133342406.
2. Portanova J, Irvine K, Yi JY, Enguidanos S. It isn't like this on TV: revisiting CPR survival rates depicted on popular TV shows. Resuscitation. 2015;96:148–50. https://doi.org/10.1016/j.resuscitation.2015.08.002. Epub 2015 Aug 19.
3. Yan S, Gan Y, Jiang N, et al. The global survival rate among adult out-of-hospital cardiac arrest patients who received cardiopulmonary resuscitation: a systematic review and meta-analysis. Crit Care. 2020;24:61. https://doi.org/10.1186/s13054-020-2773-2.
4. Andersen LW, Holmberg MJ, Berg KM, Donnino MW, Granfeldt A. In-hospital cardiac arrest: a review. JAMA. 2019;321(12):1200–10. https://doi.org/10.1001/jama.2019.1696. PMID: 30912843; PMCID: PMC6482460.
5. Hagberg G, Ihle-Hansen H, Sandset EC, Jacobsen D, Wimmer H, Ihle-Hansen H. Long term cognitive function after cardiac arrest: a mini-review. Front Aging Neurosci. 2022;14:885226. https://doi.org/10.3389/fnagi.2022.885226. PMID: 35721022; PMCID: PMC9204346.
6. Sandroni C, Cronberg T, Sekhon M. Brain injury after cardiac arrest: pathophysiology, treatment, and prognosis. Intensive Care Med. 2021;47(12):1393–414. https://doi.org/10.1007/s00134-021-06548-2. Epub 2021 Oct 27. PMID: 34705079; PMCID: PMC8548866.
7. Secher N, Adelborg K, Szentkúti P, Christiansen CF, Granfeldt A, Henderson VW, Sørensen HT. Evaluation of neurologic and psychiatric outcomes after hospital discharge among adult survivors of cardiac arrest. JAMA Netw Open. 2022;5(5):e2213546. https://doi.org/10.1001/jamanetworkopen.2022.13546. PMID: 35639383; PMCID: PMC9157268.
8. Wachelder EM, Moulaert VR, van Heugten C, Verbunt JA, Bekkers SC, Wade DT. Life after survival: long-term daily functioning and quality of life after an out-of-hospital cardiac arrest. Resuscitation. 2009;80(5):517–22. https://doi.org/10.1016/j.resuscitation.2009.01.020. Epub 2009 Mar 17.
9. Ballentine JM. Pacemaker and defibrillator deactivation in competent hospice patients: an ethical consideration. Am J Hosp Palliat Care. 2005;22(1):14–9. https://doi.org/10.1177/104990910502200106.
10. Quill TE, Barold SS, Sussman BL. Discontinuing an implantable cardioverter defibrillator as a life-sustaining treatment. Am J Cardiol. 1994;74(2):205–7. https://doi.org/10.1016/0002-9149(94)90107-4. PMID: 7726890.
11. Karlawish J. Assessment of decision-making capacity in adults. 2023. https://www.uptodate.com/contents/assessment-of-decision-making-capacity-in-adults. Assessed 19 February 2023.

Hospice Care Education for Patients and Families

17

Healthcare providers working with patients with terminal disease should be well versed in the basics of hospice care and able to provide a general overview of hospice care to patients and their families. Remember, death is not the surprise ending of a human life. All patients who do not die suddenly will be eligible for hospice care at some point in their lives.

> **Objectives When Providing Hospice Education to Patients and Families**
> - Present important hospice facts.
> - Describe hospice philosophy.
> - Discuss approach to hospice care.
> - Discuss the location options and cost of hospice care.
> - Discuss the next steps for patients and families ready for hospice care.

Present Important Hospice Facts

When moving patients and families through the Hospice Care Arc, listen carefully for concerns or fears that reflect common misconceptions about hospice held by the general public and many people working in the medical field. Address any concerns or misconceptions immediately by presenting important hospice facts because untended fears remain an obstacle to hearing what is being said.

Hospice Fact 1: Hospice Care Can Be Provided for Weeks or Months, not Just Days

Often, when people are asked "What does hospice mean to you?", they will visibly cringe or articulate concerns indicating that they believe the patient is not close to dying, such as "Oh well, I'm not ready for hospice" or "She's not there yet."

© The Author(s), under exclusive license to Springer Nature Switzerland AG 2024
A. Shaw, PA, *The Arc of Conversation*,
https://doi.org/10.1007/978-3-031-70495-6_17

A helpful follow-up question is as follows:

- "When you think of hospice, how much time do you think a person has left before passing?"

This investigation allows people to provide an answer that might reveal their belief that hospice care is only for the final few days of life.

Regardless of the timeframe provided by the answers to this question, which can range from "Just a few days" to "six months," offer the following commentary.

- "Hospice is a Medicare benefit intended to provide patients and families *at least* six months of comfort care and quality of life at the end of life. However, there is no absolute limit for the length of time patients can remain in hospice care. When we consider hospice care, we tend to think of six months left of life. Some patients will live longer than six months, while others will not. Ideally, we would identify the exact moment when each patient meets hospice criteria, giving patients and their families the most time to benefit from hospice care."
- "Hospice patients are regularly requalified, or 'certified,' for hospice care. To continue to qualify, patients must show some objective or measurable decline, such as weight loss, worsening symptoms, or disease progression resulting in an increasing need for care."

At this point in the conversation, patients and families often ask for prognostic information, inquiring, "I know you can't know for sure, but can you tell me how much time you think I might have left?" This question can be difficult for people to articulate, reflecting a vulnerability (and bravery) in the face of existential fear that most of us believe we will never have to face. Tend to the emotional content of this question first, expressing compassion and empathy and providing the reassurance that,

- "You're right; none of us can know how much time a person will have left."

Then, address the humanity in this question, providing the reassurance and insight patients and families seek about how much time they may have left to focus on the things that matter most and support their sense of self, family, purpose, and love.

- "But we can know when a patient has reached a point in their life when their time is likely limited and further treatment options will not likely improve their health or delay the progression of their illness. Knowing this can help patients and families make decisions that allow them to focus on what matters most—expressing and experiencing love. For each person and family, that might look different. It might mean planning a holiday celebration or family gathering, tidying up practical affairs, or inviting relatives or friends to say their goodbyes before it's too late."

This is a humanistic, patient- and family-centered approach to providing prognostic information.

Remember never to provide specific prognostic information, such as, "You have two weeks left." Such specificity reflects an arrogance that is off-putting to patients and families, is usually incorrect, and risks offending personal beliefs about who or what is ultimately in charge of the end of life. It also risks setting up expectations that are likely to be wrong.

Prognosis should only ever be described by a range of time, such as "hours to a day(s)," "days to week(s)," "weeks to month(s)," or "months to year(s)," delivered compassionately and humbly and with the disclaimer, "While we can't know for sure, I worry that you are at a point in your journey where you may have just days to week(s) left," adjusting the range to align with the prognostic expectation. This allows room for human error and for patient and family spiritual or religious beliefs to be supported while also acknowledging the humbling reality of disease progression and end-of-life decline. See Chap. 5 for more information on prognostication.

For patients with little time left, it is very supportive to recommend that they consider encouraging anyone who wants to visit to do so as soon as possible. Families are often dispersed across the country, and those far away are often not kept in the loop on patient diagnosis and decline. Articulating this recommendation supports most people's end-of-life desire to focus on the things that matter most. A compassionate way to make this suggestion is to provide the following response, adjusting the recommendation to align with the prognostic estimate.

- "With where you are in your journey, I recommend reaching out to any family you would like to visit with to encourage them to come and see you as soon as possible. Although I hope you have many weeks left, we cannot know. You might encourage them to visit within the next few days to week(s)."

For patients on the cancer and organ failure trajectories, where decline can occur precipitously or at any subsequent hospitalization, recommendations for visits sooner rather than later are usually appropriate.

While prognosis can be challenging, and although patients at the end of any disease trajectory can experience rapid decline and death from even innocuous-appearing causes, such as urinary tract infections or respiratory infections, it can also be reassuring to patients who likely have more time left to be provided with this information.

- "I want to provide you with some reassurance that I don't think you're going to pass away imminently, meaning I don't have reason to believe you will die in the next week."

Hospice Fact 2: Medications that Contribute to Comfort Are Continued When a Patient Goes on Hospice Care, Though Some Others May Be Stopped

Many patients will respond to the inquiry of, "What does hospice mean to you?" by sharing the worry that all the patient's medications will be stopped. Some providers assume this is true as well and stop all medications before sending a patient to hospice. This is not recommended and can lead to an acute worsening of symptoms. Unless the patient is very close to passing and is unable to swallow pills or take anything by mouth, hospice teams should be deferred to regarding decisions about discontinuing medications. The following commentary can be helpful in providing accurate information about hospice medications.

- "Because the goal of hospice care is to keep people comfortable along their journey, the hospice team will continue medications working to control symptoms of disease that patients bring to the end of their lives. This includes medications helping to manage the patient's mood."
- "There are some medications that are typically discontinued, like blood thinners, given the risk that a fall could pose to a patient at the end of life. Decisions about whether to continue or stop medications are made for each patient individually by the hospice team, which will carefully consider the patient's disease mix and how best to keep them comfortable."

Whenever a medication is stopped, an explanation that makes reasonable medical sense should be provided to reassure patients and families that the decision to stop the medication is in the patient's best interest and is not being done merely because hospice care does not provide life-prolonging interventions. The explanation that a medication is being stopped because "hospice doesn't use medications to prolong life" is never appropriate and should not be articulated. This is callous, unkind, and insensitive and leaves people feeling like the medical community is giving up on them.

Rather, an explanation that is compassionate, reassuring, and reasonable should be provided, such as,

- "Some medications that are designed for long-term benefit can reasonably be stopped. An example is cholesterol medications. Because these medications provide benefits over many months and years, they can be stopped safely for most patients receiving hospice care. Other medications can increase risks to patients at the end of life. For example, blood thinners in patients who might fall can lead to life-limiting brain bleeds or other internal bleeding events. Insulin use in patients with type 2 diabetes who are not eating very much can also be problematic, leading to hypoglycemia—a very low blood sugar level—which can lead to a diabetic coma and death. For these patients, unless they have a history of very high blood sugar levels that caused symptoms or led to hospitalizations, we typically recommend that they stop their insulin. Also, pricking a finger multiple times daily to check blood sugar levels is uncomfortable, and hospice care is focused entirely on patient comfort."

Reasonable explanations like this make people feel that decisions about their medications come from a caring place.

Hospice Fact 3: Morphine Is not Used to Help People Die Faster on Hospice Care

The idea that morphine is used to help people die on hospice likely derives from the temporal connection between someone with severe agitation or pain finally being made comfortable and their passing soon after. Clarifying this connection can be helpful.

- "Commonly, people assume morphine is used to help people pass, but that is not legal, and that is not how morphine is used in hospice care. This idea probably comes from the observation that when patients with severe pain or agitation are finally made comfortable with appropriate medication, their bodies seem willing to let go."
- "Rather, morphine is used for comfort care."
- "Morphine is started at very low and safe doses in patients who were not previously taking any narcotic. Patients on hospice should not worry about overdosing because narcotics are started at very low doses and increased slowly."

Hospice Fact 4: People Receiving Hospice Care Can Remain as Active as Their Health and Strength Allow

The idea that people must be bed-bound or required to stay at home or in a facility when they are enrolled in hospice care is undoubtedly a confusing one. The following brief commentary can be helpful.

- "Just like chemotherapy or surgery, hospice is merely *an approach to medical care*. There are no restrictions for patients on hospice care; however, if a patient plans to leave the geographic area within which their hospice team works, it is wise to communicate travel plans to the hospice team, who can guide what to do if a medical concern should arise while traveling."

Many patients who experience a high level of function at the beginning of their hospice journey will not notice much of a difference between their life before and after hospice enrollment, other than the fact that they will not have to worry anymore about going to the doctor or managing many of the details of their care such as prescriptions, equipment, and personal care. Providing this reassurance can be helpful and is another way of painting a picture of what hospice care will be like for patients and families.

- "Because you are experiencing a high level of function still, being able to walk and visit with friends and go out for dinner and to church, you likely won't notice a real difference from your life right now to when you transition to hospice care. The nice thing will be that the hospice team will come to you, allowing you to focus on living your life and spending time as you please with your loved ones."

Hospice Fact 5: People Can Choose to Leave Hospice Care Whenever They Wish

A similar misperception is that once a patient is in hospice care, they must remain in hospice care forever. The following commentary can be helpful.

- "Hospice care can be **revoked** at any point. Should a patient decide that they no longer want to be in hospice care or, should the patient experience a critical injury that needs to be addressed in the hospital, the patient's insurance coverage for curative medical care can be reinstated. Should the patient choose to go back on hospice care again in the future, that is allowed, as long as they meet hospice criteria at that point."

Hospice Fact 6: People Can Eat or Drink as Much as They Like on Hospice Care

Sometimes, people report a belief that food or drink will be limited to patients receiving hospice care because "nourishment is life-prolonging." The following commentary can be helpful.

- "Food is an essential aspect of our quality of life, around which we build family traditions and holidays. Because food is important to comfort and well-being, patients can eat and drink whatever they want while receiving hospice care. Patients with swallowing issues are also welcome to eat and drink, as long as they understand the risk that doing so might entail."

A guiding principle of hospice care is allowing patients to pass peacefully without efforts being made to prolong their lives. Tube feeding, for instance, is not encouraged in hospice and is often not initiated or continued for patients receiving hospice care. Some patients, of their own accord, might choose to stop eating or drinking, but hospice providers will never instruct families to withhold food or liq-uid from patients who want to and can physically receive it.

Remember that the word "palliative" means to relieve suffering without curing. The goal of palliative and hospice care is to relieve pain and suffering without the use of interventions intended to cure disease, which often are ineffective or even harmful at that point. *Palliative treatment does not mean no treatment.* Treatment that controls symptoms and adds to patient and family comfort and quality of life is welcome and can even be "aggressive" in the sense that it vigorously works to reduce pain and other distress quickly.

In many cultures, cooking and serving food is an essential expression of love. Many people worry that a person who is not eating at the end of life is suffering from hunger pain due to starvation. Providing a compassionate, reasonable, and caring medical explanation that a declining appetite is a normal aspect of the end of life is a meaningful way to validate and honor people's love, concern, and advocacy for one another. A supportive approach encourages family members to offer, but not force, food or liquid, explaining that patients at the end of life have less energy for the bodily functions involved in eating and digesting food. The following explanation can help.

- "Many families worry that their loved one is suffering from hunger pain at the end of life when their appetite starts to decline. At the end of life, it is natural to eat less as the body is declining and as its ability to digest and translate nutrition into healthy skin, muscle, and bone declines. The body naturally has less energy for digestion, and the appetite declines in line with that process. We don't believe patients experience pain and hunger, and this process is different from starvation."
- "It's okay to offer food and drink to your loved one, but if they refuse, that's okay and natural. Forcing food or liquid can lead to other problems, like nausea, constipation, or fluid overload, which can lead to weepy skin or edema (swelling in the legs), which can be painful. When patients are no longer interested in eating or drinking, providing a little moisture to the mouth and protecting the lips with lip balm can provide comfort."

Such explanations are very supportive of the need for family members to feel that they are doing everything they can to ensure the comfort and dignity of their loved ones at the end of life.

Describe Hospice Philosophy

Once concerns and misconceptions about hospice are presented, the following overview of hospice philosophy should be provided to patients and families.

- "Like chemotherapy or surgery, hospice is just an *approach* to medical care. Hospice care is an approach to care that focuses entirely on keeping people comfortable."
- "To receive hospice care, patients must meet hospice criteria, meaning their disease must be advanced enough that we worry that their time is limited. Patients and families must also be 'hospice minded,' meaning they are ready

to allow nature to take its course and want to focus on quality of life and comfort until the patient passes."

- "Hospice care is a shift from using medical care to fix or cure disease to live longer—a focus on *quantity of life*—to a focus on *quality of life*. Hospice care provides the soft landing patients and families want at the end of life. Importantly, it allows patients to avoid unwanted hospitalizations at a time in their lives when hospitalizations are an otherwise expected part of disease progression for those who don't have the necessary care and support to enable them to remain comfortably at home."
- "Hospice care allows patients and families to focus on the things that people say that matter most, including spending time with family, friends, and pets in their familiar surroundings."
- "Hospice care is a Medicare benefit intended to provide patients with *at least* six months of comfort care and quality of life at the end of life, but there is no absolute limit for the length of time patients can remain on hospice care. To continue to meet hospice criteria and receive hospice care, patients need to continue to show some objective or measurable decline, such as weight loss, worsening symptoms requiring more comfort measures, or progression of disease resulting in an increasing need for care."
- "When we consider hospice care, we think of patients who likely have about six months of life left. Some patients will live longer than six months, while others will not. Ideally, we would identify the exact moment when each patient meets hospice criteria, giving them and their families the most time to benefit from hospice care."
- "Again, the entire focus of hospice care is on keeping patients comfortable so that they can pass peacefully, without pain, and with dignity."

Discuss Approach to Hospice Care

To support patients and families in deciding about hospice care, it is beneficial to paint a picture of what hospice care will look like. Provide the following overview of the approach to hospice care.

- "I'd like to paint a picture of hospice care so you can get a feel for how it will work. This can be helpful in making your decision."
- "Hospice is different from the approach to care most of us experience for most of our lives, where we seek medical care to identify and fix a problem. With hospice, our entire focus is on managing symptoms and ensuring patient comfort so that the patient can pass peacefully and with dignity when their time comes."
- "When patients transition to hospice care, their Medicare and insurance will be converted to the Medicare hospice benefit. (Most Medicaid programs and many commercial insurance plans offer a hospice benefit if the patient is not yet eligible for Medicare.) Remember that hospice care is intended for people who are ready to allow nature to take its course. For that reason, hospice

coverage will not pay for the interventions intended to cure disease. For instance, the hospice benefit will not pay for ER visits, ambulance rides, hospital admissions, ICU stays, trips to rehabilitation facilities, most physical and occupational therapy, workups including labs, imaging, and other tests, and curative interventions like surgeries or other procedures. Patients on hospice will no longer see their specialty providers or primary care provider unless the primary care provider is also their hospice attending provider."

- "Rather, all of the patient's care on hospice will be delivered by the hospice team and the attending hospice provider."
- "Most patients in the United States are in their own homes at the end of life. And most can start and complete their hospice journey at home. For patients who receive hospice care at home, they will be supported by a hospice nurse, who will come to their house about once a week, or more frequently if needed, to assess patient symptoms, assess caregiver concerns, deliver medications, and educate the caregiver on when to administer them. The patient and family are further supported by certified nursing assistants (CNAs), who can come to the house to help with bathing, skin care, wound care, etc. A social worker, bereavement counselor, and chaplain are also part of the hospice team, available to provide spiritual, emotional, and mental health support. Finally, hospice volunteers can be arranged to assist with household chores or visit with the patient while the main caregiver takes a break."
- "Very importantly, families can access the hospice team 24 hours a day, seven days a week. If there is a sudden change in patient symptoms or an urgent concern, caregivers can contact the on-call hospice number at any time of the day or night. A nurse will triage the call and try to get things situated over the phone, but if needed, they send a nurse to the house, no matter what time of day or night, to help get the patient and family comfortable. This is the mechanism by which hospice teams can ensure that patients can remain at home at the end of life when it is typically only a matter of time for a body that is declining to develop symptoms that would lead to another hospitalization without this type of support."

Discuss the Location Options and Cost of Hospice Care

The following description of where hospice care can be received and how it is paid for helps alleviate many patients' and families' worries about the end of life.

- "Most patients in the United States, more than 95%, receive hospice care at home or wherever they live at the end of their lives. 'Home' can include nursing homes, assisted living or continuing care facilities, or private residences. When patients are at their private home on hospice care, the family is responsible for providing most of the care for the patient. The hospice care team acts in a support role to guide caregivers and to provide medications to ensure patient comfort. Still, the hospice team's visits, including the nurse and CNA visits, are intermittent and limited, maybe just a few hours a week. Families caring for a loved one at home with hospice care are responsible for providing most of the care that the patient needs."

- "Medicare covers the entire cost for patients to receive hospice care at home, including the cost for the nursing and attending provider visits, the CNA visits, and the cost for medications and any equipment needed to care for the patient. At the end of our lives, all of us will eventually get to a point where we are bedbound, and Medicare will cover the cost for a hospital bed to be delivered to make caring for the patient easier. The hospice team can also supply equipment like oxygen or a bedside commode."

- "For families who cannot be there around the clock with their loved one, they may need to hire extra support from a home care agency to provide care to their loved one. Medicare does not cover the cost of this extra support. Sometimes, Medicaid will cover the cost of additional support for patients enrolled in certain programs. Long-term care insurance also sometimes covers this support and the Veterans Administration (VA) also often provides some of this support to veterans. The hospice team can help families navigate these considerations."

- "For many patients, it is not possible to remain at home at the end of life. Perhaps their spouse is elderly or experiencing medical issues of their own. Perhaps the patient lives alone. To safely remain at home with hospice care, patients need to have someone who can care for them, and when patients become bedbound, they need someone to be there with them around the clock to ensure their comfort, safety, and hygiene. For patients without this support at home, there are different options for where end-of-life care can be received."

- "Some communities have a dedicated hospice facility. Patients can be placed in nursing homes and other care facilities. In these situations, Medicare covers the same costs it would cover at home, including the nursing and attending provider visits, CNA visits, medications, and equipment. Medicare does not cover the room and board fee to stay overnight at a hospice center or care facility. The hospice care team can assist with figuring out the cost involved and whether the patient's insurance, long-term care policy, VA benefits, or Medicaid might help cover the room and board fee."

Discuss the Next Steps for Patients and Families Ready for Hospice Care

Following the provision of this overview of hospice care, check in with patients and families by asking the following:

- "I know that was a lot to go over. Do you have any questions?"

After providing time for their consideration and response, follow up by asking the following:

- "How are you feeling about this conversation?"

This open-ended question allows patients and families to articulate their emotions, fears, concerns, and wishes. People ready for hospice care typically respond by saying something like, "That sounds good. I think that's what we want."

For patients ready to transition to hospice care, the next step is to encourage the patient and family to select the hospice agency they would like to enroll with. Referring providers cannot legally limit patient and family choice to only one option. Thus, becoming familiar with the hospice agencies serving your area, including their reputations and quality metrics, is essential to ensure that patients and families have the information they need to make good choices.

Once the patient and family have selected the hospice agency they want to work with, let them know the next steps, being prepared to make an efficient and effective referral on their behalf. Inquire with your organization to understand this process ahead of time. The following response is an example of how to help patients and families feel supported through this transition.

- "If you're ready to transition to hospice care, once you have selected the hospice agency you would like to work with, the next step will be for me to communicate your readiness and qualifications to that agency. They will then reach out to you to schedule an appointment for enrollment. You don't have to do anything; just be on the lookout for their call. Most typically, they will come to your house for the enrollment visit, and at that point, you will have their support going forward."

Assisting with a smooth transition to hospice care is an important aspect of patient- and family-centered care at the end of life.

For hospitalized patients, arrangements should be made for the hospice agency to meet the patient and family at home upon discharge. An effort should be made to reduce the time that patients and families are without the support of hospice care at home as much as possible, for patient symptoms and caregiver needs can quickly evolve, leaving patients without hospice support at home with no other choice than to return to the hospital again for care.

For patients and families who are not yet ready for hospice care, provide reassurance and validation, letting them know that

- "There is no urgency. Please take whatever time you need to make your decision. There is no right answer, only the answer that is right for you and your family."

Index